MEMOIR
of a
PANDEMIC

FIGHTING COVID FROM THE FRONT LINES TO THE WHITE HOUSE

BRETT P. GIROIR, MD

TEXAS A&M UNIVERSITY PRESS

COLLEGE STATION

♾ This paper meets the requirements of ANSI/
NISO Z39.48-1992 (Permanence of Paper).
Binding materials have been chosen for durability.
Manufactured in the United States of America.

Library of Congress Cataloging-in-Publication Data

Names: Giroir, Brett, author.
Title: Memoir of a pandemic: fighting COVID from the front lines to the
    White House / Brett P. Giroir.
Other titles: Joseph V. Hughes, Jr. and Holly O. Hughes series on the
    presidency and leadership.
Description: First edition. | College Station: Texas A&M University Press,
    [2023] | Series: Joseph V. Hughes Jr. and Holly O. Hughes series on the presidency
    and leadership | Includes index.
Identifiers: LCCN 2022052470 (print) | LCCN 2022052471 (ebook) | ISBN
    9781648431586 (cloth) | ISBN 9781648431593 (ebook)
Subjects: LCSH: Giroir, Brett. | United States. Office of the Assistant
    Secretary for Health—Biography. | Government physicians—United
    States—Biography. | COVID-19 Pandemic, 2020—United States—Personal
    narratives. | COVID-19 Pandemic, 2020-—Political aspects—United
    States. | COVID-19 (Disease)—Government policy—United States. | COVID-19
    vaccines—Government policy—United States. | Medical
    policy—United States—Decision making. | LCGFT: Autobiographies.
Classification: LCC RA644.C67 G57 2023 (print) | LCC RA644.C67 (ebook) |
    DDC 362.1962/4144—dc23/eng/20221114
LC record available at https://lccn.loc.gov/2022052470
LC ebook record available at https://lccn.loc.gov/2022052471

To my wife, Jill, who stood by me and independently contributed to our nation's pandemic response from day one and without whose encouragement and support this book would never have been written.

And to the officers of the US Public Health Service (USPHS)—my brothers and sisters in uniform—who have served as America's health responders since 1798. During COVID-19, USPHS officers were deployed around the world and throughout our nation, from the *Diamond Princess* in Japan to US nursing homes, alternate care facilities, drive-through testing sites, and tribal nations. Their efforts saved countless lives, and their critical importance to our nation—past, present, and future—should never be forgotten. Bravo Zulu!

Contents

Preface

Over one million Americans have lost their lives to COVID-19. Four hundred and twenty thousand of these died under Pres. Donald Trump. But despite effective vaccines, diverse therapeutics, mature supply chains for testing, and a new administration, as of December 2022, an additional 660,000 Americans have died from COVID-19 during the Biden presidency. Every American wants to know why.

Most people now realize that campaign rhetoric and political scapegoating do not actually solve problems. Ending this pandemic is not as easy as stating we are going to "shut down the virus," or replacing a president, or "following the science," which we in the Trump administration did at least as well as the Biden administration is now doing. Every day I am questioned by people from all walks of life and political affiliations. They seek transparent and unfiltered information about why the pandemic continues to ravage our nation over two years after it began and, most importantly, how the United States can ensure that "this never happens again."

The unfortunate fact is that our human species has been, is, and will remain vulnerable to pandemics, even more so now because of both natural and human-influenced factors. The success of our responses will always be dictated by the adequacy of our public health and societal preparations *before* a pandemic begins, the individual capabilities and relationships of our national leaders, and the inevitable politics of the day. Whether the next novel infectious disease arises spontaneously from nature or begins as an intentional bioweapon attack by adversaries, the United States' current institutions and leadership structures have proven wholly incapable of preventing or effectively mitigating another pandemic.

The United States remains vulnerable, and I would argue that our nation is *much more vulnerable* than most high-income nations, as the COVID-19 pandemic demonstrated. Our vulnerability stems in part from the freedoms we uniquely enjoy as Americans and our natural opposition to their infringement, even during a pandemic. While citizens of many other nations freely accept involuntary GPS tracking and warrantless searching of church records for the purpose of contact tracing, Americans are not likely ever to accept such measures. At least I hope we never do. The United States is also uniquely vulnerable because of our overall poor baseline health status; for example, nearly half of Americans are clinically obese, and our life expectancy before COVID-19 was far below the average for peer countries. Our outcomes during COVID-19 almost exactly mirrored our national "preexisting condition" of poor health and lower life expectancies.

From the Centers for Disease Control and Prevention (CDC) and the US Food and Drug Administration (FDA) to the White House and the World Health Organization (WHO), it is time to demand reforms that will keep our nation biosafe in the twenty-first century. Many of these reforms stem directly from lessons learned during COVID-19, but we first have to get past the delusion that there are simple answers, that dollars alone will remedy our deficiencies, and that a pandemic like this one will never happen again. It almost certainly will happen again—it is a matter of when, not if.

The purpose of this book is to venture beyond the political rhetoric, inaccuracies, reputation salvaging, and oversimplifications that have dominated the airwaves and bookshelves. Here, I recount the major events in the Trump administration's pandemic response *as I personally witnessed them*, from the front lines on cruise ships and makeshift hospitals to the Situation Room in the White House. As one of the physicians on the White House Coronavirus Task Force, I am certainly motivated to add to the historical record, but I do not intend for this book to be an exhaustive and comprehensive history of the entire response. Rather, I endeavor to provide the context of several key inflection points and operational initiatives, the personalities and the conflicts involved, the intense debates about strategy and guidance, and the intersection of science and politics in the decision-making processes that led ultimately to our national strategy—for better or worse.

Implementing a response to a previously unknown, highly contagious, and evolving virus for which there were no vaccines, diagnostics, or therapeutics was itself a Herculean challenge of historic proportions. But in addition, from the first day that COVID-19 became the dominant national focus in 2020, every aspect of the response was made infinitely more complex by the politics of a presidential campaign and the tense relationship between President Trump and the media. Energized by political rancor, the media often took on the role of a sparring partner at times when the American people desperately needed more facts and less sensationalism.

All of these circumstances notwithstanding, major components of the response were successful beyond all expectations, especially given the lack of preparedness of our federal institutions prior to the pandemic. Among these successes were the dramatic evacuations of Americans trapped abroad when the pandemic began, the unprecedented public-private partnerships that led to effective vaccines and a pioneering national testing system, and the national focus on the plight of racial and ethnic minorities. But these successes were most often the result of extraordinary efforts by unlikely "heroes" both from within the government and from the private sector—individuals who showed up, accepted the call to duty without hesitation, and navigated the completely uncharted waters of a global plague caused by an unknown and adapting virus. I tell the stories of these unlikely heroes and how we relied on them because there was nobody else to rely on.

When I left DC in March 2021, the last thing I wanted to do was continue appearing on national television. Dealing with media from inside the Trump administration was enormously challenging even on good days, and occasionally it was personally hurtful. But I had always felt it was my duty and an important part of transparency with the American people to be on media as often as possible—whenever requested by any outlet, conservative or liberal. I always tried to deliver the best information we had with humility and honesty. I hoped to empower the American public to make healthy choices and remain safe—to get tested, wear a mask indoors, protect the vulnerable, move on from hydroxychloroquine to proven effective therapies, get vaccinated, or whatever the key public health messages of the day were at that time.

My relationship with the media was reasonably good, and we had a great deal of mutual respect, but I wanted my time in the media to be over—or at least to take a very long break from the camera. No more microphones, or makeup, or questions based on breaking news that were perfectly timed to surprise the "Trump guy." I never wanted to be in politics, and my time in the administration was over. I was at a stage in my professional career where I did not need to focus on my next job, so I had no reason to promote myself on air. My intention was to get back to Texas with my wife and spend time with our grandchildren. I was happy to let the Biden team own the messaging. They had won the election, and I thought a change in voice might help persuade more Americans to effectively protect themselves and their families from the virus—and most importantly, to get vaccinated. Indeed, the Biden team did have a strong start, communicating a comprehensive pandemic plan on day one of the administration. The plan was actually not that different from what the Trump administration had been implementing, but it was wrapped up in a concise package and presented authoritatively—and that was a good move by the Biden team.

But my outlook on doing national media changed because, quite frankly, I became angry and frustrated and felt a need to express myself on behalf of all those who had sacrificed selflessly during the Trump administration. As opposed to the many "on-point" messages about the pandemic from the new administration, Pres. Joe Biden and Vice Pres. Kamala Harris began stating that there was no vaccine plan in the previous administration, that there were no vaccinators, and that they inherited a mess related to vaccines when they took office on January 20. I don't know if they actually believed that or if they were just told that by their political handlers.

In either case, they were de facto rewriting history and claiming full ownership of the successes of Operation Warp Speed (OWS), the unprecedented public-private partnership that resulted in the development and distribution of COVID-19 vaccines in record time. Not only was that claim factually incorrect, but I knew immediately it would politicize vaccines to an even greater extent than they had already been and further polarize the nation along ideological and political grounds. Frustrated conservatives were going to become more alienated and distrustful, and the vaccine hesitant would be convinced that immunizations were more of a political tool than a public health necessity. And in retrospect, that was exactly what happened.

I spoke with many of my former administration colleagues who had been in leadership roles, and most were reluctant to speak up for personal or political reasons. Many were just not ready to be in the spotlight; others feared further retaliation to their careers and even their personal lives just because they had been in the Trump administration. I was not oblivious to that type of political targeting but nevertheless decided to step back in front of the cameras and tell what I knew was the real story of where we left vaccines on January 20, 2021. This is an *American* success story, started by President Trump and continued by President Biden. COVID vaccines should be a unifying force, not a dividing one. The vaccines we developed are literally saving the world.

Later in the spring and summer of 2021, messaging from the CDC became increasingly inconsistent and incomplete and even more confusing to the American people: vaccinated people could not transmit the virus, and then they could. Masks were not needed for vaccinated individuals, and then they were. Boosters would be available to everyone, but then they weren't recommended by scientists, yet they were approved by the CDC director anyway. The data about the importance and strength of natural immunity continued to be censored for no apparent reason, which further alienated the public, including many of our heroes serving in the armed forces and on the front line of the health-care response. Finally, the Biden administration announced several emergency executive orders that they stated were critical to saving lives and then took three months to actually publish the proposed rules and regulations. And so on.

I wanted to continue to do my part as a relatively objective messenger with no conflicts of interest (I don't work for Pfizer or Moderna)—hopefully reaching across party lines and staying grounded in the science. With peak hospitalizations and deaths in 2021 *topping* those of the summer of 2020, even before the Omicron variant poured gasoline on the embers, clear communication was necessary—so I found myself back on CNN and Fox News, regional and national radio, and everything in between. Again, my goal was to inform and empower the American people. The tools were there (vaccines, therapeutics, home tests), but we needed to use them appropriately in order to end the pandemic.

Similarly, I also had no intention of writing this memoir. I did not chronicle my daily activities while at the Department of Health and Human Services (HHS) because I was just too busy and exhausted to even think about doing so. My email and calendars were US government property, and I no longer had access to them. My wife, Jill, had kept some notes, starting in March 2020, but they were far from comprehensive. In retrospect, I did a lot of calls from our apartment between 9 p.m. and 2 a.m., so she had a good idea of many of the issues and characters involved, if not the specific content.

I also still have many of my meeting notes and reports, a few of which were in my files that I hurriedly packed after the January 6 riot, not knowing if I would be able to get back into my office for my last two weeks of public service. And there were some items that I made sure to keep, like my original situation report (sitrep) to Secretary Alex Azar on March 4, 2020, detailing the CDC's prediction that as many as one million Americans could die in the pandemic and Dr. Scott Atlas's testing manifesto entitled "Specific Notes on Prioritized Testing," which he delivered to me during our first meeting in Pence's office in August 2020. I thought these documents were critical for the historical record and essential to inform our nation's preparation for the next pandemic. I detail both of these original documents in this book.

Five months after leaving office, I also began to read the long-awaited deluge of books about the pandemic response under President Trump. Nearly all of these books were pieced together from multiple secondary sources, were filled with inaccuracies and unsupported innuendos, and offered only one-sided (often political) points of view (either Republican or Democrat, hate Trump or love Trump). These books did not understand or explain the complexities or the context or convey the true life-and-death drama behind the decisions and the headlines. They *couldn't* convey these essential aspects because the authors were not present in the Situation Room or the Oval Office and therefore did not experience the events personally. They did not lose sleep speaking with the vice president (VP) or governors, handling regional crises, galvanizing support from industry CEOs, or sending military airlifts across the globe to secure critical supplies. They had not laid awake at night feeling the burden and overwhelming stress of a raging pandemic that would kill another two thousand Americans the next day. I did that every single night for almost a year.

After seeing many of these books, the conversation with myself went something like this: "I do have firsthand knowledge of many of the notable events and decisions in the pandemic response. I know what things actually happened, the reasons why they happened, and the personalities and conflicts involved in the decision-making. I worked daily with the vice president and the task force and frequently with the president directly. I was personally involved in organizational and leadership changes over time. I know how we built the plane while we were flying it. And I can recount many untold stories that illustrate our shining successes as well as our frequent missteps."

So it seemed clear, despite my initial hesitancy, that I needed to write this book; Americans deserve to hear the unfiltered story, and academics and other experts need to learn from our successes and failures. My decision was reinforced when I reluctantly agreed, at the request of friends and former colleagues, to speak to a few small groups in my home community of College Station, Texas. The overwhelming response was "We had no idea. You need to write all of this down."

A month into writing, I also realized how much I needed to finish this book as part of my own healing process. I had been completely engrossed in the response, slept very little for a year, was worried constantly about the safety of my US Public Health Service (USPHS) officers, and did my best every day to provide the public with accurate information to save as many lives as possible. I had not taken incoming mortar fire in Baghdad, but I clearly had some degree of post-traumatic stress. I am sure all of us inside the pandemic response leadership were experiencing that.

In the first chapters, I describe the events, personalities, considerations, and conflicts that led up to the pandemic. Nature's "warning shots" of Ebola and H1N1 foreshadowed—and to a degree predicted—our successes and failures during COVID-19. In February 2020, we heroically rescued and repatriated Americans stranded abroad and began research on a vaccine, but we also lost precious time in implementing and scaling testing. By March 2020, we were engaged in a frenetic scramble to salvage the response because the traditional bureaucracies of government were failing—and they would have failed no matter who was president at the time. I was designated the "testing czar" because the failures of the CDC and the FDA were continuing and actually getting worse, and these failures were costing lives.

I know everything about "Jared's volunteers," individuals from outside of the government brought in by Jared Kushner (Trump's son-in-law and an assistant to the president). During their critical first week on the scene, I co-led the efforts of these volunteers from my office at HHS, where they were all camped out and joined by USPHS officers who had just returned from the *Diamond Princess* cruise ship, where they led the evacuation and repatriation of United States citizens from that COVID-19-ravaged vessel. We urgently connected with CEOs of global companies, dispatched military airlifts, and designed the national community-based testing program within forty-eight hours.

Now that I am out of the "DC bubble," I have had the opportunity to speak with people from around the country, all of whom are curious about the White House Coronavirus Task Force: "Was it for show?" "What was Tony Fauci like?" "What truly happened there and how?" So I provide an inside perspective on the operations of the task force, the personalities involved, and the interpersonal conflicts from the day I joined in March 2020 until the day before President Biden's inauguration when we disbanded. The task force included leadership from nearly every cabinet department. We debated and ultimately decided on the strategies and policies to combat the pandemic and the most important messages to convey to the American public. What happened in the Situation Room was sometimes dramatic and unexpected, but mostly it was data driven and wonkish—except for the occasional rant from Peter Navarro or Dr. Scott Atlas's contrarian arguments that began the moment he was added to the task force.

All plans are obsolete when the first shot is fired, but our nation (and the world) can better prepare for the next pandemic. Technologies advance, and there are many expert panels recommending approaches to keep pace with scientific challenges, but new technologies are only a small part of the overall problems we must overcome to keep the world biosafe.

The million-plus deaths in the United States were not due to technological failures. In part, these deaths were the inevitable result of a highly contagious and deadly virus that had disseminated across the globe without warning. But many of these deaths were also due to the United States being unprepared and our nation's institutions failing us—including heralded ones like the CDC. I discuss many examples of profound CDC failures—in testing, evacuations, guidance, and beyond. The intent is not to destroy the CDC but to provide an honest evaluation that can start a process to reenvision and strengthen the CDC for pandemics we will face in the future.

In the last chapter, I recommend actionable solutions to keep our world biosafe based on the lessons learned from COVID-19—what we did right, what we did wrong, and what needs to change in order to prepare for (or hopefully prevent) the next pandemic. I focus on the urgent need for fundamental root-cause reforms in leadership structures and organizations— from the CDC to the White House, from state and national governments to the WHO. There are many actions we can take today—and can vote for tomorrow—that can help prevent the next pandemic. But even though we cannot prevent pandemics entirely, there are many actions we can take to detect pandemics early and minimize their impact. My hope is that a moderator at the 2024 presidential election debates will ask tough questions to our candidates based on my recommendations and that the future president will have substantive, heartfelt, and meaningful responses.

President Trump was no more personally responsible for the 400,000+ deaths that occurred during his term than President Biden is personally responsible for the 600,000+ deaths (and thousands more in the future) that have occurred under his administration. Could Trump and Biden have done more? Absolutely. But saying that the Trump administration "did not follow the science" is blatantly false. One popular author has blamed the American people, whom he claims did not sacrifice enough—where exactly was that author in 2020 during the pandemic? The American people sacrificed greatly, and if anyone, they are the heroes of this story—not the politicians, the apologists, the critics, the authors, or the pundits.

Political scapegoating will only provide a false sense of security and suggest easy fixes when there are none. The answer is not to have a different president, more personal suffering, or a team of Fauci clones or to ransack the Wuhan lab and others like it throughout the world. Real solutions require strengthening the global health security agenda—a global preparedness playbook already championed by the United States—and assuring that it is implemented comprehensively throughout the world. Solutions require that the United States actively addresses the growing diversity of natural and manmade threats, invests consistently in domestic public health infrastructure and preparedness, and overhauls several of the federal bureaucracies that did not live up to expectations—and will never do so absent substantial reform.

The Trump administration—including my team and I—did many things right, to an exemplary degree, but we also made mistakes that led to confusion among the American people and may have cost lives. And of course, the entire pandemic response—and certainly public health communication to the American people—was made infinitely more difficult and complex by the most divisive presidential election in the history of our country. But that was the situation, and this book will tell you exactly how I experienced the events and decisions, the personalities and the politics, the science and the myths, and the president.

Abbreviations

ACF   Administration for Children and Families (operational division within HHS)

ASH   assistant secretary for health

ASPR   assistant secretary for preparedness and response

BARDA   Biomedical Advanced Research and Development Authority, a component of the Office of the ASPR

CBP   Customs and Border Protection (federal law enforcement agency within the Department of Homeland Security)

CDC   Centers for Disease Control (operational division within HHS)

DARPA   Defense Advanced Research Projects Agency (within the Department of Defense)

DEA   Drug Enforcement Administration (agency within the Department of Justice)

DHS   Department of Homeland Security

DPA   Defense Production Act

DTRA   Defense Threat Reduction Agency (combat support agency within the Department of Defense)

EUA   emergency use authorization (can be used for vaccines, drugs, tests, etc.)

FDA   Food and Drug Administration (operational division within HHS)

FEMA	Federal Emergency Management Administration (agency within the Department of Homeland Security)
HBCU	historically Black colleges and universities
HHS	Department of Health and Human Services
IHME	Institute for Health Metrics and Evaluation (independent global health research center at the University of Washington)
LDTs	laboratory-developed tests
NDMS	National Disaster Medical System (federally coordinated health-care system and partnership of the DHS, HHS, Department of Defense, and Veterans Affairs; NDMS personnel are frequently deployed by the ASPR)
NRCC	National Response Coordination Center (at FEMA)
OASH	Office of the Assistant Secretary for Health (staff division at HHS)
ODU	operational dress uniform (blue work and deployment uniform)
OMB	US Office of Management and Budget
PanCAP	Pandemic Crisis Action Plan
PCR	polymerase chain reaction (highly sensitive molecular test that detects a virus's genetic material)
PEPFAR	The US President's Emergency Plan for AIDS Relief
PPE	personal protective equipment (including masks, gowns, gloves, and other materials necessary to protect from infection)
PPO	Presidential Personnel Office

SNF	skilled nursing facility (technical designation, frequently used interchangeably with "nursing homes")
SNS	Strategic National Stockpile
TCID	Texas Center for Infectious Disease
UCG	Unified Coordination Group (leadership structure at FEMA for the COVID-19 response)
USAID	US Agency for International Development
USPHS	US Public Health Service
WHO	World Health Organization

Key Players

Jerome Adams

US surgeon general; vice admiral, US Public Health Service

Blythe Adamson

director of quantitative sciences, Flatiron Health; private-sector volunteer to the national COVID-19 testing initiative

Amy Alving

former director, Special Projects Office at the Defense Advanced Research Projects Agency (DARPA)

Alex Azar

secretary, Department of Health and Human Services (HHS)

Rachel Baitel

deputy chief of staff, US International Development Finance Corporation; assigned to COVID-19 testing initiative

Charles (Charlie) Baker

governor, Massachusetts

Katie Bante

lieutenant commander, US Public Health Services; aide to Admiral Giroir

Tammy Beckham

director of the Office of Infectious Disease and HIV/AIDS Policy, HHS; lead, COVID-19 Laboratory Diagnostics Task Force

Sherri Berger

chief of staff, Centers for Disease Control (CDC)

Tiffany Bilderback

major, US Army; assigned to R. Adm. Erica Schwartz and the Task Force on Community-Based Testing

Deborah Birx

coordinator, White House Coronavirus Task Force

Adam Boehler	CEO, US International Development Finance Corporation
Rick Bright	director of the Biomedical Advanced Research and Development Authority (BARDA), HHS
Jay Butler	deputy director for infectious diseases, CDC
Michael Caputo	assistant secretary for public affairs (ASPA), HHS, from April 2020 to September 2020
Benjamin (Ben) Carson	secretary, US Department of Housing and Urban Development
Richard Childs	rear admiral (two star), US Public Health Service; clinical director of the National Heart, Lung, and Blood Institute's Division of Intramural Research, National Institutes of Health (NIH); commanding officer of the mission to coordinate and return Americans from the *Diamond Princess* in Japanese hospitals
Francis Collins	director, NIH
Andrew Cuomo	governor, New York
Bill de Blasio	mayor, New York City
Sumbul Desai	vice president of health, Apple
Josh Dozer	incident commander at Federal Emergency Management Agency (FEMA) for the COVID-19 response
Alexander (Alex) Eastman	trauma surgeon; senior medical officer—operations, Department of Homeland Security (DHS); lieutenant and lead medical officer, Dallas Police Department

John Bel Edwards	governor, Louisiana
Anthony (Tony) Fauci	director of the National Institute of Allergy and Infectious Diseases (NIAID), NIH
Robert Ford	president and CEO, Abbott
Brendan Fulmer	senior advisor, Center for Medicare and Medicaid Services (CMS); advisor to the secretary, HHS
Peter (Pete) Gaynor	administrator, FEMA
Newsha Ghaeli	president and cofounder, Biobot Analytics (wastewater surveillance)
Jill Giroir	wife of Admiral Giroir
Deanne Griswell	New York City emergency management commissioner
Patricia Haigwood	program analyst, Office of the Assistant Secretary for Health, HHS
Brian Harrison	chief of staff, HHS
Mia Heck	director of external affairs, Office of the Assistant Secretary for Health
Gordon Hensley	media strategist who consulted for HHS during the pandemic
Dave Hickey	president, BD Life Sciences
Larry Hogan	governor, Maryland
Debra Houry	director and acting principal deputy director of the National Center for Injury Prevention and Control, CDC
Michael Iademarco	rear admiral (two star), US Public Health Service; director of the Center for Surveillance, Epidemiology, and Laboratory Services, CDC
Jay Inslee	governor, Washington

Daniel Jernigan	deputy director for Public Health and Surveillance, CDC; member of the Unified Coordination Group, FEMA
Lynn Johnson	assistant secretary, Administration for Children and Families (ACF), HHS
Robert (Bob) Kadlec	assistant secretary for preparedness and response, HHS
Rachell Kellogg	deputy chief of staff to Admiral Giroir; lead for the nursing home testing program
Nim Kidd	chief, Texas Division of Emergency Management
Nancy Knight	rear admiral (one star), US Public Health Service; commander for repatriation mission at Joint Base Andrews, San Antonio
Larry Kudlow	director, White House National Economic Council
Jared Kushner	assistant to the president; son-in-law to President Trump
Mariana Matus	CEO and cofounder, Biobot Analytics (wastewater surveillance)
Coral May	CEO and cofounder, eTrueNorth
Tyler Ann McGuffee	associate advisor, Office of the Vice President; White House coordinator for activities and initiatives under Dr. Birx
Mark Meadows	White House chief of staff
Nancy Messonnier	director, National Center for Immunization and Respiratory Diseases, CDC
Katie Miller	press secretary for Vice President Pence

Michael Mina	assistant professor of epidemiology, immunology, and clinical pathology, Harvard University
Steven Mnuchin	secretary of the treasury
Quellie Moorhead	special assistant to the president and director of the Office of Policy Coordination
Jen Moughalian	chief financial officer, HHS
John Michael (Mick) Mulvaney	director, Office of Management and Budget, White House
Phil Murphy	governor, New Jersey
Peter Navarro	assistant to the president; director of Trade and Manufacturing Policy
Ronald (Ron) Niremberg	mayor, San Antonio
Susan Orsega	rear admiral (two star), US Public Health Service; director, Commissioned Corps Headquarters
Heidi Overton	White House fellow and surgeon
Sonny Perdue	secretary of agriculture
Gustav Perna	general, US Army; chief operating officer, Operation Warp Speed (OWS)
Rick Perry	secretary of energy; former governor of Texas
John Polowczyk	rear admiral (two star), US Navy; vice director for logistics, Joint Chiefs of Staff; lead, COVID-19 Supply Chain Task Force
Stephen Redd	rear admiral (two star), US Public Health Service; director of the Office of Public Health Preparedness and Response, CDC

Robert Redfield   director, CDC

Paul Reed   captain and then rear admiral (one star), US Public Health Service; deputy assistant secretary for health, HHS

Jessica (Jess) Roach   deputy for policy and communication, COVID-19 Laboratory Diagnostics Task Force; senior policy advisor, Office of the Assistant Secretary for Health

Brooke Rollins   assistant to the president; director, White House Domestic Policy Council

Eugene Scalia   secretary of labor

Anne Schuchat   rear admiral (two star), US Public Health Service; principal deputy director, CDC

Erica Schwartz   deputy surgeon general; rear admiral (two star), US Public Health Service; lead, COVID-19 Community-Based Testing Task Force

Marc Short   chief of staff to Vice President Pence

Jeffrey (Jeff) Shuren   director of the Center for Devices and Radiological Health, FDA

Moncef Slaoui   lead, Operation Warp Speed

Rachel Slayton   lieutenant commander, US Public Health Service; modeling unit lead, CDC

Brad Smith   director, Center for Medicare and Medicaid Innovation; deputy director, White House Domestic Policy Council

Timothy Stenzel   director of the Office of In Vitro Diagnostics and Radiological Health, FDA

Christopher Sununu	governor, New Hampshire
Timothy Templet	executive vice president of sales, Puritan Medical Products
Jessica Tisch	chief information officer, New York City
Sylvia Trent-Adams	rear admiral (two star), US Public Health Service; principal deputy assistant secretary for health, HHS
Olivia Troye	aide to the White House Coronavirus Task Force; Homeland Security advisor to the vice president
Nat Turner	CEO, Flatiron Health; private-sector volunteer to the national COVID-19 testing initiative
Seema Verma	administrator, CMS, HHS
Russell Vought	acting director and then director of the Office of Management and Budget (OMB)
Jeff Williams	chief operating officer, Apple
Chad Wolf	acting secretary, DHS

MEMOIR OF A PANDEMIC

1

My Last Day in the Situation Room

On January 19, 2021, I attended the last Trump administration White House Coronavirus Task Force meeting—in person in the Situation Room in the White House. Four hundred thousand Americans had died under our watch. I knew that number could have been much higher, but I also realized that it might have been lower. America's hopes were now on our newly authorized vaccines, developed and distributed with unprecedented speed, but also on a new administration that would have to confront some very harsh realities that it never had to face as outsiders on the campaign trail. Merely replacing President Trump or "following the science" was not going to "shut down the virus."[1] I truly hoped that soon-to-be president Joe Biden realized that fact when he made these statements repeatedly during the campaign.

The brief staff car ride from HHS headquarters to the White House had become very familiar. There was just enough time to make a short phone call and coordinate the work for that evening. Sometimes I would be at the White House for just an hour. But if the president wanted a press event or the vice president or Jared Kushner had a special assignment or new challenge, I could easily be at the White House for five hours or more. It was hard to predict on most days exactly what would happen because the situation was very dynamic—not just the virus but the politics as well.

I had a White House full-access pass, and the guards and Secret Service agents knew me well, but they still searched me per protocol. Nearly all of them had my personal challenge coin. I carefully designed it to portray the symbol of the US Public Health Service and its founding year of 1798 on one side and my admiral's flag and official Senate-confirmed position on the other. A challenge coin is a traditional military symbol of comradery, and I was honored to share my coin with the Secret Service agents, especially after all that transpired in the previous months.

But that January 19 trip to my final task force meeting was different and the closest thing to a surreal experience I have ever had. Capitol Hill was shut down, encircled by a high fence topped with barbed wire, and militarized because of the January 6 riot. There were National Guard soldiers stationed along the fenced perimeter of the Capitol and the nearby Hubert H. Humphrey Building—the headquarters of HHS, and the location of my office. Because of the January 6 riot and the heightened security preceding the inauguration, there was almost no one in the Humphrey Building—the halls were empty, dark, and echoey. I walked to work, as I had done so for nearly three years since I had been confirmed and sworn in as the assistant secretary for health (ASH). So at least I could still get to the Humphrey Building—although I had to negotiate numerous new fencing barriers and roadblocks that made my route about twice as long as normal and forced me to cross streets in the middle of speeding cars that were making the most of the near-empty roads.

For that last task force meeting, it was impossible for me to get an HHS staff car or even an Uber to the White House, but eventually, my incredibly capable aide-de-camp (Lt. Cmdr. Katie Bante, now Commander Bante) secured a ride for me and the surgeon general in a vehicle from the Department of Homeland Security's (DHS) Tactical Medicine Branch. Lieutenant Commander Bante had been by my side for the entire pandemic as my aide; she was rock solid and incredibly capable. As an environmental health officer (EHO), she was also invaluable as a technical expert in personal protective equipment (PPE) and the overall safety of my officers whom I had deployed around the nation and the globe. This would be my last day with her as well. The staff car was fully armored up and therefore oddly appropriate for the war zone that was now our capital district. The streets were empty, so DC traffic was not a problem—for once in three years!

The surgeon general and I arrived at the White House, which was also heavily guarded with an extra perimeter of high fencing and steel barricades. Lafayette Square was still a war-torn, burned-out mess from the summer 2020 Black Lives Matter protests, so the whole scene looked like something out of a World War II siege instead of our nation's seat of power preparing for a peaceful transition of presidential administrations in less than twenty-four hours.

I passed the first security checkpoint. The second checkpoint provided me with my West Wing access pass. After collecting my belongings from the X-ray chamber, I entered the White House grounds a few yards from the main entrance to the West Wing. The grounds included not only the White House proper but also the Eisenhower Executive Office Building (EEOB)—a beautiful nineteenth-century office building originally housing the State, War, and US Navy Departments but now home to the Executive Office of the President and the Vice President's Ceremonial Office.

My first stop that day—as it always had been—was the White House Medical Unit (WHMU) on the ground floor of the EEOB to get my COVID-19 rapid test—a test that my HHS team had provided to the WHMU nine months before. Ever since the early days of the pandemic, being tested was the standard protocol for anyone who would be in close proximity to the vice president or president. Needless to say, I had been tested more times than I could count by January 19, 2021. The military medics who swabbed me could see that I was an admiral, but when they stuck swabs up my nose, they had no idea I was the testing czar and could provide them with the regulatory history and manufacturing origin of every single test and swab that they were using. It was somewhat ironic and a little humorous that the testing czar needed to be tested so frequently.

Test results were available in fifteen minutes, and unless they phoned about the result, you knew you tested negative. On January 19, I was negative, as I had always been, but I never assumed that I would remain negative, since COVID had infected many colleagues at the White House and also at the Federal Emergency Management Agency (FEMA) and HHS, including most recently one of my senior civilian staff (whom I tested and diagnosed in my office). I was not yet vaccinated because by national standards, I was not a priority. I had made the conscious decision not to jump the line, although I certainly could have if I'd wanted to.

Any positive test result by the WHMU, whether my own or a staffer's (or even President Trump's), would be investigated by an epidemiology team led by a USPHS Commissioned Corps officer whom I had assigned to the White House in the spring of 2020. Before COVID, there had been no "disease detective" assigned to the White House team—which itself is a remarkable fact considering the massive infrastructure supporting the president and the risk of accidental or intentional disease transmission crippling or killing our senior-most (and often elderly) leaders. The commanding officer of the WHMU asked me to personally pick and assign this disease detective; he did not call the CDC. The WHMU knew I would provide a seasoned operator, not an academic type who might be the pick of the CDC. The WHMU wanted to protect the president and senior staff; they did not care about publishing a paper in the *Morbidity and Mortality Weekly Report* (*MMWR*), the weekly journal of the CDC.

After testing, instead of remaining on the ground floor, I went up one staircase to my favorite place to hang out prior to Situation Room or Oval Office meetings—and I wanted to do that just one more time. EEOB Room 180 is used as a basic conference room now, but it is quite historic, even though it never appears on any EEOB tours. This was Nixon's "hideaway office" where he preferred to work and where many of the Watergate tapes were originally recorded. Vice Pres. Hubert Humphrey also used this office because Pres. Lyndon Johnson kept the official office of the vice president (on the second floor of the EEOB) for himself after Kennedy's assassination. That was cool enough, but more importantly, this room was the site of a historic meeting between Vice President Humphrey and Rev. Dr. Martin Luther King Jr. that led to a significant acceleration of the civil rights movement. There are several black-and-white photos hanging in EEOB 180 to document this meeting, and sitting and working beneath those photos always affected me deeply and elevated my sense of purpose and history.

When it was near time to be in the Situation Room, I left EEOB 180 and walked down the Navy steps to soak in that striking and iconic view of the West Wing one last time. No matter how familiar the White House became or how tired and stressed I was, walking down those steps put my mind squarely in focus on the enormity of the challenges brought by the pandemic and the oaths I swore to defend our nation and its constitution not only as a senior official but also as a person wearing the uniform of our nation. Of course I was loyal to President Trump, but there was never any confusion in my mind about to what I had sworn my oath of allegiance.

I imagined that day would be the last time I ever walked those steps, so I fully experienced the moment. I then traversed the hundred feet or so past the media tents and microphone "sticks" to enter the West Wing through the lobby near the Roosevelt Room, where I deposited my electronics, said hello to the "receptionist of the United States," and went down the very narrow staircase to the Situation Room. Once there, I made final preparations with the other members of the task force before standing up to acknowledge the vice president when he entered the room. I put my Diet Coke on a coaster that had the official Seal of the President stamped on it. The napkins had the seal as well. Even the paper cups and sugar packets were branded with the White House emblem. I think I became even more keenly aware of these details because I suspected it was the last time I would experience them.

Before Vice President Pence entered, I had a flashback—one that sent a chill throughout my body. One year before, when the virus was passing through Wuhan, it might have been possible to delay its spread, or at the very least, if the CDC would have been allowed in, we could have learned about how the virus was transmitted by aerosols and by people without symptoms. That knowledge would have changed our entire early approach to mitigation and might have saved tens of thousands of lives. If I had been on the

Executive Board of the WHO, with Director Gen. Tedros Adhanom Ghebreyesus reporting to me, perhaps the CDC—or even myself as part of the WHO leadership—could have gotten into China and ascertained those facts. But that opportunity never happened because after being nominated to be the US representative to the Executive Board of the WHO in November 2018 by President Trump, my confirmation was held up personally by Senator Chuck Schumer until May 2020, long after our nation needed a seat at the table. In contrast, under Pres. Barack Obama, Dr. Tom Frieden had been confirmed for the Executive Board within twenty-four hours. My confirmation took eighteen months. During the most serious health crisis in one hundred years, the only country without a seat at the WHO Executive Board table was the United States. Senator Schumer should be held accountable, I thought, but I knew he never would be.

My flashback ended when Vice President Pence walked into the Situation Room, and I snapped to attention. The task force meeting that day was mostly a reflection on the work we had done together over what seemed to be a lifetime. Not all task force members were present because they either could not get to the White House due to fortifications throughout DC or chose not to be there for other reasons, including the fact that some had already resigned from the administration. I was never tempted to resign because I still had a job to do, and the lives of Americans depended on that. It was a simple calculus, and I thought no more deeply about it than that.

For me, it had been almost one year of near-daily White House meetings with the vice president, the task force, and often the president; late-night calls from the vice president and governors (of many different temperaments and abilities); frequent formal and informal meetings with members of Congress; private-sector engagement with industry giants like CVS, LabCorp, and FedEx; billions of dollars of investment into domestic manufacturers that I never knew existed (like those making swabs and viral transport media); working with other uniformed service personnel (US Army, US Navy, US Air Force, US Marines, US Coast Guard), who provided truly unequaled technical expertise, contracting, logistics, and heavy-lift capability; communicating with a worried but heroic American public through the filter of a sometimes biased and angry media; and negotiating the internal politics and personalities of the White House, task force, and HHS agencies. Make no mistake, the internal politics and pressures were intense, and they often surfaced—but we generally made it all work. There was no other choice but to make it work.

That last day in the Situation Room, the vice president was, well, *the vice president*. In the year that I had worked so closely with him—during historically challenging times and even through an Air Force Two bird strike and smoky emergency landing—he had always remained respectful of everyone, gracious, level-headed, principled, and quick to give credit to others. I felt I knew the VP very well, and he frequently called me after hours on my mobile phone to discuss a specific problem or just to check how things were going in a particular state or region. Occasionally, he just called to thank me for effectively communicating the public message on an evening news show.

Vice President Pence had high expectations for all of us because of the truly existential threat to our nation from the virus itself but also from the Draconian responses in some states and cities that threatened our economy and compromised our individual rights without justification. Those extreme responses also threatened public health—if people couldn't eat outside at restaurants, many of them would order takeout and cram all their friends in their small apartments. I witnessed that daily from my Navy Yard apartment in Washington, DC. It was amazing how many people I would see packed and partying in a crowded apartment—because they could not eat outside, and even the rooftops of the apartments (a safe outdoor space) had been closed. That was absolutely insane from a public health point of view, and those kinds of restrictions just plain beat people down every single day.

Increased feelings of loneliness and despair, suicides, drug overdoses, heart attacks, and missed cancer screenings—these were also real-world consequences of "infection control" that did not take into account our human emotional fragility and need for socialization during the pandemic. Some of those social interactions could occur virtually, but Americans quickly learned that Facebook did not substitute for hugging your children, visiting grandparents in assisted living communities, or holding the hand of your dying mother.

We all knew that Vice President Pence had our backs and would support us in any way that he could. He was the type of leader who never had to "point to his stripes" because we all wanted to follow him, and conversely, he respected and always incorporated (and generally followed) our scientific and medical advice. Respect and fondness for Vice President Pence were shared by all the task force doctors, including Dr. Fauci and Dr. Deborah Birx, until the end. On that day we again expressed our gratitude to the VP for his leadership and support. We were also quietly imagining the living hell he had just been through since January 6 and likely before that fateful day, but he never let that show outwardly. Never. He always remained respectful to President Trump, no matter what. I had been in the Oval Office with Pence and Trump many times during some tough debates, and there was no question in my mind that Pence had the toughest job in DC.

President Trump did not attend that last task force meeting. He had mostly disengaged from the task force since the early summer, and we had only rarely briefed him in person during the last half of 2020. Scott Atlas, who had been somewhat of a Scud missile aimed at Birx and Fauci, was also back at his Stanford institute three thousand miles away after resigning from the White House six weeks earlier. Those of us who remained had become a very tight and effective team over the long year. We all knew we did our absolute best to save as many lives as possible, but we always questioned what we could have done differently. I still question that almost daily. I had slept very little in months, but that was not because I had any guilt about my efforts—it was just the constant challenge of trying to do just one more thing, make one more call, fight one more battle with the Office of Management and Budget (OMB), do one more CNN hit, or start one more initiative in order to save additional lives. It took two months after the end of our administration before I actually had a restful night of sleep. Even though I was officially out of the fight, I kept waking up instinctively planning the next intervention against the virus multiple times every night.

On the next day, January 20, 2021, after the inauguration of President Biden, all of us in that task force meeting would be gone except for Fauci and perhaps my colleague in uniform, Surgeon Gen. Jerome Adams, whose official term would last well into the Biden administration. But Jerome was fired the morning of the inauguration without warning. I suspect that this was in retaliation for Trump firing then Surgeon General Vivek Murthy three months into Trump's term in 2017, well before I became the assistant secretary and Murthy would have reported to me. But with Jerome having young children and a wife being treated for recurrent metastatic cancer, you would think that a few weeks' notice would have been appropriate. But apparently not. Politics again over public health, and this time politics was much more important even than simple compassion for an individual serving in uniform and his family.

Just as awful, R. Adm. Erica Schwartz—the incredibly capable career officer and then deputy surgeon general who had been the transition lead for HHS into the Biden administration—was also casually informed by a mid-level Biden staffer that she would not become acting surgeon general, as was customary for a deputy surgeon general until a new surgeon general was confirmed. She was going to be replaced immediately by another officer. So much for a smooth transition for the USPHS Commissioned Corps in the middle of our largest deployment in history and a global pandemic still destined to claim hundreds of thousands of American lives!

I still question the wisdom of firing the two most senior uniformed USPHS officers without cause, both of whom are African American, when the number-one priority was getting African Americans and other underserved minorities vaccinated. I wonder what would have been the media response if Trump had fired, without warning or reason, the two highest-ranking USPHS officers, both of whom were African Americans, and temporarily replaced them with white officers. When Biden did it, it went completely under the media radar.

After the task force meeting, the DHS tactical vehicle returned me to the Humphrey Building. My office was packed up and mostly moved out. It seemed like yesterday that I'd moved into that office; the three years went by in a flash. I was wearing my service-dress-blue uniform, the appropriate uniform for a meeting with the vice president. I hadn't just *worn* the uniform; I'd *lived* the uniform, and every officer in the USPHS will affirm that fact. It was the honor of my life.

That day, as was the case every single day of the pandemic, I walked home to my apartment in the Navy Yard near Nationals Park. Normally, I would change clothes in my office and walk home in civilian clothes or sometimes wear my operational work uniform on the way home. But on January 19, I walked home in my service-dress-blue uniform; it was my last day on active duty, and that is the way I wanted to end it. I loved my time in the corps and felt completely bonded to all my fellow officers; I knew I would miss them and our service beyond description—and I still do. I walked past the National Guard soldiers deployed from distant states and posted around the capital. I could see from their faces that they did not understand why an admiral (they undoubtedly thought I was a US Navy admiral) was walking through the "DC war zone," with barricades and razor wire, in a dress uniform, but they went about their routines and performed their thankless jobs. God bless them!

My wife, Jill, met me halfway home so we could walk together, as was our custom. We had done so every day during the pandemic—at all hours of the day and night. We felt safe, but I always had two doses of Narcan, bandages, and a battlefield tourniquet in my backpack—and occasionally, I actually had to use them on people who were overdosing or fell down and cracked their heads. This would be our last walk—and one of the only ones that was not interrupted by a call from a governor, a senator, a FEMA regional representative, an industry CEO, or even the vice president. Gov. Phil Murphy from

New Jersey seemed to know exactly when I was walking home, whatever time it was, and frequently called me. Independent of politics, he was one of the most collegial, capable, and respectful public officials with whom I had worked, and he had a great team around him. But for this walk home, I had turned in all my electronics to HHS—so after working 24-7 to combat this pandemic for over a year, I was off the clock.

I was done—well, mostly. The Biden team had been talking to me intermittently since the election about staying on in some form after the inauguration to further assist in the transition. They even offered me a nonexecutive temporary government job within the office I previously led as the assistant secretary. Of course I refused that offer. Not only was it insulting and a bit clueless about the organization and its leadership, but it would have been unworkable for the new assistant secretary and surgeon general. An obvious alternative would have been a temporary advisory position in the White House, which I would have accepted for the good of the country.

I was certain that the multiple transition meetings and highly capable team I had left in place would make my presence unnecessary. But the Biden team asked me to stay, voluntarily, in DC until the end of February, and that is what I did—without a position or pay—just in case Biden might need me for anything. Ending the pandemic and saving lives was my only focus, and if I could help the country do that, I wanted to do so. I had spoken to Jeff Zients—Biden's COVID task force coordinator—several times after the election, and he seemed like an organized and reasonable guy. Moreover, Jared Kushner personally called me and said that Zients was capable and could manage operations well. Jared also thought I should stay and help if asked. It was the appropriate thing to do, and Jared supported it. Secretary Azar also supported it. I have no idea what President Trump would have thought, and I did not ask. But in the end, I was not called to formally help the Biden team after the inauguration. At least that left time for me to reflect on the incredibly unlikely circumstances that put me in the Trump administration in the middle of a pandemic and a year filled with the most daunting challenges I had ever faced.

2

From the Department of Pediatrics to the Department of Defense

My pathway to January 19, 2021, in the Situation Room of the White House was anything but predictable. In fact, the most common question people ask me is "How did a pediatrician wind up leading an office at the Defense Advanced Research Projects Agency (DARPA), a top-secret defense department agency developing futuristic national security technologies?" Once taking that leap to DARPA in 2004, I became fully involved in preparedness for bioweapons attacks and natural pandemics. Becoming the ASH in a future administration was not expected or anticipated, but it became much more likely after my DARPA experiences.

I grew up in Marrero, Louisiana—a small town near New Orleans. My mother was a police officer, and my father worked in the oil fields of south Louisiana and was also an officer in the police reserves. I spent my summers on the bayous and marshes hunting, fishing, and thinking I would grow up to join the military or perhaps teach guitar. My first band was in sixth grade, and we had a few underage gigs at local bars.

My parents always stressed education and books (which is why I can't work on cars), and they sacrificed greatly to send me to a Jesuit high school in the big city. It was a long commute—initially with three city buses and a river ferry—but the Jesuits' focus on personal integrity and academic excellence truly changed me forever. I did well in school, won the high school national debate championship, and excelled in the Marine Corps Junior ROTC, where I led the drill team. We used demilitarized M14s, not the "toy guns" that many other schools used—and I still have the scars on my arms from the iron rifle sights to prove it.

I was the first person in my family to attend college, so I really did not understand what college was all about—and certainly not the application process. I naively applied to only two schools and wound up attending Harvard. I had world-renowned professors, like E. O. Wilson (a pioneer in the biology of behavior), John Rawls (perhaps the most influential philosopher of the twentieth century), and Archibald Cox (former US solicitor general and Watergate prosecutor), but it was not a nurturing environment, to say the least. I met my future wife, Jill, when I was a sophomore and she was a senior in high school. I was a judge in one of her debate rounds at the Harvard National High School Forensics Tournament in 1980.

I did well at Harvard and had published three scientific papers in the field of immunology with my roommate by the time we graduated. The Ivy League had a lot to offer, but I was ready to get back to the South, closer to my family, and attend a school where medical students received practical hands-on training in addition to book learning. I was hungry for the opportunity to deliver babies, suture knife wounds, assist in surgery, and put in breathing tubes. The University of Texas Southwestern Medical Center (UTSW) in Dallas, with Parkland Hospital for clinical training, checked all my boxes. The academics were not all that difficult, but the volume of material was daunting. Medical school was physically demanding beyond anything I had previously experienced, but it did not compare to the challenges of residency and fellowship.

After four years of medical school and seven years of postdoctoral training in pediatrics and critical care medicine/trauma, I joined the faculty at UTSW as a pediatric critical care physician and research scientist in 1993. It was what I had worked for my entire life—to have the privilege of caring for sick children and their families while also leading a laboratory research group in discovering new ways to save more lives. People who do both clinical work and laboratory science are called "physician-scientists," and being a physician-scientist defined my persona. UTSW was replete with physician-scientists who were legends in medicine, not the least of whom were Joe Goldstein and Mike Brown, both awarded the Nobel Prize in Medicine during my third year of medical school for their pioneering work on cholesterol metabolism, which has saved millions of lives.

My focus was on severe, acute, life-threatening infections in children and how to prevent these infections from progressing to irreversible shock and death. I trained under many national leaders in pediatrics and infectious diseases, like Dr. George McCracken and Dr. Dan Levin, and then did my postdoctoral training with a true pioneer in the field of the innate immune response, Dr. Bruce Beutler, recipient of the 2011 Nobel Prize in Medicine. I had no thought of doing anything else except treating patients and performing cutting-edge research in my lab. I certainly never imagined I would eventually be sitting in the Oval Office with the president of the United States leading a major component of the national response to a global pandemic.

But then my entire world changed on a dime.

Severe infections in children became a terrifying news headline in the early 1990s when North Texas was struck by an outbreak of meningococcal disease. This disease is caused by bacteria, not viruses, but is contagious if a susceptible individual has close contact—often through saliva—with a person who is colonized with these bacteria. Although this disease is commonly called "meningitis," the deadliest form occurs when bacteria spread widely throughout the bloodstream and do not remain confined to the coverings of the brain. Instead of seeing one or two cases per year, we were treating thirty children with meningococcal disease each year in my ICU. The victims were generally either toddlers or college students—both groups shared a lot of saliva with their peers.

Some children died within twelve hours of their first symptoms; others lost arms or legs from gangrene. The sheer number of kids with catastrophic cases that we were helpless to save left my team with emotional scars. We did everything to improve outcomes, including leading global clinical trials testing new treatments. In the end, it was not so much new therapies that saved lives but early recognition and aggressive treatment in specialized centers that made the difference. Either way, more children went home to their families—and that is really all that mattered.

PUBLIC HEALTH AND NATIONAL SECURITY

As part of our clinical research, I began a collaboration with an outstanding physician, former US Army medical officer, and patriot, Dr. Patrick Scannon, who had founded a biotech company, XOMA, near San Francisco. Pat and XOMA courageously supported our work and collaborated with my team in order to save these children. What I did not know at the time was that Pat was part of an elite scientific futurist group affiliated with DARPA, an organization I had never heard of at that time. The group thought my experiences with meningococcemia might yield insights that could help the United States prepare for biological and chemical weapons attacks and perhaps even a future pandemic caused by an unknown virus. It was very prescient, looking back.

I had never served in uniform but had always desired to contribute in a patriotic way to our nation, so I jumped at the opportunity. After several interviews and intense background checks, I joined this DARPA-affiliated scientific group (called the Defense Sciences Research Council, or DSRC) in 1998. The sixteen-member DSRC included some of the most prestigious scientists and engineers in the United States, including George Whitesides from Harvard and Haydn Wadley from the University of Virginia. I definitely felt like the dog that caught the bus, but I was going to contribute as best as I could.

Our first assigned study was to define an approach to decontaminate critical infrastructure after an anthrax attack. The standard at that time was decontamination with formaldehyde followed by incineration—and that was not going to do if the National Archives was sprayed with anthrax spores. That study led to the development of chlorine dioxide as a gaseous decontaminant, which was used successfully to sanitize the Hart Senate Building and several post offices after the 2001 anthrax ("Amerithrax") attacks. Our work was making a difference at the national level, and it felt good to be part of that.

I later chaired or cochaired a number of year-long studies, including universal medical countermeasures to bioweapons, agricultural bioterrorism, and enhancing human performance for combat. I also was recruited for other related opportunities, including a two-year program within the Department of Defense for twelve young academics under the mentorship of retired four-star generals and admirals to prepare us for future civilian service to the Department of Defense or intelligence agencies. I even became a member of the Planetary Protection Panel at NASA, working on protocols to ensure we don't accidentally bring some nasty space life back from Mars when we return Martian soil and rock samples to earth.

So while being a full-time academic faculty member in Dallas and treating children in the ICU, I was also spending months per year with the armed forces: with US Marines on full-fire combat exercises at Twentynine Palms, on US Navy destroyers and aircraft carriers, and on US Air Force KC-135 Tankers doing in-flight refueling of combat aircraft. We even did time at Fort Bragg and with the SEAL Teams during their training. I did not know how many pediatricians had top-secret clearances, but I was definitely one of them. I was living two separate lives that had very little intersection. People at the hospital only knew I went away for periods of time and did not talk about what I was doing. The title of my first grand round was "The Public Health System *Is* a National Security Issue"; in retrospect, it must have been clear to everyone that my interests were not just confined to the children's hospital.

DARPA is the most important organization that almost no one has heard of and even fewer understand. Begun by Pres. Dwight D. Eisenhower in 1958 after the Sputnik launch, the mission of DARPA is to assure the United States will never again be technologically surprised and, more importantly, that we will instead be that agent of surprise to the rest of the world.

The impact of DARPA cannot be overstated. The organization is responsible for entirely new scientific fields, such as most of the modern semiconductor industry, stealth materials and design, GPS technology, and the invention of ARPANET (now known as the internet). DARPA is small (about one hundred people), is organizationally flat, and has a large budget (~$3 billion annually), the most flexible in the US government. The entire culture is focused on world-changing innovation. Program managers and office directors come to DARPA from all walks of life—academia, national laboratories, the military, the private sector, and even nonprofits. But one can only be at DARPA for four to five years by design. The specific intent is that the people who work there never have to worry about risking their careers because they don't have careers to protect in the first place. This philosophy is extremely effective for avoiding bureaucratic inertia and slow decision-making. There is no penalty for failing—just for not being ambitious enough. As we frequently joked, at DARPA, if you don't invent the next internet, your grade is a B.

After years of work on the DSRC, in October 2003, I was asked by the DARPA director (Tony Tether) to leave my "dream job" as a physician-scientist and formally join DARPA full time—where I would not have a career but would have one hell of an opportunity to change the world.

This was a very dark time for our war fighters in Iraq and Afghanistan, with many young Americans being killed or maimed by improvised explosive devices (IEDs) and rocket-propelled grenades (RPGs) exported by the Iranians. In addition to biological warfare defense, I would also spend considerable effort improving war-fighter protection, battlefield medicine, training, resilience, and survival. It was a difficult decision to leave Dallas and my tenured academic position, but Jill and I agreed that the sacrifice for our family was for an important cause—our military needed us, and there was no way we were going to say no. So with the full support of Jill, I joined DARPA as the deputy director of the Defense Sciences Office (DSO), number two to Steve Wax—a highly experienced and respected materials scientist who was very savvy to DC and the Pentagon. Both he and Tether were great mentors, and three years later, when Steve's tour at DARPA was completed, I became the office director for DSO, the first physician in DARPA's history to hold that position.

My office was most known for programs like Revolutionizing Prosthetics, led by a military officer and physician-scientist, Colonel Geoffrey Ling. Through his constant insistence on success and disregard for conventional wisdom, Ling's program developed the first true brain-controlled bionic arm for amputees, changing the lives of wounded warriors forever. My office also fielded the first-generation microair vehicles that saved countless American lives in Iraq and Afghanistan by enabling over-the-horizon intelligence at the platoon level.

But my office was also heavily focused on biological warfare defense and preparedness for natural pandemics. We focused on both because the effects of bioweapons and natural pathogens can be the same—and so are most of the medical defenses against them. We devised an entire suite of initiatives under the overall program name Accelerating Critical Therapeutics. Our goal was bold: to develop the capability of providing one hundred million doses of a vaccine or treatment within twelve weeks of detecting a novel pathogen. While that goal is still not fully realized in 2022, we made tremendous progress in only a few years.

I recruited Dr. Michael Callahan, a top infectious disease and disaster physician from Harvard and Massachusetts General Hospital, to inspire and lead major components of this initiative, including a program entitled Accelerating Vaccine Manufacturing. Michael would show up many times in highly significant roles over the next fifteen years after I recruited him to DARPA, including in the *Diamond Princess* superspreader event and in air evacuations of Americans from the front lines of COVID-19. He is one of the heroes of US preparedness and response—but you are not likely to see him on CNN. And if you ever do see him on CNN, you can be sure there is a potentially catastrophic global crisis in the making.

DARPA continued with these important initiatives after I left the agency in mid-2008. In 2013, DARPA awarded Moderna, then a new company, with $25 million to research and develop mRNA-based medicines and vaccines. This work was eventually transitioned to the Biomedical Advanced Research and Development Authority (BARDA), an HHS component loosely modeled on DARPA. BARDA's main role was to sponsor the advanced development of such innovations so they could become authorized by the FDA and purchased for the US Strategic National Stockpile (SNS). BARDA initially funded Moderna to develop a Zika virus vaccine, but both DARPA and BARDA knew that Moderna had a platform technology that could be applied to any number of emerging infections—including a new pandemic. And as we now know, this company would eventually supply hundreds of millions of doses of a safe and effective vaccine against COVID-19.

The NIH deserves significant credit for the basic science it funds, but the American public should realize that other organizations, like DARPA and BARDA, often take the high-risk academic science and make something practical out of it—accelerating benefits to Americans by decades. I never heard Francis Collins or Tony Fauci mention DARPA when they spoke of the Moderna vaccine. In general, that omission was very consistent with the NIH habit of taking all the credit—even when undeserved—and thus most of the congressional funding.

By the end of 2007, I knew my time at DARPA was coming to an end. But after four and a half years at DARPA, my academic career as I knew it was also over. I was struggling like many others at DARPA had done before on how to reinsert myself back into "normal society" once my DARPA tour was over. Nothing quite compares to being at DARPA, working with the brightest people on the planet; "hair on fire" with almost no red tape or budgetary limitations; passionate about defending the United States against adversaries, saving US troops, and changing the world. But I did not want to fall into the self-destructive spiral of believing DARPA would be the best professional time in my life and then lamenting that fact for the next several decades.

Unexpectedly, I had become interested in an area that I had never thought about as a physician. I knew that a potential vaccine could be discovered through modern scientific methods within weeks. The problem was no longer the *discovery*; it was the scale-up of manufacturing to hundreds of millions of doses within a short period of time. And, of course, that was exactly the situation the United States faced with COVID-19. It took only two weeks to develop a candidate vaccine. The remaining months were dedicated to industrial manufacturing, clinical trials, and FDA approval.

Since mid-2008 (and this is still mostly true today), vaccines have been produced in biological systems. For influenza, the system is a fertilized chicken egg that is artificially infected with a live flu virus. For other vaccines, it is an immortal cell line that is genetically manipulated and grown in huge stainless-steel fermenters holding as many as five thousand gallons of cells growing in nutrient liquid ("media"). In 2008, manufacturing facilities were essentially custom-built for every single product at a cost of $500 million to $1.5 billion each and required years of construction and validation.

The United States was never going to make one hundred million vaccine doses in twelve weeks if it took years to build a custom manufacturing facility. We needed a solution, and I decided to focus on that challenge after leaving DARPA. I wanted to pioneer the design and construction of flexible vaccine-manufacturing facilities that would cost at least ten times less and could make many different products on short notice—weeks, not years.

BTHO INFLUENZA!

Texas A&M University is in many ways a typical land-grant university, designed to provide quality education to state residents who might otherwise not have an opportunity to attend college. As a first-generation college student myself, that mission immediately resonated with me. But Texas A&M is also unique among all US universities in its military origins and the fact that it still provides more officers to the US armed forces than any other school aside from the formal military academies. The entire institution is driven by values, dedication to tradition, and profound respect for fellow and former students. A good example of tradition and respect is Silver Taps, which first began in 1898.

Silver Taps is a solemn event that occurs on the first Tuesday of the month following a student's death. And unfortunately, with nearly seventy thousand students, there is at least one death almost every month. The names, graduating classes, and academic majors of the fallen students are written on cards and placed at the base of the flagpole located at the Silver Taps Memorial. There, students frequently leave letters to the families. Then at 10:15 p.m., the campus goes completely dark, chimes begin to play from the nearby bell tower, and students gather in complete silence at the academic plaza—thousands of students! The families of the fallen Aggies are escorted onto the plaza by student volunteers. After the families take their places, the ceremonial drill team, in their crisp, white uniforms and red silk sashes (the Ross Volunteers), march slowly and silently onto the plaza. In the darkness, you can only hear the tapping of their shoes until they are right in front of you. The Ross Volunteers then deliver a twenty-one-gun salute.

Next, buglers play taps three times—once each to the north, south, and west, but never to the east because the sun will never again rise on those fallen Aggies. When I first went to Silver Taps, I was completely overwhelmed by the true love that students had for one another and the comfort provided to the families by having so many thousands come out to honor their lost children. I often reflected that if I had died during my undergraduate time at Harvard, the only student interest would be whether my death would raise or lower the grading curve. It was the opposite of that at Texas A&M.

When I was about to leave DARPA, I knew I wanted to focus on the design and construction of vaccine-manufacturing facilities. As outstanding as UTSW was as a medical school and research institution, I knew it did not have the engineering faculty or students to build the team I needed. Since I was in the University of Texas system, my first thought was to transition to a faculty position at UT Austin, but my idea to pioneer next-generation bio-manufacturing did not resonate with the UT leadership—not at all. I left my visit to Austin convinced that they thought I needed psychiatric help more than a faculty position. And maybe I did!

By chance, it so happened that after that very disappointing meeting in Austin, the chancellor of the Texas A&M University System was in town and driving to the airport. I knew little about Texas A&M, except a few "Aggie jokes," but I knew they had a dominant College of Engineering with over ten thousand students. The person organizing my trip to Austin had me catch a ride to the airport with the Texas A&M chancellor, Dr. Mike McKinney, and there was an immediate connection. Mike is a unique combination of country boy, talented family physician, brilliant administrator/executive, former Texas health commissioner and chief of staff to Gov. Rick Perry, and all-around great guy. He invited me to College Station for a visit, and I accepted.

The full story needs to be told in another book, but there was great synergy and energy at that time, led by Governor Perry (whom I had met only once prior to my visit), two regents (John White and Bill Jones), the chancellor, and a vice chancellor and confidant of Governor Perry (Guy Diedrich). The governor wanted to build biotechnology and the pharmaceutical industry in Texas but had not been able to crack the code. He and the Texas A&M leadership had just invested in another strength of A&M, the College of Veterinary Medicine, and the world's most famous veterinary surgeon, Dr. Terry Fossum. Together, they built the most capable and modern large-animal research facility in the world, which would be used to improve animal health as well as human health. It would be a draw for biotech, for sure, especially those companies focused on interventional cardiology or advanced imaging, like CT scans and MRIs. But it was clear A&M could do more, and leveraging chemical engineering for novel biomanufacturing of vaccines appeared to hit the mark. So I threw out all my UT longhorn T-shirts, and Jill and I became Aggies.

Governor Perry had faith in the concept, in the project, and in Texas A&M. We put together a multidisciplinary team of faculty and industry partners and developed a design for a fully flexible, first-in-class biomanufacturing facility that would revolutionize the industry, improve biosecurity, and also bring new jobs to Texas. The state supported the project with $50 million from its Emerging Technology Fund, and we were off. We kept BARDA and other US agencies informed, but we did not ask them for anything. Depending on Texas was much more certain than trying to deal with federal bureaucracies.

The new facility, which we audaciously named the National Center for Therapeutics Manufacturing (NCTM), was truly groundbreaking. Although the NCTM structure was the size of a football field, it was completely flexible inside—so flexible that the clean rooms themselves were on air bearings so they could be literally pushed around the facility (like air-hockey pucks) to reconfigure process lines. The clean rooms were connected to utilities (electricity, water, etc.) through quick connections first used in the oil industry. Inside the clean rooms was flexible disposable process equipment. It was actually so successful that the journal *Nature* wrote an editorial that stated, "The future of the US government's biodefence strategy sits in a warehouse in rural Texas."

In March 2011, while the NCTM was still under construction, BARDA issued a request for proposal (RFP) to "establish U.S.-based Centers for Innovation in Advanced Development and Manufacturing (the 'Centers') as public-private partnerships that share facility construction costs, facilitate development and manufacture of medical countermeasure (MCM) product candidates, ensure domestic vaccine and other biopharmaceutical manufacturing surge capacity in an emergency, and provide workforce development training programs."

These centers would be required to incorporate flexible technologies to make a number of products at various scales and also to provide a massive scale-up for flu vaccines in case there was a sudden pandemic, like H1N1 just two years before. It seemed my predictions to the chancellor years earlier were correct, and biomanufacturing was now a national focus supported by billions of federal dollars.

Our team was in a good position to respond to this RFP, although the idea of an academic institution being a prime contractor for a dozen subcontractors, including the global pharmaceutical giant GlaxoSmithKline, was totally unprecedented. In our favor, we knew that other proposers only had PowerPoint presentations; we had a pioneering fully flexible biomanufacturing facility, the full support of a powerful state, and a built-in workforce from the university. It was a brutal competition, but in June 2012, three contracts were awarded by BARDA: one to Novartis, one to Emergent BioSolutions, and a $285 million contract to our team at Texas A&M. The contract also had a long tail of potential task orders that could total well over $1 billion.

Fast-forward to 2020. Although the US government did not adequately support the ongoing operations of these centers, both Emergent and Texas A&M were nonetheless sufficiently prepared and ready to respond to the COVID-19 pandemic. Both centers received task orders for COVID-19 vaccines. The Texas A&M center received a $265 million task order to reserve capacity and prepare for manufacturing the Novavax vaccine.

Another tradition at Texas A&M is "beat the hell outta," or BTHO. Texas A&M BTHO football rival Alabama. They BTHO breast cancer. They BTHO Hurricane Ike. And in honor of our 2012 BARDA contract, there was even a maroon T-shirt that read, "BTHO Influenza."

I stayed at Texas A&M in various roles until May 2015. Governor Perry was no longer in office; there was a reorganization of the university and a new president, and I was reorganized out of my job. I loved the students, former students, and faculty; the administrative leadership, not so much. But I still live three blocks from campus and continue to interact with and mentor students. The university president who asked me to resign is no longer the president.

The biomanufacturing center continues to grow and is now approaching one thousand employees thanks to the persistence of Texas A&M's new commercial partner, FUJIFILM Diosynth. Biotech has exploded within Texas, catalyzed by this Texas A&M center; research and innovation in the major medical centers of Houston, Dallas, and Austin; and novel state-funded programs like the Cancer Prevention and Research Institute of Texas (which invests $300 million per year into cancer research, new cancer companies, and recruiting superstars to Texas). It is nice to see a plan come together. Eventually, I hope that Rick Perry receives the credit he deserves for this tremendous success.

It was hard for me to leave an institution that I had grown to love and that ultimately educated both my daughters and my son-in-law after his nine years in the US Army and two combat tours in Iraq. But things happen for a reason. I was welcomed with open arms by the adjunct faculty of Baylor College of Medicine, stayed on the board of directors of the Texas Medical Center (the largest and among the most prestigious medical districts in the world), mentored young companies at the new Houston accelerator called TMCx, and became CEO of a Baylor College of Medicine spinout company that promised to help children with infections after bone marrow (stem cell) transplant. Most of these kids were cured of their cancers but could die from a common virus because their immune systems had not yet recovered. We were able to change that, and it felt great.

I had no idea that Trump would win the election and that I would ultimately leave Texas for a position in DC. Again.

3

The Trump Team Calls

Like most Americans, I followed the presidential campaign in 2016. But I was personally not involved. I voted early because on Election Day, I was scheduled to be the keynote speaker at an investor conference in Barcelona, Spain. Attending were many of the richest and most influential families in Europe and their family financial offices. My task was to explain recent breakthroughs in science—like new treatments for treating cancer—so that these families could become more informed about investing. I always liked translating science to nonscientists, which is fortunate because that is what I would do every day during the pandemic. Since each family was required to have at least $1 billion in assets to attend the conference, I hoped they would become more interested in investing in innovative new therapies for a wide range of diseases. I also hoped that much of that investment would be in small US companies.

Jill and I watched the election returns, but because of the time difference in Europe and my early morning keynote, we went to bed early. I imagined it might take days or weeks before the election results were final. However, the next morning, right before my keynote, with everyone at the conference watching CNN on big screens, Trump was declared the winner. The audience was silent and completely shocked. They had not anticipated, in their wildest imagination, that Trump would win. The conference moderator actually walked up on stage, announced the results of the election, and asked (perhaps rhetorically), "Who could actually vote for Trump?" My wife and I both raised our hands. I raised mine a little sheepishly, but not Jill—she went for it.

My keynote went well, but the main topic of the conference—at breaks and dinners and cocktails—was the US election. The Europeans actively talked to Jill and me about our reasons for voting for Trump. They were not only polite but increasingly empathetic. They had heard all the potential downsides of Trump but none of the upsides. The Europeans appeared to have open minds, or at least their poker faces were much better than I expected them to be.

I had not thought much about the possibility of returning to Washington, DC, in 2017 because, quite frankly, I did not believe Trump would win. In contrast, Jill stated that she knew Trump would be victorious from the moment he came down the escalator with his wife, Melania, to announce his candidacy. But even Jill was a little shocked.

I am not sure if Rick Perry called me or I called him, but we talked the day after the election. It was clear to me that Perry was going to be a cabinet member. My bet was that he would become secretary of defense, given his past service in the US Air Force and absolute dedication to those in uniform. In fact, he dedicated much of his time—and even opened the governor's mansion—to military personnel transitioning to civilian life, especially those suffering from traumatic brain injury and post-traumatic stress. Perry knew I was willing to serve and said he would provide my name to the Trump transition team at the appropriate time.

Everything was quiet for weeks, so I did not hold out much hope. Then on December 28, 2016, I received an email from Blake Masters, then president of the Peter Thiel Foundation, who had received my name from Geoff Ling, a retired US Army colonel and physician who was an extraordinary program manager in my office at DARPA and the driving force behind the DARPA bionic arm.

I did not understand the inner workings of the Trump transition team, but there was clearly a group led by Peter Thiel (founder of Palantir and PayPal and board member for Facebook). He and his closest colleagues were identifying and screening people for technical positions that would eventually require a presidential appointment or nomination. There is an important distinction here: a political *appointee* needs only to be supported by the presidential transition team and ultimately the president. A *nominee* is someone whose name the president sends to the Senate, after vetting by the transition team, for the arduous process of confirmation for a specified position.

Blake Masters emailed me at noon on December 28, 2016; I responded at 1:10 p.m., and we had a call twenty minutes later. It was a very positive call, and we discussed several positions in the Department of Defense, intelligence agencies, DHS, and, of course, HHS, including the CDC director position. I would have been willing to serve in any number of positions, but my true love was public health, and that was also my career, and thus my top choices were in that domain within either HHS, DHS, or the Department of Defense. Within HHS, I thought my background and qualifications were a good match for either the ASH (assistant secretary for health), the ASPR (assistant secretary for preparedness and response), or the surgeon general. I had always told my wife that I would go back to DC if asked to be in any one of those three positions, but that seemed far-fetched; now it seemed possible.

I learned that Bob Kadlec was already in the works to be the ASPR, and I was fully supportive of him in that role. Bob and I had worked together intermittently since my first days at DARPA in 2004. He was uniquely qualified for the ASPR job and was the perfect choice. On January 4, I heard back from Blake. Their internal team had reviewed my credentials and discussed my interviews, and they were recommending me (to whom, I don't know) to be either the assistant secretary for health or the surgeon general. I was very excited about either possibility.

It was again totally quiet until January 16, 2017, when I received an email from Trae Stevens, another colleague of Peter Thiel and a partner in one of Thiel's ongoing enterprises. He was given my curriculum vitae by Rick Perry and was contacting me about a potential national security position. I did not know if that meant I was out of the running for surgeon general or assistant secretary or if this was an unrelated opportunity based on my long involvement in the classified world. After we spoke, I continued to stand by.

My other big supporter was Dr. Ron DiPinho—former president of MD Anderson Cancer Center and world-renowned cancer physician and scientist. I don't know Ron's politics, but he was influential across party lines and frequently spoke to the Thiel team. I had known Ron for several years, and most recently, I had served on his MD Anderson Cancer Center Moon Shots Program advisory board. It was extremely valuable to have someone of Ron's scientific stature and personal integrity support my nomination. I wanted to be selected for my experience and capability, not my political ideology or campaign activities, and Ron could vouch for me.

It was quiet again for another month until February 19, when Bob Kadlec put me in touch with Thomas DiNanno, who had been officially positioned on the "landing team" for DHS. Thomas was working to advance Bob's candidacy to be the ASPR within HHS. Because the ASPR was responsible for the medical and public health defenses against terrorist attacks, it did not surprise me that DHS was weighing in on the ASPR position. Thomas asked me if I was on the administration's radar yet, and I responded with "It is hard to tell," since it had already been almost two months since my original call with Blake Masters. I did learn that there was an online form that needed to be filled out for anyone seeking a political position. That was news to me. I complied and was finally "officially" in the system. Then more waiting.

On March 9, a senior advisor in the White House Office of Presidential Personnel (PPO) called and requested I fill out two simple forms and submit them: the first was a one-page bio and the second was my five-year salary history. Next step: meet with the PPO, and that meeting was scheduled in DC at the Eisenhower Executive Office Building for March 26, 2017. I was nervous because I had no idea what to expect. At DARPA, my position was nonpolitical, so I did not have to go through any of this. The interview was anticlimactic, to say the least. I met three members of the PPO team for a total of thirty minutes combined. At the end of the meetings, they admitted that they needed to lay eyes on me to make sure I neither was crazy nor had any obvious fatal flaws. I understood that and did not regret for a moment the long trip for a thirty-minute smell test. It was now clear: the president was considering me for the assistant secretary for health position within HHS, and that was incredibly exciting.

On March 31, I received a code to enter information into the e-QIP (Electronic Questionnaires for Investigations Processing) system. This was my formal background check and would serve as the basis for a security clearance. I was very confused because I already held a top-secret clearance through the Department of Defense and had just undergone a routine reinvestigation two months earlier. I had filled out the same forms, an investigator interviewed me, and as per protocol, that investigator talked to my family, my friends, my neighbors, and many other contacts in search of dirt that could make me a national security risk. I supplied all my financial information to ensure I would not be a target for spies due to a gambling addiction or other financial problems. I swore to the investigator that I had no girlfriends or boyfriends and did not engage in any anti-US activity.

Unfortunately, my recently renewed top-secret clearance was not sufficient for the PPO, so the entire process started again. This time, however, instead of being handled by a contracted private investigator, FBI special agents conducted the investigation. The special agent assigned to my case was located in the Bryan, Texas, office, which was a few miles from my home. She had recently transferred from Virginia and was incredibly thorough with me and all my close contacts over the previous ten years. I am not sure if she did many investigations of this type, but it was clear she took her work seriously. No stone was left unturned. My neighbors must have thought that I was involved in some type of questionable activity with the FBI poking around so thoroughly. I assured everyone that I was not in trouble—or at least not the kind of trouble they were worried about me being in!

There were also financial and political disclosures as onerous as the national security clearance disclosures. The PPO and then the Senate committee that would conduct my confirmation hearings (the Senate Committee on Health,

Education, Labor, and Pensions, or HELP) wanted to know everything about me financially and politically: my campaign contributions, every mutual fund and stock interest, every employer, every board of directors or science advisory board, every volunteer position, every social club, and basically everything else. I did not have an accountant or beltway consultant, so Jill and I did these on our own. We were seriously afraid to miss something or put something in the wrong category—I was sure it would be interpreted in the worst possible light.

At the same time that I was completing the financial forms in the first week of April, I received a call from HHS Secretary Thomas "Tom" Price, recently confirmed by the Senate after his nomination by Trump. He had heard good things about me from Rick Perry and others but clearly needed to do his own evaluation. The call was surprising to me in many ways. Price was very kind and humble and started with the question "Why would someone who has had a great career want to come to Washington and ruin it?" I knew this was partly tongue in cheek, but there was a bit of truth to it—and also some prophetic foreshadowing about his own career and eventual untimely resignation as secretary.

Price was mostly interested in my clinical training at Parkland Hospital. He had a long history of practicing medicine at Grady Hospital in Atlanta, another legendary public-safety-net hospital. He wanted to know about my commitment to the underserved. He wanted to know about my motivation and what I hoped to achieve. I specifically told him that my primary role would be to support the secretary in developing and implementing policies that improve the health of the nation. Everything would stem from that. I wanted to be a convener and a catalyst and to develop measurable goals and then push to achieve them. And I wanted to innovate. I also said that I knew the assistant secretary for health could be window dressing, but I would only come if I could make meaningful contributions and have a voice, and he assured me that I would.

What was never asked by Secretary Price, the White House, or Peter Thiel's team were my views on any social issues. I thought for sure that I would have had to declare allegiance to a social agenda, but I was never asked. There was no "virtue vetting" for my position at that time or at any future time. And that fact was entirely opposite of many talking points about Trump nominees under consideration.

I was told that it would be many weeks before the vetting was completed by the White House, so I was surprised to get a call on April 20 indicating that the president would announce his intent to nominate me the next day, before my paperwork and investigation were complete. My nomination was to be for the assistant secretary for health and also medical director in the US Public Health Service Commissioned Corps. That meant the president wanted me in uniform, and that was my strong desire as well, given my long association with DARPA and the armed components of the military. Only about one-third of former assistant secretaries had been in uniform—most served as civilians.

I was not prepared for the sudden spotlight, nor were my family, friends, colleagues, or coworkers. But it happened. The intent to nominate was just that: not a commitment, just an intent. I interpreted this as a way to get my name into the public, just in case dirt would surface. The president could then save face before an official nomination went to the Senate. On April 21, I understood why my intent to nominate might have been expedited. On that day, HHS fired V. Adm. Vivek Murthy, the surgeon general who was a hold-over from the Obama administration. I inferred that the Trump transition team wanted to have another health professional named and on deck, since the surgeon general was fired—and I was that person, as there was no surgeon general nominee yet named by Trump.

Since I was not allowed to speak to anyone at HHS aside from a single legislative coordinator (fondly called my "Sherpa"), I prepared for my role by speaking with everyone in the broad public health community who would talk to me. Key among those organizations were the American Public Health Association, Trust for America's Health, the American Academy of Pediatrics, the American Heart Association, the Association of State and Territorial Health officers, and many others. I hired a PhD student in public health from Baylor College of Medicine, Kara Elam, who helped me put together position papers and issue analyses. She later joined my office at HHS and was a driving force behind our national human papillomavirus (HPV) vaccination campaign.

I spent extensive time speaking with the Commissioned Officers Association of the USPHS to learn details of my future service and the problems they were facing. I also spoke to Dr. Karen DeSalvo, who was acting assistant secretary for over two years in the Obama administration. Over the ensuing many months, I was able to build a public health agenda for HHS and a strategy to reinvigorate the Commissioned Corps. It was an exciting time for planning but also an incredibly frustrating time because of the endless delays in the confirmation process. The clock was ticking.

I was also very concerned about whom the president would pick to be surgeon general. The surgeon general would report directly to me. At that time, there were rumors that the pick could be a "TV doctor" or even someone who was not a physician or nurse at all. The media rumored it might even be an anti-vaxxer! I had a great sigh of relief when Trump eventually announced his intent to nominate Dr. Jerome Adams, a perfect choice in my mind—but that intent to nominate did not come until June 29.

I was officially nominated by Trump on May 25 after six months of seemingly endless paperwork.

The next step for me was Senate confirmation. I would have a hearing in front of the Senate Committee on Health, Education, Labor, and Pensions, chaired by Republican senator Lamar Alexander with Democrat ranking member Patty Murray. In addition to the extensive documents required by the committee and publicly posted, I also put together a packet of support letters from numerous individuals and organizations. I was very humbled by the support I received, especially from faculty members at Texas A&M who made it clear that I was a leader they respected and that I went out of my way to support diversity and the advancement of women faculty.

Per protocol, my Sherpa and I tried to set up personal meetings with each member of HELP so that they could speak with me privately, face-to-face, before the hearing. The position of the assistant secretary was steeped in political rancor and rhetoric. That had nothing to do with me personally, but I would be the political punching bag for the battle between the Democrats and Republicans over social issues, including abortion. There was little I could do about that except to take the punches and move on. That is exactly what Georges Benjamin of the American Public Health Association said to me; he affirmed that his team had examined my record up and down and there was nothing controversial whatsoever in my past. But as the saying goes, "Everyone at the party has a good time except the piñata," and I was going to be the piñata.

As background, the Title X Family Planning Program (which included Planned Parenthood as an awardee) and the Teen Pregnancy Prevention Program were administered by the Office of the Assistant Secretary for Health (OASH). In addition, I would be in charge of high-profile policy offices dealing with minority health, HIV, and women's health—all of which were hot-button items on both sides of the aisle. As a result, there had not been a Senate-confirmed assistant secretary for health since August 2014, nearly three years. A political fight about my position was inevitable. But I had no idea that this was going to be the case when I started the process.

Because senators frequently canceled meetings with only a few hours' notice, Jill and I spent almost five weeks in various hotels and VRBOs in DC trying to complete these meetings. This was expensive and time consuming but part of the process. It was a hazing, and I understood that. I had my first meeting (on time and on schedule) with Senator John Kennedy of Louisiana because Louisiana was my birth state. He was, in person, exactly as you see him on TV: witty with a slightly twisted sense of humor, a country-boy affect, and a Harvard-lawyer intellect. It was a great meeting and very reassuring to me.

Chairman Alexander is a Renaissance man who represented the best of the Senate. He is a brilliant, respectful Southern gentleman who had been the US secretary of education, the governor of Tennessee, the president of the University of Tennessee, and a successful businessman, just to name a few of his accomplishments. The meeting with him was uplifting, and I had his full support. I also met with many Democrats, and those meetings were generally positive as well, to my surprise. Sheldon Whitehouse is a data wonk—and I mean that in a good way. We spoke about access to health care and many children's issues. Our discussion went through numerous topics in an evidence-driven, policy-oriented fashion. I was impressed.

My most surprising meeting was with Elizabeth Warren. It was scheduled for twenty minutes but lasted almost an hour. It was clear she was probing at first to see if I was a "Trump crazy" in any way or had extreme views on political or social issues. I didn't. I was, and am, pretty straight with the science and evidence. We next discussed my background and qualifications and my motivation for the job, which also went very well. Then Senator Warren shifted her tone and overall body language and started talking about how we could work together. She knew I would be working for an administration she would vehemently oppose but offered to work on important health issues with me where we could gain alignment (and there were quite a few of those, actually). She stated that I could contact her directly, and if I needed her to "make a fuss," she said she was "very good at that as well." At the end of the meeting, she made it clear that she probably would not vote for me because I was a Trump nominee, but she would be happy to work with me once I was confirmed. I found her honesty refreshing and felt increasingly optimistic that even in the politically polarized world of DC, I might be able to work across party lines to get things done for public health. That was my sole focus.

But there were also many disappointments. I had at least three meetings scheduled with Senator Murray—all were canceled with little notice, leaving me stuck in DC twiddling my thumbs, wasting a lot of time and money. As the ranking member, Murray was key to my getting an affirmative vote in her committee and thereafter being confirmed by the full Senate. But I was only able to meet with her on my fourth attempt, and it lasted about three minutes in her office as she was running out to a Senate vote.

In retrospect, I think she really did not want to meet me because at my hearing on August 1, 2017—which was a joint hearing with other HHS nominees (Jerome Adams, Eleanor McCance-Katz, Lance Robertson, and Bob Kadlec)—Senator Murray went for the Trump administration's jugular from the moment her mouth started moving. My wife, who was sitting behind me trying not to have any reactions or facial expressions, later recounted that she started sinking in her chair and having palpitations because of the intensity of the attacks. There had often not even been formal confirmation hearings for these positions in the past, as noted by Chairman Alexander. Most of the time, qualifications were reviewed on paper, and the nominees were voted out of committee and sent to the Senate floor for confirmation. But Senator Murray insisted on a public hearing, and we understood the reason—politics.

Senator Murray began by openly challenging whether we would put science and facts over politics. I found this very condescending and insulting, since all of us had spent our careers doing just that. Murray again grilled us about whether we would do the right thing even if there was political pressure from above. Again, only a senator could get away with those types of self-righteous questions in front of people who had actually spent their careers at the bedside helping people every day.

Then she attacked President Trump and Secretary Price directly. We all took incoming from her. She wanted to know whether we would stand up to the administration's positions. At that time, none of us had had the opportunity to discuss or understand the administration's positions (since we were not allowed to converse with anyone at HHS). And of course, if we disagreed with a policy, we would debate that internally, not in front of senators or the media. She complained about the president firing the surgeon general and that this showed his disrespect for science. (Trump kept him for months into his administration, but Biden would later fire Jerome Adams on Inauguration Day—did Murray ever complain about Biden's firing of Jerome Adams?)

Directed specifically to me, she said she was deeply concerned about actions in my future office and the "attacks on women's health and the rights of women" and that Trump had appointed "radical anti-choice" zealots to my office. I think Murray meant that the appointees were "pro-life." In addition, Murray stated that these appointees were continuing their "ideological attacks on women."[1] I felt it hard to understand how Murray could accuse women appointees of conducting ideological attacks on women. But she was the ranking member, and making accusations and impugning character was her prerogative, especially for Trump nominees.

In response to questions, I affirmed my commitment to all the issues that she was concerned about, including the importance of the Teen Pregnancy Prevention and Title X programs. I stated my commitment to work with her and all the members and to do an independent assessment of the data and draw my own conclusions. I pledged to elevate science over politics, which I later would do every day during the pandemic. I supported the critically important services provided by Title X clinics like performing cervical cancer screening. I affirmed that I would "implement the laws passed by Congress and given to me faithfully and as they are intended." I stated that "if there were restrictions passed down to me, I am obliged to follow the law." I specifically stated that my intent was to provide all of these critically needed Title X services across the board in an affordable and accessible way to all who sought them. In retrospect, I could not have given more agreeable answers to her questions and challenges.

We were all passed out of committee the next day. Many Democrats voted against me and my fellow nominees. Bernie Sanders—a member of the committee—never met with me and did not show up for the hearing, but he voted against me anyway. That seems very irresponsible, but I guess by that time, he was too busy to engage with the nominees. We were clearly not his priority. And besides, he already knew he would oppose nearly everyone associated with Trump—no matter their qualifications. Senator Al Franken called me after the hearing when I was on a layover for a flight back to Texas. He yelled at me for many minutes over the phone for not coming out against the administration—how exactly was I to do that in a Senate hearing, especially since I had not been allowed to even converse with the administration over specific policies? But I did get many Democrat votes, and I appreciated them.

On August 3, my four colleagues who were at the hearing with me were confirmed by voice vote in the Senate. I did not get a vote because Senator Murray insisted that I have a roll-call vote on the Senate floor. Apparently, I made a mistake by saying, "I would follow the law," and Murray subsequently announced (despite my qualifications and record) that she was "unconvinced Dr. Giroir would be willing to stand up to this administration's ideological attacks on women in a key leadership role at HHS." This was again political theater, with no basis whatsoever. Demanding a roll-call vote might permanently kill my nomination because at the time, Democrats could demand thirty hours of debate before my vote, which was more time than the Senate was in session during any given week. And the Republican Senate leadership was not going to waste a week on a single assistant secretary with so many federal judges waiting to be confirmed. Judges were the priority, and the Democrats knew it.

I was indeed the piñata; this was politics over public health. Delaying my confirmation delayed many progressive public health programs. And what Murray never realized is that I was perhaps the most socially liberal person in a senior role at HHS and that if she really cared about her issues, she would have had me in office as soon as possible. But it was "get Trump" at all costs. There would be more of that from the Democrat senators in the future.

But to my amazement, my nomination eventually began to shake loose. It was no longer about women's issues. My nomination was being held hostage in exchange for HHS providing an internal memo about the Affordable Care Act to Democrat members. The Democrats got their memo, and it looked promising for me to be confirmed by voice vote on the last day of the Senate session prior to the holidays in December 2017. My team said it was all *done* and my name was on the list. I was extremely excited to finally get in the game and start contributing. My wife and I were listening to the proceedings on C-SPAN, and they began reading the list of names that were confirmed by acclamation. My name was supposed to be on the list, as were many others awaiting confirmation. But Schumer decided at the last moment to block many of us again—just to disrupt the Trump administration and his agenda one more time. The senators went home for vacation, with the nation still not having a person confirmed as the senior public health policy official. Inexcusable.

If that weren't bad enough, Schumer had the option to leave my nomination where it was, ready for a vote on the Senate floor in the New Year. That was the custom. But he did not choose that. He sent me—and many other nominees—back to start the process all over again for the new Congress. The president had to renominate me (which he did). I had to fill out all the onerous Senate paperwork again (which I did). Fortunately, the committee decided not to hold another hearing and passed me back to the entire Senate once the paperwork was resubmitted. Eventually, at the end of January, I was right back where I started on August 3 the year before. But I had given up hope of ever being confirmed. Jill and I started planning for a different future.

Then on February 7, 2018, I received a call from my Sherpa that something might happen in the Senate. She advised me to listen to C-SPAN, which I had spent hours upon hours doing over the past months. I turned the TV on, and within five minutes, my name was read—just like that—and I was confirmed unanimously by voice vote. *Done.* No explanation but six months delayed from when I should have been in DC along with my other colleagues.

So in retrospect, was it good for public health to delay my confirmation? Aside from my role during the pandemic, I led HHS initiatives related to substance-use disorders and mental health, advocating for treatment instead of incarceration. I led the Ending the HIV Epidemic in the US initiative and put highly qualified career physicians and scientists in leadership roles in my office—replacing many of the marginally qualified staff who were either newly appointed or left over from the Obama administration. I started a global coalition to fight sickle cell disease in the United States and sub-Saharan Africa. I must have done a few things right because I received several nonpartisan awards during my term.[2]

The political theater of Senate confirmation repeated itself again for my nomination to the Executive Board of the World Health Organization within the Department of State—that time with potentially catastrophic consequences for the emerging COVID-19 pandemic. It is truly ironic that the Trump administration was always accused of putting politics ahead of science. None of us in science roles did that—ever. But it was clear that the ones criticizing the loudest, including Senators Schumer and Murray, were the prime offenders—far worse than anyone I had seen within the Trump administration.

On the evening of February 7, 2018, I was confirmed by the Senate. We did not have a place to live in DC or any other arrangements. I immediately resigned from all my professional positions and divested all my stocks so I would have no perceived conflicts of interest. Jill and I flew to DC on February 14, 2018, and stayed at the Hampton Inn in the Navy Yard. We celebrated Valentine's Day (we had actually met on Valentine's Day in 1980) at a neighborhood seafood bar and prepared for our adventure. The next morning, she looked for an apartment as I started work at HHS.

Early on February 15, I was sworn in as the sixteenth assistant secretary for health and admiral in the USPHS Commissioned Corps. I later admitted that one of my first goals was to determine if Valerie Huber—the person already in the chief of staff role—was really an activist fanatic as the Democrats and media portrayed her to be. It would have been really unfortunate to fire my chief of staff (a political appointee) during my first week, but I would have done so if needed. I was surprised, pleasantly, that although she clearly was highly principled on certain social issues, Valerie was very rational, talented, and collegial. She very soon demonstrated her willingness to modify some of her policy proposals once I presented a physician's point of view. We became great colleagues and were both made better by working with each other.

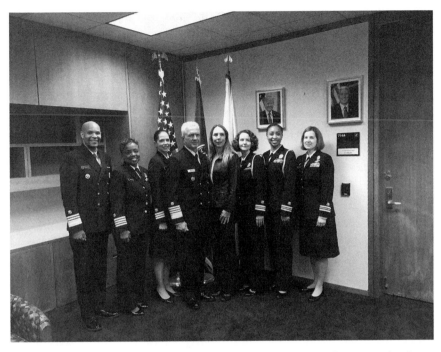

Photo with Surgeon Gen. Jerome Adams; my wife, Jill; and USPHS officers immediately after my swearing in as assistant secretary (personal photo).

On February 21, I held my first all-hands meeting in OASH, during which I laid out what was probably the most progressive public health agenda in the last three decades, including the nine words that would guide our policy development: health for all, health by all, and health in all. I outlined new programs for improving vaccination, including those that protect against the overwhelming majority of HPV infections, and how we would reduce the number of HIV cases by 50 percent within three years. We would focus on prevention and early intervention and battle historic disparities by using the US Public Health Service officers as change agents. We would have a particular focus on the social determinants of health, especially adverse childhood experiences that destined children for the development of chronic physical and mental disorders decades later. It was an exciting time, and the entire office was buzzing with enthusiasm and activity.

My effectiveness would ultimately depend on the secretary and his view of the role of the assistant secretary for health. As such, I was very concerned about my first meeting with Secretary Alex Azar, not for any personal or policy reasons but because Price was no longer the secretary. I had no idea if Azar actually wanted me in the role (he did not pick me) or if he would value the position of the assistant secretary. I did not suspect at the time that Azar had little regard for the ASH position. In his prior experience, the ASH was mostly ceremonial, traveling around the public health circles but not meaningfully engaged with HHS initiatives or the secretary.

A few things were clear about Azar from that first meeting, and I appreciated all of them. Azar had an incredible intellect, and he had a mastery of all the complex issues across the vast policy expanse of HHS—from access to care and insurance, to drug pricing, to influenza and pandemic preparedness, to human services for children and families, to the wide variety of social issues, including religious conscience and the Title X abortion provisions. I should have expected he would be that smart given his academic pedigree and the fact that he clerked for Supreme Court Justice Antonin Scalia. But you never know. Despite his intellect, he always and humbly asked for honest feedback and input to improve himself and his leadership. He took feedback from "almost peers," like me, but also from young staffers who supported his legislative agenda or communications platforms.

More important to me was the fact that he knew how to run "the building." Azar had previously served as the general counsel and then deputy secretary under Pres. George W. Bush. He knew what could get done and how to do it. As much as I liked Secretary Price personally, his learning curve would have been steep—Azar essentially knew everything about how this behemoth of an agency, with ninety thousand employees and a $1.4 trillion budget, operated. Azar was also disciplined about execution because he knew that was where we could fail—not in the ideas or strategy but in the practical execution.

Azar respected the fact that I was a physician-scientist, and he needed someone like me on the core team because both he and the deputy secretary were lawyers. They were both cognizant that there were many areas where they had little knowledge—especially scientific and technical areas. In other words, they "knew what they didn't know," and that is rare in DC. Equally important to our relationship was that I had no interest in his job or any other job. That was not the case for at least two of his senior division heads. I was an assistant secretary, meaning quite literally that I was there to "assist the secretary." Naturally, I had my own policy priorities, but those were secondary to supporting my boss. He trusted me, and I never let that trust down.

We hit it off very well, and I never learned about his prejudices about the ASH position until at least a year later, when it was no longer relevant. In any case, he acted in the exact opposite way—giving me more and more responsibilities within the department. I soon became a "go-to guy" to organize initiatives for the secretary and, when needed, to help turn around bad situations. It made sense because that was the intended role of the ASH: to manage large efforts within the Public Health Service agencies, which include the CDC, the FDA, the NIH, the HRSA (Health Resources and Services Administration), and others. My first such assignment came very early, on March 29, 2018, when the secretary dual-hatted me as his senior advisor for mental health and opioid policy. The opioid epidemic was raging, and while there were interesting approaches discussed around the department, there wasn't a metric-driven comprehensive plan that crossed agency boundaries, and there was also very little accountability. I changed that immediately by bringing people together and defining objectives and strategies, complete with deliverables, timelines, and metrics. And we started to make quantifiable progress against overdose deaths—which lasted until the pandemic began.

Azar tapped me for many other assignments, including dealing with the issue of classifying (or not) kratom as a controlled substance regulated by the Drug Enforcement Administration (DEA). This was proceeding in a hell-bent way without his (or my) prior knowledge at the time. Kratom is a botanical that is used for pain relief by millions of Americans, but certain components of the plant have opioid-like properties. Azar later asked me to assist in gaining a scientific understanding of fetal tissue research, providing him and the White House with objective facts about the consequences of banning such research. I also served for a time as the senior adviser for the CDC and the HRSA, when those agencies (especially the HRSA) were hitting rough spots with leadership and budgets.

In late 2019 when it was clear that the acting FDA commissioner Ned Sharpless was not going to be nominated by Trump for the permanent position and it was possible that the Democrats in the Senate would not confirm Stephen Hahn because they liked Sharpless, the secretary asked me to become acting FDA commissioner—which I did. I was not going to "break any dishes" while there, but in eight weeks, we implemented some major policies and programs, and side by side with Azar, we were able to convince the president to allow us to proceed with enforcement against kid-friendly flavors in e-cigarettes (like bubble gum). That was a major win that we never thought would happen because of the powerful tobacco industry lobby and its vocal public campaign—but in the end, Trump did the right thing for public health as he had done many times before during my short tenure.

The bottom line is that I had a reputation for problem-solving, so when it became clear that the CDC and the FDA were not meeting expectations in the pandemic response, the secretary turned to me to coordinate change. Right before the end of our term, Azar wrote me a note and called me his "indispensable man." I appreciated that kind and generous note because of who wrote it. Azar's leadership remained a critical stabilizing influence throughout the pandemic response. And, of course, without Azar, there would not have been OWS, and we would have suffered hundreds of thousands more US deaths.

4

Nature's Warning Shots:
H1N1 and Ebola

The risk of infectious disease outbreaks is real, and these outbreaks are inevitable given the interconnected nature of the world we live in. An outbreak anywhere becomes a threat everywhere.[1]

For the last two thousand years, the history of our species *is* the history of pandemics: plague, cholera, smallpox, influenza, HIV/AIDS, Ebola, SARS (severe acute respiratory syndrome), MERS (Middle East respiratory syndrome), and now COVID-19.

In 165 CE, Roman soldiers brought a virus (likely smallpox or measles) back from campaigns in the Near East; between five and ten million Romans, one-third of the population of the Roman world, died over the next fifteen years. Between the years 541 and 543 CE, an estimated one hundred million inhabitants of the Roman Empire died during the "plague of Justinian," made possible by the rapid spread of the disease through new Roman trade routes. Nine hundred years later, the Black Death (caused by the same organism) wiped out nearly one-third of the entire European population and continued with successive waves until the early eighteenth century. The Black Death was ultimately defeated by the control of rats and fleas, quarantine, and other basic public health interventions. Smallpox killed five hundred million people over one hundred years, including three hundred million in the twentieth century alone, before it was officially eradicated in 1980 by global vaccination and isolation of the last cases. Compared to these previous threats to the very existence of humanity, COVID-19—as horrific as it is—pales in comparison.

Unfortunately, the risk of pandemics has actually increased over time. The world is now interconnected in ways previously unimagined. A man infected with Ebola in Liberia can arrive in Dallas within twenty-four hours. Tens of thousands of potentially COVID-infected people flew from Wuhan to dozens of countries, seeding hundreds of locations, before travel restrictions were even contemplated. It is true, more than ever before, that an outbreak *anywhere* in the world is a threat *everywhere* in the world.

Pandemic risk has also been heightened by our increasingly close contact with animals, especially in remote environments like rainforests and caves. This contact raises the risk of animal-to-human crossover infections. In addition, cultural practices in which numerous exotic wild animals are brought together in close quarters with one another and humans, like in some wet markets, greatly increase the chances of a virus spreading from animals to humans. Perhaps more concerning, these practices enhance the chances of genetic recombination (sharing genes) among diverse animal viruses to create entirely new pathogens never before seen on the planet.

Finally, scientific advances in genetics and molecular biology make it possible for humans, intentionally or nonintentionally, to create Frankenstein pathogens that could be catastrophic. Today, even in a modestly sophisticated laboratory, it is relatively easy to piece together a bit of one pathogen with a bit of another pathogen. For example, one could take a gene that allows for the infection of humans (as opposed to only animals) and move that gene into a pathogen that is resistant to a drug. The result would be a new human pathogen that evades drug therapy. Once created, the bug could be further evolved in the laboratory to be even more infectious over time.

In this regard, in my opinion, it remains more likely than not that the origin of COVID-19 was the Wuhan Institute of Virology (WIV), despite the fact that there are no obvious "fingerprints" of direct human tampering with this virus. What is more plausible is that the virus was originally obtained from a wild bat and then evolved within the lab to be highly infectious to humans. Then through an accidental infection of one or more laboratory staff, who may have initially been asymptomatic at the time, the virus spread locally and then exponentially across the entire globe, resulting in the deaths of millions of people.

Perhaps the most compelling argument supporting the hypothesis that the SARS-CoV-2 virus (the virus that causes COVID-19) was accidentally released from the Wuhan lab is that it was highly infectious among humans from the start. That degree of immediate infectivity is unprecedented for an animal coronavirus and in sharp contrast to the two most recent severe coronavirus outbreaks: SARS (2003), which originated in bats and spread to humans through palm civets sold at Chinese wet markets for food, and MERS (2012), which originated in camels on the Arabian Peninsula. Both of these diseases required years of occasional transmission from animal to human before the viruses were ever significantly transmitted from human to human. And when they did spread among humans, they did so at a much slower pace than the COVID-19 virus has.

Although no one predicted the COVID-19 pandemic specifically, the fact that a respiratory virus caused another pandemic in our lifetime was not a surprise. It was not a matter of if but when. If two thousand years of human history was not enough of a warning, nature fired many recent warning shots—the two most relevant were the 2009 H1N1 influenza pandemic and the African Ebola outbreak in 2013–16 and its subsequent US cases. Both had lasting effects on our national approach to preparedness, mostly for the better. But we also ignored many lessons that needed to be learned, lessons that might have saved tens of thousands of US lives in 2020 and 2021.

H1N1 2009

Influenza viruses mutate slightly from year to year. These mutations are relatively small but significant enough to leave many people vulnerable to infection by the mutated influenza strain. As a result, every year millions of Americans become infected with the flu and thousands die. The 2017–18 flu season, for example, resulted in over 500,000 hospitalizations and 61,000 deaths in the United States alone.

People infected with influenza can spread it to others up to six feet away, primarily by droplets when sneezing, coughing, or talking. It is also possible to spread the flu by touching an object that has the flu virus on it (like a doorknob) and then touching your nose or mouth. Because the flu mutates slightly from year to year, we need annual flu vaccines to keep up (at least in part) with these mutations. But even without annual flu vaccines, some people have immunity because they had been infected with a similar flu virus in the past—perhaps many years or decades before.

Occasionally, however, the influenza virus undergoes a major mutational shift that results in a very different virus for which few humans—if any— have any preexisting immunity. This major mutational shift is often due to a genetic recombination (sharing of big pieces of genetic material) between two or more flu viruses. When such a major change happens, there is a high risk of a global pandemic.

The 1918 influenza pandemic was the most severe pandemic in modern history (at least until COVID-19), infecting one-third of the world's population (500 million people) and killing an estimated 50 million, including

675,000 Americans. The origin of the 1918 virus is still debated, but it likely originated from a natural bird influenza virus, which jumped to humans either directly or through an intermediate host like a pig.

The influenza virus is known for its ability to jump from animals to humans in a short period of time, and thus we are always worried about potential flu pandemics. The 1918 virus was so mutated that few if any humans had immune protection. With no vaccine to prevent its spread and no antibiotics to treat secondary bacterial infections, the mortality rate was 2.5 percent, approximately ten times greater than the fatality rate for COVID-19.

In the spring of 2009, ninety-one years after the 1918 pandemic, the world was hit with another novel influenza strain, likely originating in northern Mexico after circulating for years in pigs before finally jumping to humans. H1N1 was "new" to the scene, and we paid the price. The eventual burden of disease for H1N1 was striking, with global estimates as high as 700 million to 1.4 billion people infected and over 280,000 deaths.[2] At least 80 percent of the deaths occurred in people *less than* sixty-five years of age, including many young pregnant women. This is in sharp contrast to typical flu seasons for which at least 80 percent of deaths occur in those *over* sixty-five years of age. A possible explanation is that older people could have been infected with a flu virus decades earlier, and that provided some protection against 2009 H1N1; younger people were not alive decades earlier and thus were completely vulnerable.

Of historical note, the first identification of the H1N1 pandemic strain in the United States was accomplished at the Naval Health Research Center in San Diego, California, on April 13, 2009, using an experimental diagnostics tool that was developed through DARPA support.[3] We will get back to that later, when we detail how the United States needs to modernize our infectious disease surveillance system.

Despite all-out efforts by the US government, the 2009 H1N1 pandemic was both disheartening and terrifying. From April 2009 to April 2010, the United States experienced more than 60 million cases, over 274,000 hospitalizations, and at least 12,000 deaths—many among young adults. Despite years of "preparation" and tabletop exercises, our national response was overall a dismal failure. Ron Klain, President Biden's current chief of staff, summarized his assessment in a pandemic policy summit held in May 2019: "A bunch of really talented people were working on it but did every possible thing wrong. . . . Sixty million Americans got H1N1 in that period of time, and it's just purely a fortuity that this isn't one of the great mass casualty events in American history. It had nothing to do with us doing anything right; it just had to do with luck."[4]

Part of this statement is absolutely correct. If the 2009 influenza had the mortality rate of the 1918 virus, 1.5 million Americans would have died—more deaths than we have had for COVID-19. Some say we dodged a bullet in 2009—but many say otherwise. A more accurate statement was that nature shot us squarely in the chest, but this time she was shooting a BB gun and not a .45-caliber semiautomatic pistol.

But this "near miss" was not entirely the fault of the federal medical experts because there were technical barriers that prevented an effective response, especially with respect to manufacturing and distributing a new vaccine. Unlike the COVID-19 mRNA vaccines developed under OWS that are manufactured by relatively rapid chemical processes, the 2009 influenza vaccines (and most influenza vaccines still today) rely on growing a weakened version of the circulating flu virus in fertilized chicken eggs—hundreds of millions of fertilized chicken eggs obtained from pathogen-free chicken flocks raised in specialized conditions using disinfected food, water, and bedding. The flocks are cared for by workers in PPE (to protect the chickens, not the workers), and the flocks must undergo testing every week. Fertilized eggs must be incubated for about ten days to start the chicken embryo growing. Then each egg is individually inoculated with the influenza virus (by a needle poking a hole in the egg). The virus grows for several days, and then the contents of the egg are extracted and painstakingly purified by many complex steps in order to provide the flu "antigen" component of the vaccine.

Even after purification, the antigen still needs to be combined with an immune stimulator (called an "adjuvant") to create the final vaccine. This process produces safe and generally effective vaccines *but takes many months to manufacture at scale.* This time-consuming, multilayered, complex process explains why flu vaccine manufacturing generally starts in January so that we have vaccines available in your local pharmacy by September. Starting manufacturing this early also means that sometimes experts at the CDC and the WHO pick the wrong flu strains, which means the vaccine for that year is mostly a bust.

In 2009, the pandemic strain was first identified in April; as such, the first vaccines became available in October but were not widely available until November. To put it bluntly, the vaccine supply became sufficient about the time when the pandemic was over. If H1N1 was more severe, millions of Americans would have died.

This experience led the US government and specifically BARDA, a division of the Office of the ASPR at HHS, to make historic investments in new vaccine-manufacturing technologies and platforms (to transition out of chicken eggs and into more modern systems). In 2012, my team at the Texas A&M University System in collaboration with several commercial and non-profit partners was awarded a $285 million contract to develop the Center for Innovation in Advanced Development and Manufacturing to ensure vaccine-manufacturing capacity for public health emergencies—especially pandemic influenza. Emergent BioSolutions in Maryland and Novartis in North Carolina also received awards. As a result of this infrastructure, both Emergent BioSolutions and Texas A&M participated in the COVID-19 vaccine response to various degrees.

Although OWS deserves enormous credit for the COVID-19 vaccine success, that success was built on at least two decades of investment into vaccine research and infrastructure, including mRNA vaccine technology, mainly by the US Department of Defense and the Department of Health and Human Services.

Unfortunately, the 2009 pandemic did nothing to prepare the United States for the development and scaling of diagnostic tests, and thus we were caught flat-footed when COVID-19 hit. The reasons are pretty straightfor-ward and understandable in retrospect. Although the flu virus changes from year to year, clinicians can use the same diagnostic test(s) every year. There were dozens of FDA-approved influenza tests already available in every health clinic to diagnose H1N1. And conveniently, these tests were mostly "rapid tests," with results in minutes, available at nearly every point of care in the US health-care system.

A more subtle point is that testing for influenza is generally seen as optional by physicians. If in the middle of flu season a person develops fever, chills, aches, and a cough, that person is clinically diagnosed (even without a laboratory test) with influenza and treated with an oral antiviral medica-tion like Tamiflu. People with these symptoms are advised to stay home to avoid spreading the disease, practice good handwashing, and exert care when coughing or sneezing so as not to contaminate surfaces or spread droplets. And the opposite is also true—if you do not have fever, chills, aches, and a cough, you don't have the flu. And if you feel entirely well, you *definitely* don't have the flu. But that is not the case with COVID-19. People can be entirely asymptomatic or have only very mild symptoms and still have COVID-19 and be highly contagious.[5]

What about testing for H1N1 at the CDC? Although the CDC approached the 2009 pandemic as an "all-out" emergency response, it was actually operat-ing in its comfort zone related to diagnostics. All doctors' offices, clinics, and hospitals already had rapid flu tests, so there was no need to send samples to the CDC for sophisticated molecular tests.

But occasionally, to assure that the same H1N1 virus was still circulating (and not replaced by another flu virus), the CDC and state public health labs performed some molecular tests. Therefore, on May 1, 2009, the CDC began shipping test kits to 120 US public health labs and 250 international public health labs for this purpose. But the total number of test kits shipped by the CDC was only one thousand (with one thousand tests per kit)—nothing like the hundreds of millions of tests required during the COVID-19 pandemic. Moreover, the total number of tests actually performed at the CDC was only five thousand over six weeks—far fewer than needed even in the first days of the COVID-19 outbreak when the CDC had a monopoly on testing. But even those five thousand tests set a record for the CDC—multiple times greater than the total number of tests performed at the CDC in any previous flu season.[6]

In terms of lessons learned, H1N1 led to significant changes in our national preparedness for vaccines, but it had no effect whatsoever on our preparation for widespread testing. And that is one reason, among many, why the CDC and public health labs—as well as the federal government in general—were entirely unprepared to meet the challenges of testing for COVID-19.

EBOLA HITS TEXAS

Eight months after the first case of Ebola was reported in Guinea in December 2013, the WHO declared the West Africa Ebola outbreak a public health emergency of international concern, meaning that there was a significant risk of international spread. Global cooperation was urgently needed. By the time West Africa was declared "Ebola-free," there had been more than 28,600 cases and 11,325 deaths, almost all in three countries: Guinea, Liberia, and Sierra Leone.

In contrast to influenza and COVID-19, the Ebola virus is difficult to transmit from person to person. Ebola transmission requires very close contact with body fluids, like blood, feces, or saliva. It is not transmitted by respiratory routes (coughing or sneezing), and one must be quite ill with Ebola to have enough virus to be highly infectious—and the sicker you are, the more virus you have. Excluding the very rare cases of transmission in semen months after an acute Ebola infection, there is no transmission of the Ebola virus from a person who is asymptomatic.

In 2014–15, officers of the USPHS Commissioned Corps engaged in over eight hundred deployments to the West Africa region with the mission of providing direct medical care for health-care workers who had been infected with Ebola. This was essential to stopping the African outbreak because without doctors and nurses, many more patients with Ebola would have died. But more importantly, without functioning hospitals, sick people would have remained in their homes and communities, and that would have caused significantly more urban spread. This mission of the USPHS, mostly unnoticed by Americans, stabilized the medical response in the entire region and resulted in President Obama awarding the entire Commissioned Corps a Presidential Unit Citation (the highest unit award to a uniformed service) for "extraordinary courage and the highest level of performance in action throughout the United States Government's response to the Ebola outbreak."[7] Many of the officers in this response became essential leaders during COVID-19, and their experiences in the most austere environments of Africa made them exceptionally prepared for the challenges faced in 2020.

Over 5,500 miles away from West Africa, it only took a single case of Ebola in Texas to nearly paralyze the United States. On September 15, 2014, Thomas Eric Duncan of Monrovia, Liberia, rushed a seven-month-pregnant neighbor to a hospital in his home country after she collapsed. When she was turned away from the hospital, Mr. Duncan carried her back to her apartment, where she soon died. Perhaps unbeknownst to Mr. Duncan, his neighbor died of Ebola—not a pregnancy complication.

On September 20, while he was still without symptoms, Mr. Duncan caught a commercial flight to Dallas to visit his girlfriend Louise and his son. He had met Louise in a refugee camp fleeing a brutal civil war and fell in love but had been separated from Louise and his son for nearly two decades. Louise and his son were able to obtain a visa to live in the United States, but Mr. Duncan was denied. They were finally going to be able to reunite as a family, or so they thought.

Mr. Duncan developed a fever and generalized symptoms on September 24, nine days after his encounter with his neighbor in Monrovia. He was screened in the emergency room of Texas Health Presbyterian Hospital in Dallas but was sent home. On September 28, he returned with more severe symptoms and was admitted in critical condition, isolated, with all hospital staff employing Ebola precautions as outlined by the CDC: PPE, face shields, masks, shoe covers, and other precautions. On September 30, the Texas State Public Health Laboratory in Austin and the CDC Viral Special Pathogens Branch both confirmed that Mr. Duncan was infected with Ebola.

On October 1, I received a call from then governor Perry. Serendipitously, I was in Dallas, a couple of miles from the hospital, undergoing an annual physical exam at the Cooper Aerobics Center. My home was two hundred miles away in College Station, and I had only packed a pair of exercise shorts and a T-shirt. The governor told me that we had a confirmed Ebola patient at Presbyterian and that I needed to join him for a meeting with CDC officials, the commissioner of the Texas Department of State Health Services (Dr. David Lakey), and the medical and nursing staff at Presbyterian. We would then do a press briefing to provide assurance that we had the situation under control. I jumped off the stress-test treadmill, ripped off my electrodes, drove to NorthPark Center shopping mall (a mile from Presbyterian Hospital), bought clothes off the rack at Macy's, and put them on. I then raced to the hospital to meet the governor and the team that he had assembled.

I immediately became fully involved. Governor Perry announced that I would lead a newly created Texas Task Force on Infectious Disease Preparedness and Response, the objective of which was to assess and enhance the state's capabilities to prepare for and respond to pandemic disease, including the disease we were now facing: Ebola. Although there were many long-term goals that we later fulfilled with a complete report to the governor, the task force functioned operationally as the state policy oversight committee to provide expert, evidence-based assessments, protocols, and recommendations to the incident managers on the ground in Dallas.

My task force assisted in all aspects of the emergency response in coordination with Dr. Lakey and the county judge.[8] We also provided state-level coordination (on behalf of the governor) with the CDC and the secretary of HHS, who at that time was Sylvia Burwell. In retrospect, Perry's move was incredibly insightful. While the response was ongoing, he specifically tasked our group with not only assisting and providing top cover as needed but also being a "learning organization" to detail all the successes, failures, and gaps so that we would be better prepared in the future.

Our work started immediately on October 1 and was 24-7 until the crisis was over in Texas on November 7. In that first meeting at Presbyterian Hospital, it was clear that the CDC representatives were going to provide valuable expert assistance but assistance that was extremely limited in scope. The CDC was not in charge of anything (we initially thought they would be) but instead would only consult and support epidemiological investigations performed by state and local health authorities. This was my first realization that the CDC had essentially no authority to impose health policies on state and local governments and very little willingness to assume any responsibility or accountability whatsoever. In our federal system, with public health authorities mostly reserved for the states, the role of the federal government and the CDC was limited to consultation and guidance, with rare exceptions. This of course was not well understood by most Americans and certainly not the media throughout the early COVID-19 response.

On the ground in Dallas, the handful of CDC staff sent from Atlanta were truly "disease detectives," but they were *only* disease detectives. They had no experience in appropriate donning and doffing of PPE, no advice to the clinical team about how to actually treat Mr. Duncan, no knowledge of available experimental therapies or how they could be accessed, and no experience and little understanding of the unified command structure that is the organizational framework for any emergency response. Worst of all, many of the standing recommendations from the CDC about Ebola screening and care were proven wrong—dangerously wrong.

At that time, the CDC proclaimed that any major US hospital could care for Ebola patients. That assessment turned out to be tragically incorrect and nearly cost the lives of two nurses infected with Ebola while caring for Mr. Duncan. Presbyterian is a first-class community hospital in the middle of Dallas, part of a superb health-care system, with top physicians and nurses trained at some of the best institutions in our nation. But that single Ebola case overwhelmed the staff and, due to stigma and fear, closed down many of that hospital's essential services to the community. All of a sudden people were not showing up for emergency services or cancer screening; we were going to lose more people from this type of collateral damage than from Ebola itself.

The CDC PPE recommendations were inadequate and inferior to the standards used at Ebola treatment centers, like Emory and the University of Nebraska. In fact, when the outside teams from elite Ebola centers arrived, they said something like, "You aren't really using the CDC recommendations for PPE, are you?"

And the screening algorithm for Ebola patients published by the CDC was wrong. If a patient did not have a high fever, that patient was not further screened for Ebola. The question about whether he had been in Africa came only after the presence of a significant fever. This was crazy, and we changed it immediately in Texas. The first question should have been, "Have you recently traveled to Africa or been exposed to an Ebola patient?" If that answer was yes, then it really did not matter how much fever that person had; they needed to be isolated and tested.

The CDC did, however, have well-trained and equipped regional centers for Ebola virus testing; this was important because normal hospital labs don't have the materials and reagents to test for Ebola. But the CDC had not thought through the transport of blood specimens to the testing centers or back to the CDC (which often involved many hundreds of miles). This proved a major issue, since commercial carriers decided not to allow the transport of these specimens on their aircraft or in their trucks. That decision was irrational and contrary to their usual practice of transporting potentially infectious human material, but they were exceptionally concerned because Ebola was involved. So how could we get the diagnosis made when we could not transport the specimens? The CDC had no immediate answers. We wound up using state aircraft to transport every sample individually for several hundred miles during the early response. It was not sustainable, but it was a work-around that temporized the problem.

Contact tracing and follow-up were important and fairly easy for a disease where patients were always symptomatic. But although only 177 contacts required tracing and monitoring during the entire Texas outbreak,[9] this proved to be a formidable task because the CDC lacked digital tracking tools and a common operating picture that could be shared among the many stakeholders. Literally, copies of spreadsheets were faxed around at the end of the day to inform everyone about the health status of contacts. Years later during COVID-19, there was no possibility that the United States was going to be able to contact trace millions of people, most of whom had no idea how or when they became infected.

In terms of medical countermeasures (drugs to treat sick Ebola patients), BARDA (the responsible agency at HHS) was no help. It took several days just to get their staff on the ground in Dallas, and they had very little information. There were no new medicines available for Mr. Duncan, or at least that is what BARDA officials told me.

The CDC provided no practical guidance on decontaminating Mr. Duncan's apartment. I happened to be in the operations center with the incident commander when the commercial decontaminating crew entered Mr. Duncan's apartment. The crew obviously had no experience with Ebola and, from what I could tell, mostly performed cleanup after bloody murders or drug busts. The crew only had a few brand-name cleaning solutions with them; nothing was certified for the decontamination of Ebola. The CDC was not at all helpful, but I had a lot of experience in decontamination (probably more than the CDC did) from my DARPA days working on anthrax—so we proceeded in real time. Given the set of facts on the ground, I instructed the cleanup crew to rip out nearly everything in the apartment, bag the contents, load them in a truck, and bring them to a certified incinerator to have them vaporized. That was as much for public confidence as it was for infection control. Who would really volunteer to brush their teeth in the sink that was recently used by a sick Ebola patient?

Despite the heroic efforts of the medical team at Texas Health Presbyterian Hospital, Mr. Duncan ultimately died of Ebola on October 8, 2014, one week after Rick Perry's initial phone call to me. Even his death presented unforeseen challenges. Most urgently, there was no direction from the CDC about the disposal of Mr. Duncan's remains. Mr. Duncan was not just an Ebola patient; he was a human being who was infected while trying to assist a desperately ill neighbor, suffered through a civil war and refugee camp, was separated from the love of his life for decades, and had hopes for a normal family that were shattered by the virus. But we still needed to make a decision about the body and his burial. All of us knew that Ebola was often spread in Africa through the ritualistic burial custom of kissing the dead on the mouth. Although we knew that would not happen in Texas, what about the risks to undertakers? Or what if some lunatic (or rational terrorist) decided to dig up his body and use it as a bioweapon? The CDC did not provide any direction, so we consulted the experts at the Galveston National Laboratory, who were among the most knowledgeable in the world about Ebola (and other horrific infections). When the Galveston experts told us that the Ebola virus could stay infectious even within a corpse for perhaps weeks, we decided to cremate the body instead of a burial. It was a very difficult decision but one that we had to make.

During the course of Mr. Duncan's treatment, two of his primary nurses also became infected with Ebola despite the use of PPE. The first nurse was diagnosed only two days after Mr. Duncan's death and the second only a few days after.

When the nurses became infected, I was beside myself. I called BARDA (Dr. Robin Robinson, the BARDA director, and many others within BARDA) looking for medicines and specifically ZMapp—a promising cocktail of monoclonal antibodies manufactured in tobacco-like plants that was undergoing clinical trials in Africa at the time. Dr. Robinson assured me that there were no doses available for our nurses and, indeed, had nothing else to offer even on a compassionate basis. I could not believe that. How could that be? Did they not think that we might actually have Ebola cases in the United States and save at least one dose of something—anything—for compassionate use? So I called the manufacturer of ZMapp, Kentucky BioProcessing (KBP) in Owensboro, Kentucky, and inquired about the availability of doses. Miraculously, they said they had enough supply available in their freezer to treat one or perhaps two patients!

I was amazed that Dr. Robinson, BARDA, or anyone else could not offer anything to help the nurses, send an inquiry to the manufacturer, or try to hustle doses back from trials in Africa. But we had found doses in Kentucky, and I asked KBP if we could retrieve the doses from them. They agreed. The last thing I wanted to do was to involve the CDC or BARDA, who would likely delay treatment because of bureaucratic processes or a myriad of other reasons. So we didn't tell them. We never told them.

At the time, Dr. Scott Lillibridge was on the Texas A&M faculty; he was a true pioneer in US biodefense preparedness and response and a former USPHS Commissioned Corps officer. Scott had led the CDC's response to the anthrax attack and had done a superb job with that difficult mission. Everyone knew he was the real deal. Scott agreed to personally retrieve the ZMapp from Kentucky and bring it back to Dallas.

But how would we get to Kentucky (a fifteen-hundred-mile round trip) under the radar from the government and the hysterical press? I then made what was, in retrospect, a very strange call to one of our Texas A&M University System regents, Mr. Jim Schwertner. The regents were the governing board for the entire Texas A&M University System, which consisted of eleven universities, a health science center, and seven state agencies. Jim was also a prominent Texas cattleman who piloted his own private jet. He was a true modern cowboy, in the best of ways.

I explained the situation to Regent Schwertner, who immediately volunteered to fly the mission himself so that Scott could bring ZMapp to our stricken nurses. Regent Schwertner and Scott brought a small red Igloo cooler back to Dallas containing the precious treatment, and under appropriate research protocol and consent, it was made available to one of the nurses. I wanted to tell this story, which has never been told, to emphasize how important individuals are to any emergency response, even when they are outside of the traditional federal bureaucracies. It is also a sobering example of how a federal response system may look great on paper but falls woefully short when facing day-to-day operational realities.

Even more striking than the ZMapp issue with BARDA were the frequent operational missteps of the CDC. For example, before her official diagnosis of Ebola, another nurse who had treated Mr. Duncan asked the CDC if she could fly on a commercial flight to Ohio and then back again to Texas. At the time of her proposed travel, she was registering a low-grade fever.

The CDC—amazingly—allowed her to take those commercial flights because she was not at "high risk." OK, what? An ICU nurse taking care of an Ebola patient spikes a fever right at the exact time she would start coming down with Ebola—and the CDC lets that person fly on a commercial airliner? Sometimes common sense needs to be a part of decision-making, and it clearly wasn't then. Following the flights and the national public outrage that erupted afterward, CDC Director Tom Frieden said they would no longer allow people being followed as a contact to fly (or do similar activities). Did he and his twenty thousand staff at the CDC really not think about that beforehand?

Even pets were not immune to the Ebola emergency in Texas. One of the nurses, while symptomatic, had slept with her pet dog—an adorable Cavalier King Charles spaniel named Bentley. Although there had been no reported transmission of Ebola to dogs or from a dog to a human, Ebola had been shown to be transmissible to dogs in a laboratory setting. Indeed, Spanish health authorities decided to euthanize a pet that was exposed to a patient incubating Ebola just one week earlier.

We asked the CDC for a recommendation, and a spokesperson said they would not test the dog but that "any decisions about the dog would be between the owner and Texas or Dallas County health officials."[10] That was not very helpful to us.

We decided we would not euthanize the dog but instead quarantine him for twenty-one days and test him for Ebola at appropriate intervals. So that is what we did: we placed Bentley in a comfortable room that met all animal care standards. But who would care for him? Until a Texas A&M veterinary emergency response team could arrive at the scene several days later, we called Dr. Tammy Beckham, who was a veterinarian and director of the Texas A&M Veterinary Diagnostic Laboratory. Aside from being qualified as a veterinarian to assess Bentley's health, she was a former US Army officer who had worked with the most dangerous pathogens on the planet at Fort Dietrich, Maryland. Tammy was not afraid of this situation, so she drove the two hundred miles from College Station to Dallas and cared for the dog for several days until the formal teams could arrive. Bentley remained well throughout his quarantine and always tested negative for Ebola. He eventually had a heartwarming reunion with his person later in the month.

Six years after this event, Tammy wound up in Washington, DC, working again with the military on chemical and biological defense for Central Command (Iraq, Afghanistan, Pakistan, and neighboring countries). I immediately recruited her to HHS to lead the Office of HIV and Infectious Disease

Policy. She was magnificent. And when COVID-19 hit, I appointed her to lead the Laboratory Diagnostics Task Force at FEMA. Much of the successes in testing are due to her efforts, which I will detail later.

Ebola ended in Texas when we decided to transfer both nurses (who were actually in stable condition by then) to specialized facilities at the NIH and at Emory. The staff at Presbyterian Hospital had been under enormous stress. Many of them were under quarantine, they were caring for their colleague nurses with Ebola in their ICU, and the community was suffering because of a lack of access to their hospital. Most of all, it was clear by that time that Ebola patients should never be cared for in a hospital that is not specifically designed for these types of patients and that does not have the specific advanced training required to keep its staff safe.

Governor Perry and I called HHS Secretary Burwell from the Texas governor's office. Initially, she resisted our plan to transfer the patients out of Dallas, but then she understood that this was not a request; it was the communication of a decision that we had already made. In all fairness, after a short discussion, she understood our situation and supported it. She was collaborative, cordial, and to a large degree empathetic. We proceeded from there with the transfer, and both nurses remained stable and survived without any lasting consequences, to my knowledge. The CDC eventually caught on, and the entire approach to Ebola hospital care and screening changed after this episode.

In summary, the lessons were clear. The overall federal response and coordination with state and local authorities did not meet expectations. Cuts in hospital preparedness funding, the lack of actual operational drills and readiness, and the absence of clear actionable guidelines from the CDC led to vulnerability across the nation. The CDC was, and remains, the world's leader in knowledge of epidemiology and disease investigation but displayed very little operational capability. This was no fault of the tremendously talented and dedicated professionals who work at the CDC; rather, it stemmed from how the CDC as an organization had bloated into a vast bureaucracy with a mission set that crossed all health-care domains, from Ebola to obesity to addiction to family planning. What the CDC did, it did well. But we had expected much more during Ebola, and the CDC did not—and could not—meet those expectations.

Messaging was also a tremendous challenge. Even though the CDC and Texas officials were able to eventually align talking points, so-called experts regularly populated the cable networks and spouted opinions that had no basis in reality, causing far too much alarm. If it bleeds, it leads. And that was true for Ebola. I was on CNN and Fox News many times, along with many other colleagues, trying to provide honest and transparent information—but it was a constant struggle against the alarmists and some self-serving academics seeking fame. My Texas A&M team actually went out one day and bought a tie for me to wear for TV interviews, specifically purchased because the tie resembled a maroon one Tony Fauci frequently wore for CNN. They thought I would look more credible; I thought it was hysterical. It is even funnier now. I still occasionally wear that tie (the most expensive tie I own) for CNN and Fox News appearances about COVID-19.

In retrospect, it is not surprising that when COVID-19 emerged in early 2020—on a hundred-million-fold scale compared to Ebola in Texas—the CDC was not capable of providing the leadership or operational response that the nation desperately needed. We should have seen that coming. I should have anticipated that for sure. And the same issues with messaging and public trust became even more important, especially given the partisan personalities involved and the ongoing presidential campaign.

As challenging as they were, H1N1 and Ebola were cakewalks compared to what we would face beginning in January 2020.

5

The Pandemic Begins

WE LEAVE NO AMERICAN BEHIND

In early January 2020, I received a call from Lynn Johnson, the assistant secretary in charge of HHS's Administration for Children and Families (ACF).[1] Lynn and I had worked closely together on the southern border crisis to assure appropriate care and placement for unaccompanied children after they were turned over to HHS by US Customs and Border Protection (CBP). She had the right mix of idealism—truly wanting to make the United States the best place to be a child—and pragmatism, knowing how to get things done and whom to call if she needed assistance. Although Lynn is one of my favorite people, I hated getting calls from her—because every call meant there was an imminent crisis. On January 2, I knew it couldn't possibly be the southern border again, but I was completely unprepared for what was about to transpire.

Just three days earlier, the initial reports of an unknown respiratory illness causing pneumonia in Wuhan had surfaced to the World Health Organization (WHO). But it was not until January 4 that the WHO tweeted that "#China has reported to WHO a cluster of #pneumonia cases—with no deaths—in Wuhan, Hubei Province. Investigations are underway to identify the cause of this illness."[2] It was decided appropriately—but I don't know by whom—that Americans in the hot zone needed to be brought back to the United States. Given that so little was known about the reality on the ground in Wuhan, it was clear that when these Americans arrived back on US soil, there would need to be many decisions regarding quarantine sites and duration and who would ultimately be in charge of various aspects of the operation.

It was my understanding that ACF was the lead federal agency (LFA) once Americans had actually stepped foot on US soil, and therefore ACF would be responsible for providing temporary assistance and shelter once they arrived. Later on, there were many debates about whether the CDC was in charge under their authority to quarantine people returning to the United

States, but Lynn answered the call for action a lot faster and more operationally minded than the CDC did. And I trusted her.

Specifically, Lynn requested help from the USPHS Commissioned Corps to support the return of US citizens from Wuhan and for our officers to provide just-in-time training in infection control for ACF staff who would be on the ground at repatriation sites, likely military bases. Within hours, the ACF also requested the deployment of additional officers to provide more operational staff at repatriation sites.

Although my response was of course yes, I had a sinking feeling inside of me. Eighteen months earlier, the Office of Management and Budget in the Executive Office of the President had sought to eliminate the USPHS Commissioned Corps, which was founded in 1798 and whose members, in military uniform, protected the health of Americans since 1889. Our service was in the middle of reorganization and modernization. We had implemented new standards for deployment readiness and physical fitness—these were life-saving in retrospect. But we had no funds for advanced training and only a minority of our officers were prepared to appropriately utilize PPE, including N95 masks. You can't just put an N95 on and go take care of highly infectious patients. For safety, there must be a certification that the mask fits and that essentially 100 percent of the air breathed in and out is filtered by the mask. No air can leak around the edges of the mask or else the protection against the virus goes down dramatically. Masks come in different sizes and shapes, and not all masks work with all people.

My first responsibility was to protect the health and safety of my officers, and that was going to be a challenge. I immediately spoke to R. Adm. Susan Orsega, director of Commissioned Corps Headquarters (DHQ), and we made plans. Rear Admiral Orsega was a seasoned veteran and a nurse practitioner who had extensive experience performing clinical trials on Ebola vaccines in Africa. She was the right person in the right job at the right time. Her only response was "Yes, sir. I got this."

I received the official request for deployment of USPHS officers in support of ACF on January 9, 2020, and deployments began on January 27 to Anchorage, Alaska; March Air Reserve Base in California; and Travis Air Force Base, also in California. On February 2, we deployed additional officers to Travis Air Force Base, to new quarantine facilities at Lackland Air Force Base in San Antonio, and to Dobbins Air Force Base in Marietta, Georgia. On January 27–28, we deployed more officers to support the assistant secretary for preparedness and response (ASPR, Dr. Bob Kadlec) in various roles, including logistics and information management. Our officers were already

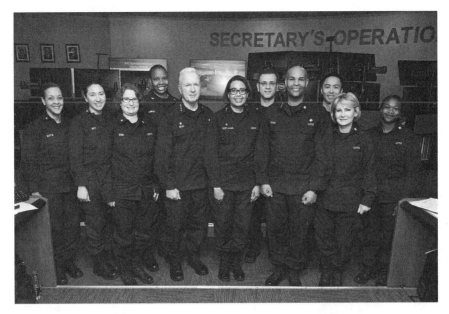

USPHS officers staffing the Secretary's Operations Center at HHS headquarters with Admiral Giroir, Vice Admiral Adams, and Rear Admiral Trent-Adams (personal photo).

staffing the Secretary's Operations Center in HHS headquarters in Washington, DC. We were fully in the fight.

On January 28, the Department of State conducted the first flight from Wuhan, landing at March Air Force Base on January 29. For some reason, the CDC had initially only requested that the repatriated citizens voluntarily remain at the military bases for seventy-two hours. I have no idea why only seventy-two hours and why it was voluntary. But on January 31, the CDC changed their approach and issued a mandatory fourteen-day quarantine order for all Wuhan repatriates. By February 7 under the leadership of Dr. Kadlec, we had completed four additional flights, repatriating and quarantining a total of 808 US citizens from Wuhan. All citizens were released from quarantine by February 20.

My primary role was to assure that the corps could meet all deployment requests. That would eventually mean the deployment of literally every officer who could deploy—over two-thirds of the corps. Those who did not deploy were already on the front lines providing care to COVID patients in the Indian Health Service or the Bureau of Prisons or other agencies. If these individuals deployed to Texas or Japan, there would literally be no one to take care of the people they served, so we kept these frontline clinicians where they were for the duration of the pandemic.

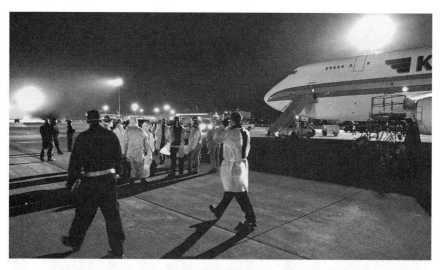

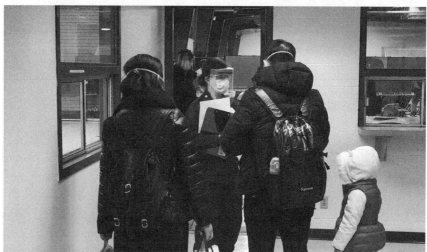

Flight unloading Americans from Wuhan and health screening of passengers by a USPHS officer (personal photos).

On February 3, I wanted to send a clear message about the severity of the pandemic to every agency where USPHS officers worked and to the general public who saw our officers on the street and in their communities. So I issued an order instructing all officers (whether deployed or not) to wear their operational dress uniforms (ODUs) until further notice. This was a major departure from standard procedures because we typically only wore these uniforms during active deployments to hurricanes, wildfires, Ebola in Africa, national security events, and other similar crises.

Our 6,200+ officers stationed throughout the world would undoubtedly be asked about this noticeable change in uniform, and I wanted the message to be clear: "This pandemic is serious, and our officers are already responding. It is crunch time." Consistent with my order, I frequently showed up to the White House "inappropriately" dressed in my work uniform, not my business attire (service-dress-blue uniform with a tie and jacket). Truth be told, the president actually liked it that way, and so did I.

The repatriation mission from Wuhan—like nearly everything else accomplished by the Trump administration—was reflexively criticized by media and political pundits for whatever reasons that could be found or fabricated. They completely disregarded the unprecedented nature of this complex rescue operation.

There were real issues concerning who was "in charge," as pointed out in a US Government Accountability Office (GAO) report released in April 2021.[3] But this was the first time that HHS was called upon to bring back this number of US citizens in the early stages of an infectious disease outbreak. There was no playbook, no matter how many times you hear critics complain that we did not follow the Obama administration's. That playbook mostly consisted of phone numbers in order to assemble an even bigger bureaucracy than the one that was already failing—the playbook was no help. To my knowledge, it is also true that the Trump administration had not planned for evacuating Americans from foreign countries during the early stages of a pandemic, but neither had any other administration. That was not part of any plan, but in retrospect, it should have been.

To complicate matters, there were a number of agencies with overlapping statutory authorities that needed to gel in an unprecedented way. The Department of State was responsible for organizing and implementing the activities on foreign soil. ACF was the lead agency when citizens arrived back inside the United States. The CDC supplied technical support and also had the authority to issue quarantine orders for international arrivals. The ASPR office was the lead for the entire operation, by statute, and deployed an incident command team to March Air Force Base on January 31. The Office of the ASPR ran the Secretary's Operations Center, our command-and-control center for the response, and also had the authority to activate the National Disaster Medical System (NDMS). In addition, there were always complex interactions with state and local health authorities, mayors and county judges, and local media. The response of the local community directly affected not only these first missions but also our overall response during the remainder of the pandemic.

Repatriation occurred to Department of Defense military bases, but many in the armed forces had never seen a USPHS Commissioned Corps officer before. And while soldiers and airmen were perfectly happy charging a hill against enemy gunfire and artillery, a pandemic virus was something totally different and singularly unnerving to them. Nonetheless, all in uniform—USPHS officers and armed forces personnel—immediately formed cohesive and integrated teams. We were a badass joint fighting force, but this time on a mission against an invisible enemy.

There were real issues concerning infection control early in the repatriations, especially at March Air Force Base during the first mission—but these issues were remedied quickly by leaders like USPHS Capt. Paul Reed, whom we deployed early (and often) because of his unique experience in humanitarian operations. Paul and I had worked shoulder to shoulder on the southern border unaccompanied children (UAC) crisis, and I knew he would provide sound leadership and expertise on the ground. He was also a pediatrician, so we immediately saw eye to eye. Despite the scale of operations and its complexity and at a time when little was known about the virus, the repatriation missions were accomplished without any disease transmission to US civilian or uniformed personnel or to other repatriated citizens. That was truly remarkable. In retrospect, this was just a small victory in a raging war, but it was important to everyone involved, especially the Americans we brought home and their families.

CDC QUARANTINE STATIONS

Within days of my call from Lynn Johnson, I also received a call from Dr. Anne Schuchat, deputy director of the CDC and former rear admiral in the USPHS Commissioned Corps. Ann and I had a very good relationship, and I respected her judgment, experience, and temperament. This was not her first rodeo. Ann gave me an appropriate heads-up that the CDC would be requesting USPHS officers to deploy in support of quarantine stations at eleven airports. Again, the answer was yes, but I could not help but be somewhat perplexed why the CDC, with nearly twenty thousand employees and contracted staff, needed fifty uniformed officers to deploy to quarantine stations. These fifty officers all had important "day jobs" at the FDA, the NIH, the Indian Health Service, or the Federal Bureau of Prisons. But nonetheless, I immediately informed Rear Admiral Orsega, and she and her staff expertly rostered teams according to our recently modernized deployment protocol.

A week went by, and the crisis deepened, but no official request came from the CDC. I inquired. Another week went by. Finally, on January 19, I received an official request from the CDC for the deployment of officers to support screening at CDC-led quarantine stations at (or near) airports and international crossings and to provide clinical guidance to health-care providers managing patients being evaluated and treated for COVID-19.

Those two weeks were wasted because the CDC could not figure out how to provide travel orders for my officers (a necessary legal step for active deployment) and, more importantly, could not deliver the N95 mask fit testing needed for deployments. The CDC finally suggested we deploy officers to Atlanta, have them trained, bring them back to DC, and then deploy them to wherever they needed to go. This was not going to work, so Rear Admiral Orsega found other ways to provide this training either in Washington, DC, or immediately on-site once officers were already deployed. Finally, we began deploying for this CDC mission on January 24—a mission that lasted until April 10, 2020.

THE *DIAMOND PRINCESS*: DÉJÀ VU ALL OVER AGAIN

On January 25, 2020, a symptomatic passenger departed the *Diamond Princess* cruise ship in Hong Kong and soon after tested positive for COVID-19. There were another 3,700 passengers and crew on that ship, which subsequently made six stops in various ports before returning to its home in Yokohama, Japan, where it was not permitted to dock. No one was allowed to disembark. Japanese authorities quarantined passengers to their cabins, but the crew continued to perform their tasks, circulating among passengers and undoubtedly spreading the virus everywhere. Among the passengers and crew, 712 tested positive, 381 were symptomatic, 37 required intensive care, and 9 would eventually die. This was the definition of a superspreader event, and many Americans were on that ship. We needed to rescue those Americans and bring them back home from Japan.

To support the return of US citizens from the *Diamond Princess*, Bob Kadlec (ASPR) formally enlisted the assistance of two veteran infectious disease and disaster medicine specialists—Drs. James Lawler and Michael Callahan. Michael had worked with me at DARPA and had been involved, in one way or another, with nearly every major infectious disease outbreak in the world for the past two decades. The same for Jim. Although these docs had all the credentials of the CDC experts, they had one thing most CDC staff did not have—actual frontline clinical experience treating patients in the most extreme environments. Michael and Jim were more than academics—they were operators. Seasoned operators. If there was an equivalent of SEAL Team Six for public health, they would have led it.

Michael had actually inserted himself into Wuhan in early January and even made it inside Wuhan hospitals to help treat patients. He clearly warned Bob Kadlec and me that the virus was not only severe but highly contagious via the respiratory route. So on February 12, when I deployed USPHS officers to Tokyo for the *Diamond Princess*, I knew that Michael and Jim would provide the on-the-ground expertise to keep my officers safe and bring all Americans who could be transported back home without incident. We were in daily contact, so Bob and I had good situational awareness back in DC.

With Dr. Kadlec and the ASPR team again in overall command, Americans from the cruise ship would be flown back to the United States, where they would remain in quarantine for fourteen days at either Travis or Lackland Air Force Base. In total, 329 people were flown to these bases. Dr. Lawler flew with 151 passengers to Lackland, and Dr. Callahan flew with 167 passengers to Travis.

When Lawler and Callahan arrived back in the United States, they sent a memorandum for the record to both Dr. Kadlec and me. These two docs don't even get their heart rates elevated in a war zone taking care of Ebola patients. But they were quite animated at that moment—because of the lack of operational know-how and clinical inexperience of CDC staff. Their memo for the record was dated February 18, but their email was transmitted just after midnight on the morning of February 19. In the email, they stated that CDC staff had engaged in "inadequate self-protection, contamination of biocontainment cold zones on aircraft, and disruption of medical care of ill and severely ill patients during ASPR medical evacuation of *Diamond Princess* passengers. . . . This was not the CDC of the old days. There was no DISMA training or familiarity with incident command system (ICS) or mass casualty care. No MDs to take patient sign off. An epidemiologist attempted to do triage so I overruled them and fortunate too; two of CDC 'well and ambulatory' are doing poorly in the ICU."[4] The memo itself provided additional details about the inadequacies of CDC leadership during the evacuation:

> Throughout our experience, our CDC colleagues appeared to read directly from a script developed in the absence of first-hand clinical observation and did not allow for deviation based upon additional information, direct experience, or (most egregiously) the best

medical assessment of an experienced infectious disease physician who had been providing care for these patients for the better part of 36 hours. We feel that these arbitrary decisions based upon protocol put people at risk and did not serve the best interest of the patients involved.

In addition to clinical decisions, CDC personnel appeared to be oblivious to the unique environmental risk of an enclosed aircraft with close to 200 people, many of whom were likely to be infected, in close quarters during the flight for more than 10 hours. The passengers by necessity had free range of the aircraft and were using portable toilet facilities at the rear of the aircraft. CDC officials did not consult the State Department team or infectious disease clinicians about our assessment of risk but instead proceeded to board the aircraft and conduct operations in only thin gowns, gloves, faceshield, and facemask (that appeared to be an N95).

We both think that this level of PPE was grossly insufficient due to the high level of contamination that likely existed on the aircraft. This may have put CDC personnel and other responders on the ground at risk. In addition, CDC personnel routinely transgressed boundaries of containment, moving into "cold" areas of the aircraft where flight crew worked. It is important to note that the handoff of Flight 2 to the CDC officer in Omaha proceeded quite differently and smoothly, in part due to the established personal relationship developed over the course of quarantine operations at Camp Ashland.

I am not aware that the CDC's actions actually resulted in harm to any patients or staff during these flights, but they might have. In any case, there was no better illustration of the fact that the CDC did not have the capability to provide what the United States needed at that moment. The CDC had evolved little—and perhaps devolved in its operational readiness—since Ebola in Texas six years earlier. The operational deficiencies and insular, academic nature of the organization were evident to clinicians and to HHS leadership and would be a recurring theme in the response—especially related to COVID diagnostic testing during the "lost month" of February.

SICK AMERICANS STILL IN TOKYO

Although 329 Americans were evacuated to US bases, my officers reported back that 55 Americans remained hospitalized in Japan, some in critical condition on maximal life support and scattered in hospitals throughout the Tokyo region. Although the State Department assured HHS—and me personally—that these individuals were well coordinated and cared for by the embassy staff, I did not know how many diplomats had a medical degree, much less any training in infectious diseases or ICU care.

I immediately thought about what I would want if my family member was in a foreign hospital with a new virus and on life support. I would demand much more than diplomats working on the issues, knowing full well that their primary objective was to avoid causing a "diplomatic scene" that might offend their host country or violate some norm of behavior. To save US lives, I wanted people who were medically skilled but also creative and innovative and, yes, even willing to break protocols on occasion if needed. I imagined that is exactly what the families of the stranded Americans would want as well. It was truly a dire situation, and there was *no way* we were going to leave Americans alone in Japan without trying to send in the cavalry—the Public Health Service cavalry.

So Rear Admiral Orsega and I decided to leave a small but elite contingent of USPHS officers in Tokyo after the rest of the team demobilized back to the states. These individuals were hand-picked because of their expertise and personal fortitude.[5] But the team was in dire need of a senior physician, preferably a flag-level officer (meaning a rear admiral, one or two stars), because of the complexity of the situation and the occasional need for official rank when dealing with Japanese ministries and our own US embassy.

It was Rear Admiral Orsega who suggested the exact right person to lead this mission—R. Adm. Richard Childs. Rear Admiral Childs was an assistant surgeon general, an internal medicine specialist, and the clinical director for research at the NIH's National Heart Lung and Blood Institute. He served as the chief medical officer for the USPHS Ebola response in Africa in 2014. Aside from these medical credentials, Rear Admiral Childs was a critical thinker, comfortable with complexity and handling crises, and not afraid to bend rules to save lives. I put myself in the shoes of Americans in Tokyo hospitals—wouldn't it be nice if the top doc from an NIH institute flew around the world to help me? So that is exactly what we did.

Rear Admiral Childs and his executive officer (Cmdr. Julie Erb-Alvarez) worked with the Japanese Health Ministry and the US embassy to first track down all the patients, who were scattered among twenty-five different hospitals. They assembled the medical records and X-rays for all Americans, reviewed them, coordinated care and assured it was at the highest level, and personally communicated with family members back in the United States.

The reason why Rear Admiral Orsega and I sent such an incredible team was *not* so much to carry out a specific mission but to determine what needed to be done and then implement a plan to accomplish those objectives. It was very Special Forces–like, except from a public health perspective. In Tokyo, Rear Admiral Childs by chance met a former colleague who was then at BARDA; that colleague was setting up an international clinical trial of the antiviral drug remdesivir, which eventually was proven to be safe and effective at treating COVID-19. Remdesivir was even administered to President Trump during his treatment at Walter Reed National Military Medical Center.

Rear Admiral Childs and the team, after reviewing the cases of every US citizen in Japanese hospitals, understood how desperately ill many were. In fact, ten Americans were on ventilators, and four were actually so sick that they were on ECMO (extracorporeal membrane oxygenation)—which is a long-term heart-lung bypass machine—because they essentially had no heart and lung function on their own. The Japanese doctors and nurses were doing everything possible—heroic measures, in fact—but there was no specific treatment available to combat the virus. All that could be done was to support organ function and hope the patients would recover on their own with good supportive care.

But then, in the middle of this ongoing medical emergency, another major problem suddenly arose. The senior US official in Japan, the chargé d'affaires at the US embassy, was not so pleased about these officers interacting on "his turf" without all the usual State Department clearances and protocols. He was intent on ordering my team to return back to the United States. And as the senior US official in the country, he had the power to do that. Rear Admiral Childs relayed these facts to me and stated that the chargé had summoned him to the embassy, made him shed all his electronics (like this admiral was some type of security risk), and told him that the chargé was sending the USPHS team home to the States the next day. Rear Admiral Childs appealed to the chargé's most basic instincts and stated something like, "Are you sure that this is going to pass the *Washington Post* test? The USPHS sends an elite team to help dying Americans, and the State Department sends them home?" Nonetheless, the chargé told my team to pack their bags.

What followed was a very heated set of email and phone exchanges between me (in DC) and the chargé in Japan. He accused my team of not coordinating with the Japanese Ministry of Health (which of course they did) and not getting authorization from the hospitals (which of course they also did—how else could they get access to patient records and X-rays?). He did have a point, though: my team did not seek formal country clearance from the US embassy in Japan, which was typically "necessary" for executive branch officials. I had sent my officers immediately, and on their personal passports, since they did not have official US government passports. The Americans on ventilators and ECMO could not wait for the issuance of official passports (at least a week or more in normal times) and formal country clearance. So I just sent them.

I finally stated to the chargé by email, "If you have the lead responsibility to protect Americans, you need our support to do that. Trust me." The next day, the situation dramatically changed, and the chargé became a staunch advocate for my officers and their mission. The chargé did not send my officers home, and they were able to accomplish their mission to save lives and leave no American behind. I don't have any bad feelings against the chargé—we violated protocol left and right, and in more normal times, I might have been reprimanded or fired for that. But this was a pandemic, and we did what was necessary. When the chargé realized we were just there to save American lives and had no other motives, he became fully supportive and our biggest defender. It all worked out, and I owe him a beer.

Rear Admiral Childs and his team continued their coordination and care mission but then had a crazy thought: "Why don't we try to get remdesivir for these patients?" Although experimental at that time, the drug had shown promise in previous coronavirus diseases like SARS and MERS. By working through multiple industry and US government contacts, Rear Admiral Childs was able to obtain from Gilead (the manufacturer of the drug) enough remdesivir to treat twenty patients on a compassionate basis. Ultimately, after reviewing charts and analyzing all patients, nine patients were actually good candidates for this drug and received it—five Americans and four Japanese. Remarkably, because of the outstanding care of the Japanese physicians and nurses, the medical consultations with Rear Admiral Childs and his team, and the provision of remdesivir on a compassionate-use basis, all nine patients survived. That's right—all nine elderly patients, with multiple organ failures and on advanced life support, survived.

For their truly heroic service, I awarded all officers on this team the USPHS Meritorious Service Medal with Bronze V Device for Valor, and I awarded Rear Admiral Childs the highest decoration of the USPHS Commissioned Corps, the Distinguished Service Medal with Bronze V Device for Valor. The Japanese government presented this team with a Japanese flag and

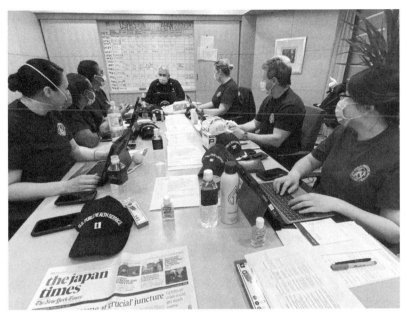

USPHS officers, led by Rear Admiral Childs, coordinating care of Americans from the *Diamond Princess* who remained in Japanese hospitals (personal photo).

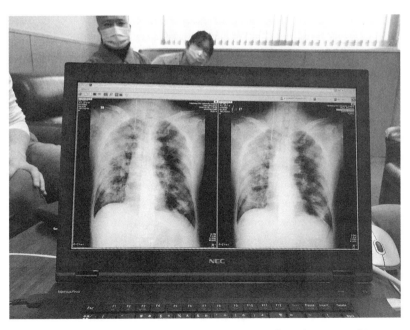

Chest X-ray showing severe lung damage in an American from the *Diamond Princess* receiving ICU care in Japan (personal photo).

expressed their enormous gratitude for assistance in saving the lives of not just the Americans in their hospitals but also the Japanese. That flag is now prominently displayed in USPHS Commissioned Corps Headquarters as a reminder to all of what it means to live out our service motto, "In the Service of Health."

JOINT BASE LACKLAND

On February 17, 151 evacuees from the *Diamond Princess* arrived at Lackland in San Antonio for their CDC-imposed mandatory fourteen-day quarantine. The CDC indeed has the authority to quarantine returning international travelers during a declared public health emergency but had not exercised that authority since the 1960s. Even for the Ebola emergency in Texas, the quarantine of returning health-care workers from West Africa was left to state and local authorities. The passengers' quarantine would end on March 2, at which time, if not ill or testing positive, they would be allowed to return to their homes. For certain, this was a "vacation" that none of these passengers would forget.

The setup in Texas was about as good as it could be. The quarantine site was secluded on the Lackland military base. The apartments were clean and fairly spacious, although aging and only as luxurious as a $49-per-night motel on an old state highway. A newly minted flag officer in the USPHS, R. Adm. Nancy Knight, who was a full-time CDC staff member, led the joint operation, which included USPHS officers, civilian teams, and armed forces support. Rear Admiral Knight was a veteran physician who had a decade of experience in Africa combatting HIV and tuberculosis (another respiratory-spread disease) and was completely capable of handling this unprecedented assignment. I was very impressed with her, as were the US Army and US Air Force officers on the base.

Because of the Texas Ebola crisis and the state's implementation of many of the recommendations of the task force I led five years earlier, Texas was one of the most prepared states for dealing with a new infectious disease outbreak. Emergency medical personnel were trained, equipped, and rehearsed. There was strong leadership from Chief Nim Kidd, director of the Texas Division of Emergency Management. We were colleagues through Texas Ebola, and we had a great working relationship, which would prove invaluable over the course of the COVID-19 pandemic. Eric Epley, another former colleague from Texas, was the director of the Southwest Texas Regional Advisory Council (STRAC), which maintained the emergency health and trauma system for twenty-two counties in that region.

If a quarantined person at Lackland became symptomatic or tested positive, that person would be transported by Eric's team to the Texas Center for Infectious Diseases (TCID) for stricter isolation. This specialty center was truly a godsend. It is a Texas public health facility designed to care for highly infectious patients with tuberculosis while undergoing treatment, often for months at a time. As such, the air-handling systems were ideal for isolating COVID-19 patients. Staff members were highly trained, motivated, and excited about this mission. And the facility was designed for long-term care, meaning that the rooms and amenities were reasonably comfortable for a couple of weeks of care and isolation.

In mid-February, my primary role was preparing USPHS officers for deployment and ensuring that our service could support all the burgeoning needs of the nation. I regularly attended meetings with Secretary Azar and Bob Kadlec, but I was not leading any aspect of the national pandemic response. Nonetheless, because so many USPHS officers were deployed and I knew all the players in Texas, I decided to do a site visit to Lackland on February 20–21 and to meet with state and local officials. What you hear in DC is not always what is happening on the ground, as I had learned all too well from the border crisis months before.

I met briefly with two of the more famous among those quarantined, young newlyweds Tyler and Rachel Torres, who were blogging about their entire ordeal, appearing on local radio, and generally providing a linkage to the thoughts of those inside the base.[6] I only spent about twenty minutes with them in a bit of an awkward situation. At that time, N95 masks were recommended for close interactions with anyone proven infected or in quarantine. But my face only fit one brand of N95 mask—for every other brand, there was significant leakage of air around the mask edges. So I would be at risk of becoming infected. Lackland did not have the type of N95 that fit me, so I talked to Tyler and Rachel outdoors through a chain-link fence, standing six feet away—the protocol at the time. I felt perfectly safe.

It appeared that everything we were hearing was indeed, and surprisingly, correct. Those quarantined were generally content, well cared for, communicated with, and listened to. With some exceptions, the attitudes and morale were very good. My officers and US Army / US Air Force personnel were doing everything they could to make the quarantine as comfortable as possible, including allowing food deliveries from the local H-E-B grocery store (my favorite place to shop!). There was no precedent for what was occurring there, but talented people working together made it work. The playbook was being written on the fly—I snapped a shot of a whiteboard entitled

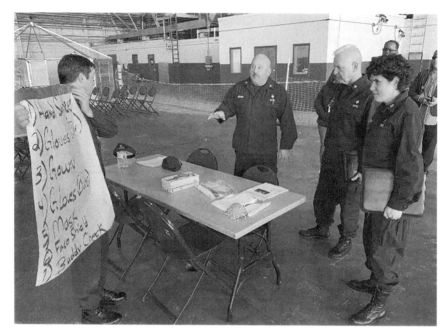

Reviewing procedures for Americans in quarantine at Joint Base Lackland, San Antonio: Admiral Giroir and Rear Admiral Orsega (personal photo).

"Swab-a-Palooza 2.0," which was the diagram to guide the next round of swabbing and testing by USPHS officers. Every passenger who consented was tested (formal written consent was required), and at that time, the test consisted of a deep nasopharyngeal swab and a throat swab, which were sent back to the CDC lab. Things were working well, and I was pleased with what I saw.

Meetings with the local officials also were positive. San Antonio mayor Ron Nirenberg was impressive—smart, insightful, asking all the appropriate questions. He looked like he could be governor or president one day. He was appropriately concerned about the safety of his citizens in the context of those being quarantined and their transport to and from the base. But he maintained a rational approach and a level head, and I was confident this whole situation was going to work out.

But I did make a statement that none of the leadership in San Antonio—or back in DC—was prepared for. My remark went something like this: "Don't worry so much about those passengers being quarantined, or their transport to the Texas Center for Infectious Disease, or their release after quarantine. Worry more about the tens of thousands of tourists that are on the River Walk in downtown San Antonio right now, especially in the bars and restaurants,

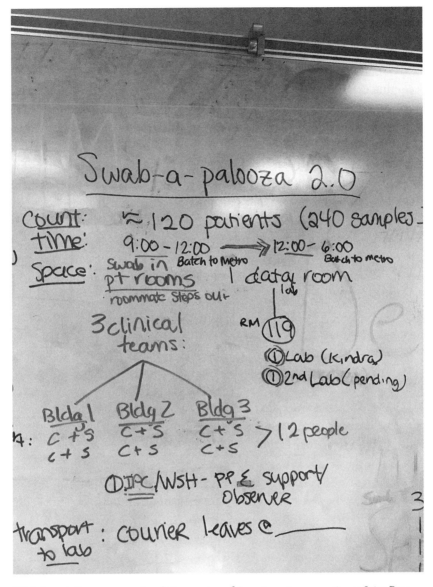

Whiteboard diagram operationalizing testing of Americans in quarantine at Joint Base Lackland, San Antonio (personal photo).

many of whom could be infected and freely spreading the disease throughout your city."

As it turned out, we now have evidence that COVID was spreading on the East and West Coasts from mid-January, six weeks before the first officially diagnosed case on US soil. Whether it was spreading in Texas when I made that statement remains unknown but is highly likely given that San Antonio is an epicenter of global tourism. COVID was an infectious nightmare, as the nation was about to realize.

I was not yet on the White House Coronavirus Task Force, but I was becoming extremely concerned about what was happening in China. Specifically, the Chinese were building alternate care facilities in convention centers because their hospitals were being overrun. I was also struck by the observations of the highly infectious nature of the virus reported by Drs. Callahan and Lawler as well as the severity of disease in hospitalized patients in Tokyo, reported by Rear Admiral Childs. Callahan and Lawler clearly stated that this was a respiratory spread and much more contagious than the CDC was describing it to be. As a result, Rear Admiral Orsega and I thought we could be facing a potential doomsday scenario in the United States. Our health-care system could be overrun, and there might be body bags on every street corner. We felt this was possible even though the average number of cases in the United States at that time was only twelve per day.

I requested that she prepare a plan for at least fifteen USPHS strike teams of one hundred officers each to be deployed across the country if US hospitals were overrun and we were forced to deliver care in high school gyms and convention centers. We did not know that this *would* happen, but we knew it *could* happen.

In medical terms, we called "the code," meaning to bring all the people to the scene immediately to save the patient. This time, the patient was the US health-care system and millions of Americans. As an intensive care physician, I also knew the best time to call the code is before the patient is in full cardiac arrest. Preventing a full cardiac arrest is always preferable to performing CPR on a person whose heart has already stopped. In our minds, we were calling the code *before* the system collapsed. By the end of February, Rear Admiral Orsega had rostered ten strike teams. I thank God we did that preparation before things got really bad in March.

SAN ANTONIO, WE HAVE A PROBLEM

Back in DC, I continued to feel optimistic about the success of the quarantine missions still ongoing across the country. But then, ten days after my return from San Antonio on Sunday night March 1, my wife told me about a tweet she had just seen from Mayor Nirenberg: "Today we learned that the CDC mistakenly released a patient from the Texas Center for Infectious Disease who later returned a positive COVID-19 reading. The fact that the CDC allowed the public to be exposed to a patient with a positive COVID-19 reading is unacceptable."[7]

Since I just visited Texas and knew everyone there for decades, I decided to get involved before this incident escalated. I reached out directly to the CDC director Bob Redfield, and we had a call at 10 p.m. so I could gain a full understanding of the situation described by Mayor Nirenberg and how to diffuse it.

I told Redfield I would get Chief Nim Kidd on the line and would then patch Redfield back in. Clear direct communication and planning among colleagues had always been key to solving problems, and that is what we were going to do. Within fifteen minutes, I had Chief Kidd and Governor Abbott's chief of staff, Luis Saenz, on the phone. They were true professionals, and I trusted them; I felt confident we could find a way to work together on a solution. It was clear that leaders in San Antonio and at the Texas state level were very upset. They had decided that they did not want *anyone* to leave isolation from the Texas Center for Infectious Diseases but also anyone to leave quarantine from Lackland. This was jolting to me and would be even more so for those Americans in quarantine, who expected their ordeal to be over within forty-eight hours.

Redfield joined the call late; I inferred that he had been on the phone with the vice president. We did multiple phone calls that night, ending at approximately 2 a.m. Despite all data about the appropriate length of quarantine and safeguards, Texas was firm that they did not want anyone released. There was considerable "fog of war" at that time, so although I disagreed with the Texas leadership, I completely understood their concerns and respected their position. Texas knew what a couple of cases of Ebola could do to the entire region; they were trying to avoid that same scenario, but ten thousand times worse, now with COVID. I got that.

Nevertheless, it was my judgment that the CDC should release everyone from quarantine when they fulfilled the requirements of the quarantine order and posed no known risk to the community. There were no medical or scientific reasons to further deny these citizens their freedom after they completed their fourteen days. If Texas wanted to take action, they would have to do so on their own and face the repercussions of the "freest" state in the union denying innocent individuals their liberty without any public health basis whatsoever.

I called HHS Chief of Staff Brian Harrison (also a native Texan) and arranged a meeting with Secretary Azar at eight o'clock in the morning.

Although I do not recall the specific details of that meeting, we absolutely wanted to resolve the issues with Texas amicably and collegially, but we agreed there was no justification for holding these passengers any longer against their will once the public health risk had passed.

I must admit that I saw it in fairly black-and-white terms: the federal authority to quarantine Americans lasted only until the time when science said it was safe. If Texas wanted to arrest these Americans once the CDC released them, let Texas do it and face the consequences. It was time to call the question, but we were not going to be intimidated or politically pushed into an unjustified federal action further denying these individuals—like Tyler and Rachel—their freedom. They had been through enough for good cause; I was not about to impose more on their lives for no reason.

Hours later, San Antonio escalated the crisis by filing a petition for a temporary restraining order in federal court to prevent the release of any passengers until they had been tested and confirmed negative or completed a twenty-eight-day quarantine (double the CDC order). Also, the mayor issued a public health emergency declaration that implied that the city could do whatever it needed to prevent passengers from leaving the base and entering San Antonio. The mayor was quoted in a city press release saying, "If the federal government will not do the right thing in this case, the City of San Antonio will use its powers so that appropriate measures are taken to protect the community from exposure to COVID-19."[8]

Of course, the federal government *was* doing the right thing, and the federal judge ruled against San Antonio, specifically acknowledging that HHS had determined that "two negative tests (twenty-four hours apart) and/or quarantine for fourteen days is sufficient to prevent transmission or spread of COVID-19. This Court has no authority to second-guess those determinations even though the Court also shares the concerns expressed by the Plaintiffs."[9]

Simultaneously, Bob Redfield had answered an interrogatory from the Texas health commissioner explaining the medical rationale for the CDC protocol and that close monitoring and release after fourteen days of quarantine was a sufficient precaution. He also explained the specific situation that occurred regarding the release of the patient from the Texas Center for Infectious Diseases while there was still a COVID-19 test pending.[10]

By Monday afternoon March 2, with the federal court decision in hand and the fourteen-day quarantine completed, the CDC staff and USPHS officers on the base walked into the compound, room by room, without masks or PPE, and informed everyone that they were free to leave at midnight as long as they showed their "rescind of quarantine" papers at the Lackland gate. This was a superb symbolic action by the CDC staff that demonstrated they were not in fear of becoming infected, so no one else should be in fear of becoming infected either. Rear Admiral Knight and her team did an outstanding job, putting their money where their mouths were—or more correctly, demonstrating with their own personal health and safety how certain they were of the science.

Tyler and Rachel, the young honeymooners, noted during their daily CDC question-and-answer session on March 2 that passengers were concerned about local authorities intervening. The CDC acknowledged that there was a risk of actions by state and local authorities. But the CDC also stated that "people who have been working on this go up to extremely high levels in the US government,"[11] and I was named specifically. I was indeed working the back channels and felt reasonably certain (but not 100 percent) that we were going to avoid a major conflict between the federal government and the state and that the passengers would be free to leave.

Redfield's last point in his letter to the Texas health commissioner acknowledged, for good reason, the state's concerns and specified that the CDC had changed its protocol to ensure that a patient with a positive test would not be released unless there were two sequential negative tests, and no one would be released with a pending test. This was a common-sense change and diffused the situation on the ground. In retrospect, much later in the pandemic, we realized that people could remain positive for COVID-19 by molecular tests for many weeks after they were no longer contagious, so the alarm about a marginally positive test was unjustified—but no one knew that then. Texas had a point and made it effectively.

The press in Texas reported the change in CDC protocol as a victory for Texas, which was fine with me, since I just wanted the issue resolved without unnecessary deprivation of individual liberties or animosity with Texas officials. There would be many more battles to fight, and we could not bust up relationships at this early stage. Tensions subsided, and state and local officials wound up assisting with the coordinated release of those quarantined. The plan was for individuals to be driven directly to the airport or leave in private cars to minimize interactions with people in San Antonio.

Tyler and Rachel had been anxiously following the unfolding legal saga and documented it in their blog. They decided to leave Lackland just before midnight on March 2 and not wait until the next morning for the "coordinated release." They exited the quarantine zone and were met by marshals who asked if they were sure they wanted to leave because they could no longer be protected after leaving the base. They were sure. Tyler and Rachel took the base shuttle to the gate, assisted by several base staff. They were picked up by friends and driven to the airport to get a rental car, cleared the Bexar County line at 1:46 a.m., and drove back to Dallas. All other quarantined passengers were gone by the end of the day on March 3. Local authorities took no actions to further detain or impede the release of the passengers.

On March 2, there were seventy-eight new cases nationally and six new deaths. We all suspected the worst was yet to come. It was ironic that everyone was concerned about a handful of potentially exposed passengers who had undergone a fourteen-day quarantine under strict CDC supervision, but no one could get their head around the fact that cases would likely soon be in the thousands.

But even I had no idea how bad it would actually become—not thousands but over 150 million infections in the United States alone—and how fast the virus would blitzkrieg across our nation. No one was safe.

6

Who's in Charge?

Bureaucracy doesn't realize when it's failing.
—House Speaker Newt Gingrich[1]

THE CDC WAS NEVER "IN CHARGE"

The White House created its coronavirus task force on January 29, 2020, with Secretary Azar as the chair. On February 26, the vice president took charge of the task force and named Dr. Deborah Birx as the task force "coordinator." Through its multiple iterations and changes in membership, the task force remained *the* overriding policy development and strategic decision-making body for the US COVID-19 response. We made decisions by consensus on issues that were submitted for consideration and prioritized by Marc Short, Pence's chief of staff. Vice President Pence always presided over the task force from the moment he took charge. When a decision needed to be made by the president, the task force briefed Trump either directly in the Oval Office or indirectly through the vice president. Early in the pandemic, the task force doctors almost always briefed Trump directly; by midsummer, personal briefings by the doctors to Trump were rare.[2]

In contrast to the strategic decision-making of the task force, there was a clear need for daily operational "command and control." Early on, it appeared to the nation that the CDC was in charge, but that was not the case. The Pandemic and All-Hazards Preparedness Act of 2006 (PAHPA) made it clear that the ASPR, under the direction of the HHS secretary (Azar), was responsible for leading all health and medical services during a public health emergency.

Without a doubt, the CDC was the authoritative source about infection control, community mitigation measures (like school closures), and vaccination, but they were not charged with (nor capable of) leading a coordinated response that included distributing resources, managing the SNS, preparing hospitals, developing and allocating medicines and vaccines, scaling PPE, coordinating evacuations, and dealing with the infinite number of other details that were part of the daily crisis response.

It was clear by March 2 that the response would be long and complicated and, more importantly, that the CDC could not be in charge—or even give the *appearance* to the American public that they were in charge. The operational deficiencies of the CDC were already obvious, and the secretary needed to make a definitive statement. Therefore, on March 2, Secretary Azar officially affirmed that Dr. Robert Kadlec (the ASPR) was the "incident manager" for the overall response, meaning that he had operational control with the appropriate oversight by the White House Coronavirus Task Force. The secretary asked me to be the deputy incident manager, and I felt that was exactly the right role for me.

Bob Kadlec had spent his professional life, in uniform and as a civilian, dedicated to emergency and pandemic preparedness. He had already led HHS responses to numerous hurricanes and earthquakes, and just months before in September 2019, Bob persuaded President Trump to sign a new executive order to better prepare for pandemic influenza. In the executive order, the president acknowledged the threat of a flu pandemic and called for urgent action to modernize rapid vaccine-response and vaccine-manufacturing capabilities and also to develop a specific plan to increase the uptake of vaccinations by Americans. I was with Bob in the Oval Office when Trump signed that order. Little did we know, we wouldn't have time to fully implement the executive order before the next pandemic would hit us.

Bob had previously led numerous exercises within the HHS and worked across department boundaries with the DHS and the Department of Defense. He valued US Public Health Service officers and knew how to use them during emergency responses. I respected Bob enormously and liked him personally. He was a straight shooter who did not look for credit, only solutions. Our history together went back to the 2000s, when I was an office director at DARPA and he was developing legislation that would ultimately create BARDA within HHS.

For Bob, there had been a few speed bumps during the repatriation of Americans from Wuhan and the cruise ships, but overall, these missions were completely successful—in my mind, a remarkable achievement. That success was due almost entirely to Bob's leadership, combined with the expertise of USPHS officers and the ASPR's disaster management teams (DMAT teams). I was very pleased and honored to be his deputy, and I trusted his leadership. I knew we would be a good team and meet the challenges head-on.

The ASPR organization was much more operationally capable than the CDC, and the ASPR had been in full response mode for months. The

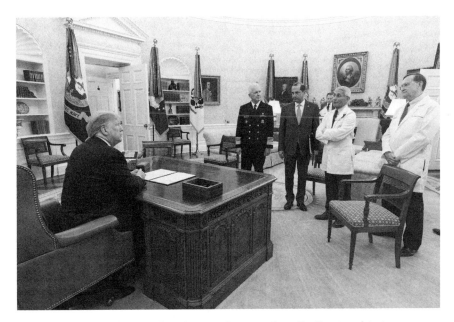

President Trump briefing by Admiral Giroir, Secretary Azar, Dr. Fauci, and Assistant Secretary Kadlec prior to signing the presidential executive order on pandemic preparedness (White House photo).

Secretary's Operations Center (SOC) was the command-and-control hub within HHS, and it had been activated under ASPR leadership since early January. The SOC went to Level 1 activation (meaning 24-7 staffing) on February 2, long before the United States had its first documented case of community transmission on February 26.

The ASPR had the long-standing Disaster Leadership Group (DLG), which regularly met to prepare for public health emergencies, long before COVID. It included senior technical and policy officials from across the federal departments and assistant secretaries. As the assistant secretary for health, I was a member of the DLG. In early January 2020, the ASPR established COVID task forces that were fully operational and provided specific recommendations for action by February 1. This fact argues strongly against the political narrative that the administration waited until March to start the response. The ASPR was completely focused on responding to COVID-19 from early January, and its operational task forces covered the following:

- *Health-care resilience.* This task force included large health-care systems throughout the country to prepare for the surge in utilization and to provide PPE and appropriate PPE guidance.

- *Repatriation.* This team was to implement and plan for additional repatriation and evacuation missions back to the United States.

- *Medical countermeasures.* This was a task force to develop vaccines and therapeutics and to improve the sharing of resources such as laboratory testing materials and models of disease.

- *Incident management.* A national-level incident management team was activated to ensure a unified planning effort.

- *Supply chain.* This task force was to understand the status of federal and state stockpiles and to enhance the availability and distribution of supplies according to needs.

- *Communications / public affairs.* This team was to ensure accurate and timely internal and external communications, messaging, and awareness.

The DLG was extremely active throughout the early stages of COVID-19. On February 7 (when there were only five new cases in the United States), representatives from HHS; the Departments of Homeland Security, Commerce, Defense, State, Agriculture, and Veterans Affairs; FEMA; General Services Administration (GSA, essential for massive-scale procurement); National Security Council at the White House; OSHA (Occupational Safety and Health Administration); and USAID (US Agency for International Development) met to establish a common understanding of the situation with respect to respiratory protection. Our discussion focused on establishing guidance to address and mitigate future shortages of PPE that could affect the pandemic response. The CDC and the FDA provided a supply-chain analysis dealing with respiratory protection, such as N95 masks and face shields. All agencies reported that they had enough supplies to fulfill their needs at that time; *no frontline teams had placed additional orders for respiratory protection equipment.*

On March 4 (when there were only 143 new cases in the United States), the ASPR issued a notice to procure five hundred million N95 masks, sending a clear message about the need to ramp up domestic production. The ASPR's modeling team was projecting hospital utilization and supply shortages even with maximum procurement, so we immediately assessed which actions could safely conserve resources.

As the deputy incident manager, my main job was to coordinate the response with CDC leadership in Atlanta. The CDC was accustomed to operating autonomously, and that could no longer be the case for the COVID response. I often joked that the CDC thought they were their own cabinet department instead of an operational division that reported to Secretary Azar. Now they were expected to follow Kadlec's leadership and be a part of an integrated team. I planned to ensure that was the case.

The people at the CDC are incredible; the organizational culture, not so much. Headquartered in Atlanta, the CDC is insular and slow, and their operational ineffectiveness was obvious to everyone. But they were also the world experts in epidemiology and infectious disease prevention, and the nation desperately needed them to excel in that role.

Dr. Redfield (the CDC director) and I were good colleagues. He understood both the greatness of the CDC and its flaws. He was actively reforming the organization. When he arrived at the CDC, it took two years to get data on the number of opioid deaths. He immediately reduced the time lag to six months and was on the path to reducing it further. Redfield also hired experts with frontline experience, like Dr. Jay Butler, the outstanding former state health official from Alaska.

Redfield and I were on great terms and on the same page. He never felt threatened and always sought and appreciated my support. As the only technical public health professional on the HHS budget council, I also fought to defend the CDC budget against the Draconian cuts proposed by the Office of Management and Budget (OMB). I was not alone in this; Jen Moughalian (the HHS chief financial officer) and even the secretary could not figure out why the OMB was so oblivious to the needs of the CDC and so many other preparedness priorities.[3]

Especially during the early days of COVID, Redfield had to be physically present in DC—650 miles away from CDC headquarters in Atlanta. He interacted daily with the secretary and White House senior leaders, including the president and vice president, and participated in all media briefings to the American public. Redfield needed to focus on these priorities; therefore, my initial job was to ensure that the leadership team at HHS knew what CDC experts in Atlanta were doing and thinking.

CDC SITE VISIT, MARCH 3–4:
ONE MILLION AMERICANS MAY DIE

My aide, Lt. Cmdr. Katie Bante, and I took the early flight to Atlanta on March 3, 2020. The schedule was tight, so it was one of the few times I took the privilege of being met on the airport tarmac and rushed to meetings in an official staff car. When I arrived at the CDC, there was indeed a beehive of activity. The infrastructure at the CDC is impressive, not at all like the drab, worn-down government buildings in DC, including HHS headquarters. The CDC had palatial entrances and shiny walkways, a high-tech conference center and museum, state-of-the-art laboratories and equipment, posh offices with great views, and, of course, an emergency response center that would make "mission control" at NASA pale in comparison. The CDC Emergency Operations Center (EOC) had literally hundreds of individuals on task, screens displaying data and input from around the globe, and hotlines to field incoming calls. I was impressed and a little in awe. Who wouldn't be?

I attended the morning CDC briefing and spent hours with their leadership. It was clear that there were some critical communication breakdowns between the CDC and HHS leadership in DC. I worked on the problem as quickly as I could.

One of my main questions was, Where did the CDC think this pandemic would go? So on March 4, I requested a private briefing from the CDC modeling group—bypassing the typical chains of command. These were the professionals who did complex statistical modeling, accounting for all the possible scenarios and assumptions at the time. On that day, we had only ninety-nine cases in a handful of states. What did the CDC think about the trajectory of the outbreak, and how should we be talking about the outbreak to the White House and the American people?

I clearly remember sitting in a small conference room at a desk that made me feel like I was back in high school when the devoted (and a little geeky in a good way) CDC modeling group started presenting their assessments. I am certain they felt great about having the assistant secretary there, interested in their work, in a direct, unfiltered private briefing. A few charts into the model, I was stunned and needed to catch my breath; I almost became physically ill.

The modelers said that their "best guess" of the eventual outcome of COVID-19 was *225,000 dead Americans*. But their model also speculated that *over one million Americans could die*, depending on the infectiousness of the virus and the ultimate case fatality rate. I had not heard those numbers before—it is not something you forget. And I did not believe that this ominous assessment was appreciated back in DC. In any case, it certainly had not been communicated to the American people.

Certainly, we had all reviewed the projected hospitalizations and deaths from a theoretical influenza pandemic, but this was the first estimate I heard specifically based on what we knew about COVID-19. When Rear Admiral Orsega and I had ordered the creation of strike teams to salvage an overrun health-care system, we thought we were being overly cautious. Now it sounded like we were actually too conservative in our fears. No number of USPHS strike teams was going to be able to fix this.

I gathered my thoughts and emotions and finished the visit. On the way back to DC, I personally wrote a sitrep for the secretary and Bob Kadlec. I specifically noted the following: the public health system was being overwhelmed in Seattle and parts of California, this situation would spread to other communities in the upcoming weeks, the CDC expected US deaths to be 225,000 but the number could be much higher, the elderly would constitute the great majority of the victims, there needed to be clear communication to the nation about the evolving status of this pandemic, and we needed to prepare the nation for some pretty extreme community mitigation steps as our only line of defense—there were no vaccines or medicines at the time.

On March 5, 2020, the day after I returned from the CDC, the White House Coronavirus Task Force highlighted the importance of protecting the elderly—consistent with the CDC view. Preliminary reports from Kirkland Life Care Center (a nursing home) in Washington State clearly indicated it was already being ravaged by COVID, so Seema Verma (administrator for the Center for Medicare and Medicaid Services) instituted aggressive nationwide actions using all the tools she had available—for example, assigning all of her nursing home inspectors solely for the purpose of improving infection control. On that same day, I approved the deployment of thirty-five USPHS officers to the Kirkland Life Care Center because its normal staff was decimated by the virus and total exhaustion. The ASPR shipped masks and gowns to Kirkland on March 10. We also prepared for potential nationwide deployments to other nursing homes. My USPHS team remained at Kirkland until April 2; they administered lifesaving medical care, triage, testing, and personal attention and compassion to the elderly. None of the officers became infected with COVID, a testament to their professionalism and proof that PPE worked. My deployed officers were extraordinarily proud and personally moved by this intense experience on the first major pandemic battleground in the United States.

At the same March 5 briefing, the task force also announced the expansion of the international travel bans, which would at least temporarily slow the spread to US cities. The vice president announced that the private sector was being engaged, especially in support of testing, but there was still a long way to go before testing would be available to the extent that the nation needed it.

And, yes, as stated by the vice president, Dr. Redfield, and Dr. Fauci during that briefing, it was true that *the overall risk to the American public at that time remained low*—but that would change rapidly over the upcoming weeks and months. I had just heard in Atlanta that one million Americans might die—somehow that fact was not captured in the statements of the task force at that briefing. I understood the need to avoid panic. But it was getting close to crunch time, and I don't believe that Americans realized how desperate this situation was going to become. And very soon.

OH MY GOD! THE PRESIDENT MIGHT GET COVID AT THE CDC

On that same morning of Thursday, March 5, having just returned from the CDC at 10 p.m. the night before, I had a 7 a.m. meeting with the secretary. He asked me to accompany him to a closed-door briefing to members of the House and Senate. Attendance was open to any member, and we knew it was critical to get everyone on the same page. The briefing was well attended and constructive on both sides of the aisle. I felt no partisan positioning behind closed doors. The secretary was able to answer all the questions, but I filled in with specific scientific and medical details when appropriate.

Following the briefings, there was a rather large press gaggle in the Capitol foyer. Fauci again stated that the risk of being infected was low, but if you were in an area of community spread, it was higher. This was an obvious point but needed to be stated. We both emphasized the higher mortality risk for the elderly and those with preexisting conditions.

I then fielded multiple questions concerning the mortality rate because I differed from the conventional wisdom published by the WHO. The WHO had stated that the mortality rate was 2–3 percent, but I knew they had a "denominator problem." Specifically, the WHO did not have complete information on how many people were actually infected, so the percentage of people dying was artificially inflated. Based on CDC data and my own estimates, I calculated that the mortality rate would eventually wind up somewhere between 0.1 percent and 1.0 percent—still incredibly dangerous, but nothing like previous coronavirus diseases that had death rates between 10 percent and 34 percent. I again emphasized that the risk of death to the elderly and chronically ill could be much higher than 2–3 percent, so Americans should not underestimate the impact of this virus.

Although there were a few probing questions, the press accepted my analysis. I think they were terrified and in shock. In retrospect, with the estimated number of COVID-19 cases in the United States being over 150 million by early 2022, the actual mortality rate of all infected does indeed fall between

0.4 and 0.5 percent—just as we had predicted. I don't want to think about where we would be if it had actually turned out to be 2–3 percent.

After the congressional briefing, I walked back to HHS and learned that President Trump was planning to visit the CDC the next day. I had the opportunity to go with the president if I chose to do so. But I had just returned from the CDC, and although it is always a privilege and honor to accompany the president, I needed to stay in DC and work on the response, especially given the dire predictions of one million deaths that had just scared the hell out of me.

A visit from the US president is always a major event, especially during a pandemic, with the virus actively circulating throughout the country. But to make matters much worse, I learned that evening that a CDC staff member had been exposed to an infected individual during a deployment at LAX. The CDC staff member came back to the CDC operations center, felt sick with a low-grade fever, decided appropriately to go home, but then returned to the CDC, where the staff member interacted closely with dozens of other staff. I could not believe that had actually occurred at the CDC! Did they not listen to themselves about exercising caution and staying home if you are sick, especially if you've been exposed to a COVID-19 patient? Nonetheless, that was the situation as it was presented to me.

Naturally (you can't make this up), the operations center was exactly where Trump planned to visit the next day. The CDC could certainly quarantine the individual staffer, but that person had already been in close contact with numerous other people at the center of CDC operations. And we were still worried about doorknobs and handrails back then, which was an entirely different concern. I also knew that the president was very spontaneous and genuinely interested in people—so it was unclear how well his staff, even the Secret Service, could wall him off from CDC personnel. Trump would do whatever Trump wanted to do. That was great about him but also truly risky in this context.

Within the next hour, my concern was raised to "DEFCON 1" when I was informed that the sick CDC staffer had been working with a DHS agent who had just tested positive for COVID. Shit shit shit shit shit! This raised the real possibility that Trump would get exposed to COVID and become infected—literally within the walls of the CDC—a possibility I could not imagine and the nation could not afford, for all sorts of reasons. Whatever credibility CDC leadership had at that time would be tanked. And, of course, Trump was up in age and overweight and would be at high risk of a serious outcome, maybe even death. It was just bad all around.

I called Dr. Nancy Messonnier, a very reliable CDC leader and close colleague, to determine if the CDC staffer had actually been tested. She did not know if the test had been done but referred me to other sources. I could not believe that a sick, exposed CDC staffer would not have had a test, so I called these other CDC sources to find out the ground truth. The sources confirmed that the staffer had indeed been tested, but inexplicably, with the president of the United States visiting the next day, the CDC had sent the test to be performed at a nearby Emory University laboratory, with an expected turnaround time of two to three days. The president would be arriving in less than eighteen hours.

Brian Harrison, the HHS chief of staff, was all over this and working throughout the night with me—we needed to get this fixed, ASAP.

Then a break—my CDC source tracked down the specimen in the FedEx box, retrieved it, and called in CDC staff that night to run the test at the CDC lab (exactly what should have been done in the first place). The result would be available the next morning. I prayed it would be conclusive, one way or the other, so the decision about the president would be easy for the White House.

At 10 p.m., I had a call with the WHMU to discuss the issue. On the one hand, we needed to protect the president. *We needed to protect the president!* This could become an assassination by COVID, and that could *not* happen. On the other hand, Trump was clear that if we were telling the American public that six feet of separation was safe, then the president wanted to "walk the walk" and not just "talk the talk." He did not want a mixed message sent to the American people, and I really respected that about him. Obviously, we could have finessed this situation by telling the media that the president did not want to interrupt the work at the CDC. But ultimately, the decision about Trump's trip was one the White House would make, not me, thank God! But I did not sleep at all that night, my head spinning with all the possible scenarios.

Early the next morning, the media was reporting that Trump had canceled the Atlanta trip. Apparently, there was a leak of information from the CDC (they were a sieve), without additional details. But at the same time, I received good news—the COVID test on the CDC staffer was entirely *negative*, and thus, the president's safety would be of no more concern than it normally was.

Trump made the trip to Atlanta after all. I thought no one would ever know about this episode, but of course, that day in the press conference, Trump was asked about the reported trip cancellation. He was very candid, as he always was. Trump said the cancellation stemmed from the fact that a person at the CDC was suspected of having COVID, but the tests turned out negative. And the president wanted to go to the CDC—so his canceled visit was "uncanceled."

But after the media feeding frenzy at the press conference, which was in large part Trump's own fault, I began to wish that the trip had actually been canceled. At that press conference, Trump called Gov. Jay Inslee a snake, stated he did not want the people on the cruise ship to be brought back to the United States because it would ruin *his* case numbers, and made a comment that became the absolute bane of my existence for the next year: "Anybody that wants a test can get a test."[4]

FROM ADMIRAL TO TESTING CZAR

During the month of February 2020, testing was a nightmare, with shortages of materials and no overall national strategy from the CDC or the FDA. The media and the public, not to mention Congress, were clamoring for more information on testing and its potential role at this stage of the pandemic.

Secretary Azar was becoming even more frustrated with the CDC and the FDA; certainly, there were political concerns from the White House, but more importantly, Azar was focused on the trajectory of infections and the potential death toll. Azar was uncertain whether he could actually trust the information he was receiving from the CDC and the FDA, not because of intentional deception, but just because the issues were complex and no one seemed to grasp the full picture. I had been working with both agencies for a couple of weeks trying to verify their testing numbers and communicate that information to the secretary so he could in turn brief the president, the vice president, and ultimately, the American people. Azar and his chief of staff, Brian Harrison, had held multiple meetings with CDC leadership and sincerely offered them whatever support they needed to improve testing and every other aspect of the CDC response.

By March 11, the secretary had enough and decided he wanted me to fix the situation—by any and all means necessary. At the time, I had no idea what that meant, but of course, I saluted and accepted the assignment. Secretary Azar had always been an insightful leader, capable, introspective, honest, and a person I trusted. He had been pushing the CDC and the FDA very hard to enhance testing but needed a person with a singular focus that he as the secretary could not provide—he did have other responsibilities, like "managing up" to the president, maintaining the entire US health-care system, and eventually, devising and leading OWS. I knew that he would, to the best of his ability, provide me with the tools and authority I needed to ultimately solve the testing crisis.

On the morning of March 12, Secretary Azar officially designated me as the coordinator of all HHS agencies with regard to testing to ensure that testing was available throughout the country and to coordinate with state and local governments and laboratories. He also indicated that the CDC director and the FDA commissioner would report directly to me with respect to COVID-19 testing.

This was a dramatic change to an otherwise immutable HHS organization chart. As the assistant secretary for health, I always had significant influence because the secretary empowered me. But since 1995, all operating divisions (the CDC, the FDA, the NIH, etc.) reported directly to the secretary (and not the assistant secretary). After twenty-five years out of the direct-reporting structure, I was now legally in charge of the FDA and the CDC with regard to all aspects of COVID-19 diagnostics. Politico first used the term *czar* in an article the next day.[5] It stuck.

The reasons why HHS needed a testing czar were complex, but it was essential to have a single point of integration and leadership. No more silos. Azar demanded swift and definitive action. And accountability.

THE LOST MONTH OF FEBRUARY 2020

On January 10, 2020, Chinese researchers published the genome sequence of the virus causing COVID-19. This was a necessary and sufficient step for laboratories around the world to develop a molecular diagnostic test—a PCR (polymerase chain reaction) test. With the gene sequence, laboratories could develop tests to detect the presence of the specific coronavirus causing the pandemic. These tests would amplify COVID genetic material and show a positive signal if the virus was present. By knowing the sequence and comparing it to other known sequences, the test would be highly specific for the pandemic coronavirus and no other viruses. The sequence was the key, and with the revelation of January 10, everyone (especially large laboratories and academic medical centers) could develop their own tests.

On January 24, the CDC finalized its test and publicly posted the protocol. This was strong work by the CDC. Publishing their protocol allowed the world to copy the CDC test design. Next, the CDC packaged their test into "kits" in preparation for distribution once the test was authorized by the

FDA. Yes, even the CDC is completely subject to FDA regulation! On February 2, the CDC submitted its request for an emergency use authorization (EUA) to the FDA. In record speed, the FDA issued the EUA on February 4. Great work by the FDA as well!

On February 6, ninety CDC test kits were distributed to fifty state public health laboratories (much like it did during the 2009 H1N1 pandemic), the District of Columbia, the Department of Defense, and repatriation sites. Every state and some large cities had an official public health laboratory that performed testing for new infectious diseases, toxins, food poisoning, and other emergencies—like this one. Although these labs are small in scale and scope, they were the first line of defense and ensured that every state and major city had testing capability.

But on the very next day after the CDC tests were distributed, it became clear that the kits were contaminated.[6]

It took until February 26 for the CDC and the FDA to devise a workaround for the contaminated tests and until March 4 for the state labs to be fully up and running with the new tests. The CDC had also arranged for a commercial supplier to manufacture kits in much larger quantities, and on March 6, these commercial test kits were delivered to hundreds of laboratories around the country. The result—we lost an entire month for COVID testing in the United States. Having that month would not have stopped the pandemic but could have been instrumental in controlling outbreaks such as those in nursing homes and meat packing plants.

In retrospect, even before the CDC test crashed due to contamination, the CDC's testing approach was doomed to failure. Their strategy was insular and relied only on state public health labs. That was an ideal strategy for Ebola or other rare infections and even appropriate for H1N1 influenza (because there were widely available point-of-care [POC] tests used by clinicians everywhere). But this approach could never meet the demands for tens of millions of tests per month required for COVID-19.

In my conversations with the CDC at the end of February, which were substantiated by an internal CDC memo, the CDC concluded that the private sector would need to be involved perhaps by August or September 2020. In retrospect, they should have been engaged the moment the genetic sequence was revealed in January. And that did not happen.

Testing required the aggressive and all-out participation of the entire private sector, especially the large labs of the American Clinical Laboratory Association (ACLA) like Quest and LabCorp. These labs needed to carry the national load, supplemented by literally every hospital and medical laboratory across the nation and even university and veterinary diagnostic laboratories. And that is exactly where we wound up, but much later.

Even Fauci clearly stated this fact during the Q and A at the March 13 Rose Garden press conference when he said, "If you want to get the kind of blanket testing and availability that anybody can get—or you could even do surveillance to find out what the penetrance is—you have to embrace the private sector, and this is exactly what you're seeing because you can't do it without it. . . . The system was not designed for what we need. Now, looking forward, the system will take care of it."[7]

But early on in the pandemic, not only were hospital, academic, and commercial labs not actively involved, they were actually *prevented* from developing their own tests by the FDA. This action by the FDA was not briefed to me or even the secretary but had a chilling inhibitory effect on test developers, especially those in academic medical centers.

FDA career staff and some political appointees had long argued that the FDA had the authority to exert premarket review (regulation) on diagnostic tests known as LDTs (laboratory-developed tests). LDTs are defined as tests that are designed, manufactured, and used within a single laboratory— like the ones that could have been used throughout the nation in January and February. After attempting to exert premarket review on LDTs beginning in 2014, the FDA decided in January 2017 *not* to finalize guidance in order to allow for further discussion and feedback from stakeholders.[8] Fundamentally, the FDA's position was that although it asserted its authority to regulate such tests, it would engage in enforcement discretion and not do so until a time of the FDA's choosing.

Unfortunately, the time of the FDA's choosing turned out to be the onset of the pandemic. As detailed in an HHS memo to Commissioner Hahn in June of 2020 that outlined the sequence of events, the FDA (without notifying the secretary, the general counsel, or presumably anyone in a national leadership role) posted on its website the following notification:

> FDA generally has not enforced premarket review and other legal requirements [with respect to LDTs]. However, LDTs for which an HHS [public health emergency] declaration justifies a need (and that potentially meet the EUA criteria) present a higher risk. This is because they are developed to diagnose serious or life-threatening diseases or conditions that not only have serious implications for individual patient care, but also for analyses of disease progression and public health decision-making. Thus, FDA requests that developers of such

LDTs submit information about their tests to help FDA better understand their design, validation, and performance characteristics.[9]

Although this website was taken down and is now untraceable, I believe the notice was originally posted on February 1, 2020, the day after Secretary Azar declared a public health emergency. HHS leadership did not even realize that this had been posted until it was pointed out to the secretary's office by a particularly outstanding newspaper reporter in the course of an investigation.

To be clear, the FDA was asserting that because of the public health emergency, laboratories were required to submit data to the FDA before a test could be utilized. This assertion imposed an onerous, time-consuming, confusing, and unfamiliar process on laboratories at the exact time we needed them to gear up. It also imposed criteria, such as the requirement that the test be successfully performed on at least five positive clinical specimens, at a time when there were actually only a small number of COVID-19 cases scattered in a few regions and no central resources from the CDC that could be used to validate the five positive clinical specimens. There was nothing magic about the CDC test that couldn't have been replicated, modified, and even improved by hundreds of laboratories across the country. But in one fell swoop of regulatory overreach, the FDA thwarted testing right at the time it was our most important weapon against the virus.

A CBS *60 Minutes* segment that aired on November 1, 2020, detailed the effects of this regulatory overreach. Dr. Geoffrey Baird, chair of the Department of Laboratory Medicine and Pathology at the University of Washington School of Medicine, claimed that they had a COVID test ready to be implemented in their laboratory but that the FDA prevented them from doing so. In the meantime, elderly patients in the nearby Kirkland nursing home were becoming sick, dying, and infecting others. There would be no adequate testing until weeks after the carnage in that facility had occurred. This void in testing could have been filled by the University of Washington, and there were similar situations where hundreds of academic and commercial laboratories across the country could have stepped in to mitigate their local outbreaks.[10] Consistent with Dr. Baird and widely reported in the media, Scott Becker, CEO of the Association of Public Health Laboratories, wrote to Commissioner Hahn on February 24. Becker stated that weeks into the response, there were no diagnostic or surveillance tests widely available to supply the state public health laboratories.[11]

To summarize, the only EUA issued by the FDA until February 29 was for the CDC test, which was contaminated and could not be used until March 4, when a work-around to the contamination was implemented. The CDC was available to perform testing at their headquarters in Atlanta during that interval, but only at a tiny scale. For example, on February 18, the CDC built a new surge laboratory that expanded testing to 350 samples (175 patients) per day for the entire country. This was less than the testing capability in South Korea at the time by tenfold—a country with only 15 percent of the US population.

In addition, testing at the CDC required burdensome paperwork and transport of the specimens to Atlanta. Testing was provided initially only for those traveling from hot spots like China or those who had direct interactions with people who were proven infected. It was not until February 27 that the CDC relaxed guidelines so that a person could be tested if any clinician or public health official suspected a coronavirus infection for whatever reason.

The regulatory bottleneck created by the FDA was only partially fixed on February 29, 2020, when the FDA agreed to allow laboratories to start using the tests they developed as long as they submitted a complete data package within fifteen days. This helped but was in no way a complete solution, since all the documentation and paperwork were still required, only slightly delayed. Nevertheless, by March 15, 2020, fifty additional tests were being used under the FDA's new policy. But oh so much time had been lost— the lost month of February.

On March 12 and 13, the FDA authorized commercial tests from Roche and Thermo Fisher Scientific on the same days they were submitted to the FDA. This was truly an inflection point because these large commercial test suppliers would churn out tests in the hundreds of thousands per month, adding up to the millions. High-throughput laboratories and major academic medical centers typically used the Roche machines, but nearly every clinical and university lab in the country had access to Thermo Fisher testing platforms—and that was exactly what we needed to massively scale testing in every state in the country.

But having tests in boxes was only a tiny part of the overall solution; I only truly realized that fact on the day I became testing czar and inherited the challenge. The next seven days would be "make or break" for testing and perhaps the nation. I realized that tens of thousands of lives were in the balance and shuddered a bit at the overall enormity of the task.

7

Seven Days in March

THE DAY EVERYTHING CHANGED

Thursday, March 12: 1,144 new US cases and 7 new US deaths.

It was my first day as the HHS testing coordinator, although there would be no public announcement of that fact until the next day. I thought I was ready for the challenge. But I had no idea what would happen over the next seventy-two hours: events that would culminate in my sharing the White House podium with President Trump on Sunday, speaking to an anxious nation at prime time.

The day started with an early morning meeting with Azar in the secretary's conference room on the sixth floor of the Hubert H. Humphrey Building. Compared to the rest of the forty-three-year-old, "Brutalist"-style building, the secretary's suite was well appointed. It was located near the center of the building, along the facade facing the National Mall and the Capitol. To enter the suite, as I did hundreds of times before, I went through a remotely locked door controlled by a receptionist and then past the secretary's armed security detail who sat in front of his office. The secretary's conference room was just down the hallway, past numerous wall-mounted photos of important events that featured the secretary with the president or other world leaders. I don't remember exactly who attended that meeting in person, but it was a small group; there were many other HHS leaders on the conference line.[1]

Secretary Azar entered shortly after I arrived; per protocol, we stood as he entered and then sat after he assumed his position at the head of the table. I was two seats down on his left side, facing the door to the conference room. I had attended these morning organizational meetings many times before, but this was my first day with the responsibility of coordinating testing. And then, suddenly, shortly after the meeting began, two individuals unexpectedly burst into the room—Jared Kushner and Deborah Birx. Unannounced visitors do not normally get past security and enter a meeting with the secretary, but this was different. They were on a mission. And they were, well, Jared and Deb.

I had not previously interacted very much with Deb, but we had appeared together several times in relation to HIV—she as the PEPFAR (US President's Emergency Plan for AIDS Relief) coordinator and I as the HHS lead for the Ending the HIV Epidemic in the US initiative, announced by the Trump at the 2019 State of the Union address. I did not fully understand Deb's role or who picked her for it, but she was indeed the coordinator of the White House Coronavirus Task Force, named two weeks earlier. That meant she had the support of the president and vice president, and that is really all I needed to know. Needless to say, Deb had a reputation for being a highly competent and confident public servant who was surprisingly savvy about DC politics and especially the HHS power structure. She also had a very realistic view of what agencies like the CDC could do and, more importantly, what they could never do.

I had spent very little time with Jared before that day (which was about to change drastically). Previously, I only worked with him when he was in a supporting role to his wife, Ivanka Trump, on initiatives like the National Youth Sports Strategy. I had also been invited to a small dinner at Jared and Ivanka's home once with Azar and the surgeon general very early in my term. There were a couple of Secret Service agents outside the home and a furtive media guy, intermittently hiding behind walls or trees and photographing everyone who went in or out of their front door. Jared and Ivanka were gracious, kind, and humble hosts, with three very adorable children who scurried in and out of the room and were not happy at all about having to go to bed midway through the evening. Sweet little Arabella, their daughter, even made little hand-drawn name cards for the evening—I kept mine on my HHS office credenza right next to my challenge coins as a remembrance of that evening and their hospitality.

In the secretary's conference room, Jared was no longer in the background. He was, after all, an assistant to the president, which in the White House ranks only below the president's chief of staff. I assumed his role was much more important than even his position denoted, since he was Trump's son-in-law. That assumption proved true. Azar seemed a little surprised by their sudden entrance but not at all flustered. The secretary was a team player, even when the team was a little ad hoc compared to his normal style of meticulous prospective planning and disciplined execution.

Jared and Deb stated that I needed to design a national system of drive-through testing sites and get them implemented in emerging US hot spots *as soon as possible.* Testing sites were starting to pop up in a few US cities, but there were no protocols, no national model, no strategic positioning, and no federal leadership or supplies. South Korea had been lapping the United States in testing because of lessons they learned after the SARS virus outbreak in their country eighteen years earlier. But even the Korean system had significant limitations, including a low throughput of patients and, at least early on, a requirement that people pay for their own testing if they wound up being negative for COVID-19.

Implementing high-throughput testing sites was the right decision. Testing was an important tool to protect the public, especially since we had no medicines or vaccines at that time. Testing was also becoming a significant political liability after Trump's "Anybody that wants a test can get a test" comment, made worse by the poor overall implementation of testing by the CDC in February. A system of nationwide drive-through sites would be a visible sign to Americans that the administration was taking action to remedy the CDC testing missteps and assuming overall control of critical initiatives that had been mismanaged by career bureaucrats. Now the president and vice president were going to provide leadership directly through the White House Coronavirus Task Force.

A week before I was named testing coordinator, Trump, Pence, and Birx had met with CEOs from major diagnostic companies including Roche and Thermo Fisher, commercial labs, and several pharmacies and big-box retailers. There was overall support for a "whole of society" approach to testing. But that general support needed to be translated into tangible national action, and, well, I was the new testing guy . . .

I left for the White House as soon as I gathered my laptop and a few documents and started the process of making this abstract concept of drive-through testing sites take shape. If successful, it would be an important inflection point in the response, but if we failed, the country would be in even worse shape, and I suspected the political fallout would be disastrous. There was actually a high likelihood of failure, but someone had to try—and, of course, be accountable. That person was now me.

It was clear that Jared and Deb—and by inference, Trump and Pence—understood that the traditional federal bureaucracies could not act decisively enough, quickly enough, or boldly enough to defeat the pandemic. This was true not only for testing but also for many other aspects of the response—from managing the SNS to vaccine development and deployment. But my role was testing, and I can speak to that authoritatively, as I personally experienced it.

The widely publicized phrase about Jared assembling people who "get shit done" is accurate. I am not sure who first used this description, but my guess is that it was Adam Boehler, who had been the director of the Center for Medicare and Medicaid Innovation within HHS and was then the newly Senate-confirmed, inaugural CEO of the US International Development Finance Corporation. He had been an extremely successful entrepreneur in the private sector and was incredibly creative—if not a little manic. As important to the story, although I did not know it at the time, Adam had been Jared's roommate during one summer in college. So there was a high degree of trust between them—and it showed.

People assigned to work on the new national testing initiative were starting to assemble in the West Wing later that afternoon and evening. Most people believe the West Wing is spacious, with accommodations for whoever is needed on a project. It is not that way at all. The West Wing is actually very small and cramped, with as many oddly placed halls and offices as could fit in the footprint of the historic building. We did find an empty office—it was Brooke Rollins's office, who was out of town at the time.[2] We crashed there and started planning. Brooke's alma mater was Texas A&M, and true to the Aggie spirit, she had a gigantic neon A&M sign against the back wall. In a strange way, that sign made me feel at home.

THINKING "OUT OF THE POD"

We started work immediately but were awaiting the arrival of a key contributor to the tactical planning process. Josh Dozer was the chief of the FEMA National Response Coordination Center (NRCC) and the deputy assistant administrator for the response. His role would soon be even more critical (after the declaration of a national emergency when FEMA became the LFA for the pandemic), but he was being looped into this new testing effort to provide a FEMA operational perspective. He did not arrive at the White House until the early evening.

Josh was quiet, calm, professional, and focused. I don't think he liked being at the White House because it was an awkward place to plan an operation. He was the kind of person for whom it was hard to decipher whether he was satisfied with the situation or completely exasperated because nobody else had a clue. Josh had a "poker face" during stressful times, and I could relate to that. As a pediatric ICU physician, I had a little of the same. The more critical and life-threatening the situation, the calmer my external demeanor became. That type of calmness is necessary to inspire confidence and also to keep an ICU room packed with adrenaline-fueled professionals focused on the task at hand: saving a life. People would frequently wonder how I kept my cool in media briefings and on TV; I think it was because it was always very high stakes, which, paradoxically, made me quiet and calm.

Josh's explanation of how FEMA operated and the massive scope of their capabilities was immediately illuminating. He clarified that the national response needed to proceed according to FEMA's model: *federally supported, state managed, and locally executed.* This was the mantra, and for good reason. Our nation is expansive and diverse, and the feds must utilize existing local mechanisms to reach into communities efficiently and effectively. This mantra was not invented by the Trump administration but instead was a long-standing tenet of national emergency response. If the federal government tried to do too much, the response would be slow and nonresponsive. But if the feds did too little, states would not be able to get the resources and guidance they needed. It was a balance. But in contrast to normal FEMA responses, this was not a short-duration regional calamity like a hurricane. This was worldwide and was going to last years.

I talked to Josh about the objective of establishing drive-through testing sites, and he immediately described the FEMA POD system. POD stands for *points of distribution.* These were used to distribute food, water, and other supplies after natural disasters like hurricanes. PODs were really a concept and a method of operation, not so much a real "thing." PODs could be placed anywhere, including parking lots. They were modular and scalable to distribute supplies to anywhere from several hundred to tens of thousands of people per day. PODs could be drive-throughs or walk-ups, or they could even accommodate mass transit.

Typically, the local emergency management agency coordinated the location of the PODs and their operation. The POD manager was responsible for the overall mission and, either directly or indirectly, the safety of all staff and personnel receiving supplies. There are support teams that manage practical aspects such as traffic control, security, and garbage disposal. The POD process was highly scripted and diagrammed, and as a result, there was an easy-to-use instruction book to minimize the risk of failure. More importantly, all of FEMA and every emergency response coordinator at the state and local levels were familiar with the POD concept. That was critical. We could not afford to reinvent any wheels.

After hearing this description from Josh, I knew immediately how to proceed. It was a critical "aha!" moment, one of many. We would utilize the FEMA POD concept for a national system of drive-through testing. But there were of course *major* differences and substantial obstacles. We would not be distributing anything but rather testing and educating sick or worried people and their families. We required specialized materials and devices, most of which were not available in the states or even in the federal SNS. We needed to deploy skilled medical personnel and perform procedures that were relatively invasive (nasopharyngeal swabs) while people remained in their vehicles. We had information-management challenges like patient identification, the logging and tracking of specimens, and biohazard shipping. We had to involve the private sector to actually perform the tests in laboratories, since the CDC was not capable of the scale we envisioned. We needed to report results in a timely fashion and provide patient education whether the test turned out to be positive or negative. And just to complicate matters even more, we had an enormous safety challenge—keeping the staff (and other patients) from becoming infected and then dealing with large amounts of biohazard waste that contained a virus that was causing a worldwide pandemic.

We were also concerned that because of the growing fear and concern about the pandemic, there could be riots, threats, or violence, especially if we turned away people who did not need a test by our prioritization scheme. And, of course, we needed to solve all of these medical and logistical problems ASAP and establish testing PODs in many sites across the country simultaneously. But aside from that, it would be a piece of cake!

We really did not have time to procrastinate or call in an advisory committee from the CDC to debate the issues. We just needed to "get shit done." We worked late into the evening at the White House and had a plan for the next day. I returned to my apartment at about 10 p.m. and met Jill, who was just returning from a trip back home to Texas. We had a new granddaughter, less than a month old; our daughter Jacqueline had almost died of a massive hemorrhage during the delivery. It was only because of the incredible team at Medical City in Dallas pumping Jacqueline full of blood and platelets and fluids and performing emergency procedures that she was still alive. We were still pretty shaken by the experience but felt blessed. I had a lot to tell Jill about that night and did, but I knew I needed to sleep. I had a 6:30 a.m. car to the White House the next morning and felt the same as I had years earlier when getting ready for thirty-six hours on call in the pediatric ICU. Jill and I both knew we were in for the long haul and that there would be no trips back to Texas for a long time.

AN AFTERNOON IN THE ROSE GARDEN

March 13: 1,317 new cases, 11 new deaths.

Early on March 13, the press began picking up that I was going to coordinate testing, and by midmorning, Politico had published an article on the anticipated new White House coronavirus push, including the new HHS testing czar. At that time, South Korea was performing about as many tests each day as the United States had done cumulatively over six weeks. Everyone knew there was a major problem with testing, and it was beginning to be the dominant topic on most national networks and within the walls of the West Wing.

People around DC were starting to panic—buying up everything they could from the local stores. The rumor was circulating on social media that the country would be *locked down* soon, whatever that meant, so people stocked up on everything from drinking water to toilet paper. It was not without justification, since we were actually very concerned about the nation's food supply; Secretary Sonny Perdue was coordinating with the CDC to ensure that Americans would be fed by keeping open meat packing plants and other critical agricultural infrastructure while safeguarding the workers. Perdue was decisive, and that gave me confidence. Jill also made sure that we were personally prepared for whatever was to come. Unlike the secretary, who has a driver and staff car to travel to and from his home and a security detail around the clock, assistant secretaries like me had to fend for ourselves in terms of personal security, transportation, and basic supplies once we left the Humphrey Building. So Jill started "fending."

That day I wore my ODU (the USPHS working deployment uniform) to the White House, the first of many days I would do so. It was protocol to wear dress uniforms to the White House, not ODUs, but this was a pandemic. Six weeks earlier, I ordered all officers in the USPHS Commissioned Corps to wear their ODUs, no matter what their assignment, to indicate our readiness to deploy and also to demonstrate the dire seriousness of our situation. So I did the same, even to the White House. My fellow officers appreciated that, and keeping their morale high amid their dangerous deployments was—and would remain—high on my agenda. The morning consisted of a lot more organizational work and gaining knowledge of which parts of the team needed bolstering.

I did not know until early in the afternoon that there was a presidential press conference in the Rose Garden scheduled for 3 p.m., with senior administration officials and CEOs of major companies, like Walmart, CVS, and Walgreens; LabCorp and Quest (the two largest national testing laboratories); and Beckton Dickinson, Roche, and Thermo Fisher (three of the largest manufacturers of

high-throughput laboratory tests). I was informed that White House leadership
wanted me on stage as well. I did not know if it was the president, the vice president, or the White House communications team who wanted me there, but it
did not really matter at that point. I only had ODUs and was far too busy to
go back to HHS and get my dress uniform. Despite protocol, the White House
organizers wanted me as I was, in my ODUs. In the days to follow, Trump
himself said he preferred me in my ODUs because it was a crisis and we were
working nonstop—he said something like there is "no time to pretty up."

Before our short briefing with Trump prior to entering the Rose Garden,
I had time to talk with many of the CEOs for the first time. I introduced
myself and wasted no time beginning discussions about public-private partnerships. For the next year, we would collaborate on a daily basis, and this
was a perfect time to start that collaboration. We met in the Cabinet Room,
just a small reception area away from the Oval Office, and talked about the
situation and plans moving forward. I thought to myself, "Holy shit! I am
definitely in the middle of this now." There was no time to be timid or hesitant. Then our entire group was herded into the Oval Office to meet Trump
and Pence. Dr. Birx was of course present and very confident in the way
forward; her confidence gave me comfort because I certainly did not yet have
a clear vision about how we were going to fix testing in the short term. Also
in the Oval Office were Secretary Azar, Center for Medicare and Medicaid
Services (CMS) Administrator Seema Verma, and Tony Fauci.

We exited the Oval Office out of the French doors that led directly to the
Rose Garden. It was an absolutely gorgeous day. The Japanese magnolias were
in full bloom, and the small trees and shrubs were just leafing out in vibrant
green. The roses were only just starting to bud, but there nonetheless was a
sweet fragrance that stuck with me. The Rose Garden was packed with reporters sitting shoulder to shoulder; there were no masks or physical distancing
back in those days. Behind the seated reporters were rows of photographers and
audio technicians. They were lined up so tight and with so much equipment,
they reminded me of a formation of soldiers in the Revolutionary War, carrying
their rifles, some kneeling while others standing, ready to point and shoot.

In contrast to the normal protocol where officials and guests would go
on stage first and await the arrival of the president and vice president, Trump
sprinted through the French doors of the Oval Office like a thoroughbred out
of the starting gate at the Kentucky Derby. He had a lot to say and was apparently ready to say it. He started speaking before everyone was even positioned
on the small stage looking out at the press. There were probably a thousand
camera clicks in the first fifteen seconds; that sound took me by surprise

and shook me a little. I had not experienced that degree of media intensity before, but after that day, it was my new normal.

I did not have a speaking role, nor did I want one. There was some good news, and I was pleased that Trump and Birx delivered it. The president declared a national emergency, which provided numerous authorities we needed for the overall federal response. The declaration also unlocked $50 billion in flexible funds. You can't respond to states' needs without a budget, and unlocking these funds was absolutely essential. But even with the new national emergency declaration, Trump still kept HHS in charge as the LFA. That would change five days later.

There was also some good testing news that stemmed from Trump and Birx's meeting with the diagnostics companies ten days earlier. Roche had just received an EUA for the first high-throughput test to enter the market. Although Roche equipment was typically used only by sophisticated laboratories in academic centers and large commercial labs, their EUA was indeed a godsend to begin replacing the low-throughput and previously contaminated CDC kits. Thermo Fisher would also receive an EUA only a few hours later, and that made test kits available to a much broader audience of laboratories. Thermo Fisher was the most important company you never heard of throughout the pandemic. With eighty thousand employees and the ability to scale any product massively, we relied on them for everything from diagnostic collection kits and PCR testing machines to freezers for vaccines. More good news: both LabCorp and Quest had begun to perform tests as well and were focusing their efforts on areas of the country where there were outbreaks. Over the next several months, these two labs carried half of the national testing load and were a major building block of our testing ecosystem. And remember, just two weeks earlier, the CDC had written that the nation would not need LabCorp or Quest until the fall of 2020. But it was crystal clear that the nation needed them immediately—and probably several weeks earlier than that day in mid-March.

Issuing EUAs for Roche and Thermo Fisher was good news for testing but not as good as the White House thought it was and certainly not as good as the media interpreted it to be. Having an assay kit in a lab is a good start but still only a small component of what was needed to actually perform a test. And at that time, all the tests were PCR tests, requiring a high-complexity laboratory with relatively sophisticated instruments and at least two or three days (if not much longer) to complete the test and report results. There were no point-of-care (POC) tests—none anywhere on the planet—that provided results in minutes, and given our experience with prior infectious diseases, it might be years before such POC tests became available for COVID-19.

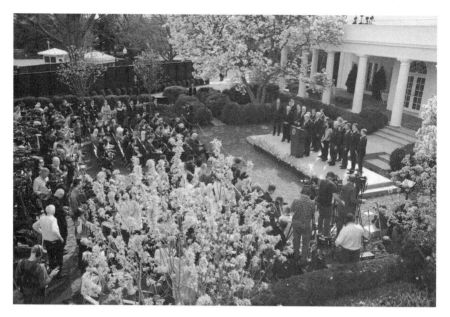

Rose Garden press briefing with the president, vice president, and CEOs from major American corporations (White House photo).

Trump remarked about how the retailers were going to have drive-through sites where people could go and be "swabbed" without leaving their cars. Well, that was true conceptually, except there were absolutely no operational plans yet for that to happen. Trump also talked about a Google "front-end website and app" so people could use their phone or computer to screen themselves and then be directed to a testing site—I did not know anything about that but later learned this was an effort that the White House was working on directly with Google.

Following Trump's remarks, Deb Birx took center stage. She presented a professional-looking graphic illustrating the process: first, it depicted how a person would use the website for screening and instructions, then the person would use a drive-through site that would test him or her and send the specimen to labs, and then the results would be posted on the website. I had not seen that graphic before the briefing. Again, all of this was possible conceptually, but there were no operational plans to turn these concepts into reality.

And then my world crashed. The vice president stated to the press and to the American people, "And for Americans looking on, by this Sunday evening, we'll be able to give specific guidance on when the website will be available. You can go to the website, as the president said. You'll type in your symptoms and be given direction on whether or not a test is needed. And then, at the same website, you'll be directed to one of these incredible companies that are going to give a little bit of their parking lot so that people can come by and do a drive-by test."[3]

Did I just hear that? I became the testing coordinator only about thirty hours before that press conference, and now the vice president of the United States is saying we would have all the information to the American people by Sunday (forty-eight hours) and an operational website?

I knew this was completely unachievable, but I also knew that I had great people working on the problems and that every resource would be made available to me by the president and vice president. What did we have to lose? Ultimately, some things turned out to be possible and others did not.

THE PICKUP GAME

Brad Smith is a young, very successful health-care entrepreneur who had just been recruited to HHS by Adam Boehler two months earlier, when Adam assumed his new role as the first CEO of the US International Development Finance Corporation. Brad took Adam's place as the director of the Center for Medicare and Medicaid Innovation (CMMI), where the future of health-care delivery was being imagined and tested through national models. Brad was a summa cum laude graduate from Harvard and a Rhodes scholar, but he was the opposite of any stereotype for a person with those credentials. Brad was confident but humble and a team player and understood complex and dynamic challenges as well as anyone I had ever met. He was also the best operations guy in the country and, more importantly, could get along with people in the White House with big egos and territories to protect. Brad was called to the White House to run operations for the new testing push and would become one of the biggest heroes of the COVID-19 response. He and I would be inseparable for the next year—starting that night.

Immediately after the Rose Garden press conference, Brad and I huddled and strategized how we hoped the next forty-eight hours would unfold. Brad would run the operations and keep people on task, breaking down barriers as they arose. I would provide the medical and scientific leadership, bring in experienced USPHS officers, and be the front person for many calls with CEOs and industry partners.

Under normal circumstances, even as an assistant secretary, my authority was limited. But not under these circumstances. I was Senate confirmed, and more importantly, Jared Kushner and Deb Birx had instructed me to get this done. It was also helpful to have four stars on my lapel for interactions with the armed components of the US military. The USPHS Commissioned Corps is indeed part of the US military, just unarmed (unlike the US Army, US Navy, US Air Force, US Marines, US Coast Guard, and the new US Space Force), and until the pandemic, most people in the armed services had never heard of us. But they quickly learned.

Brendan Fulmer was another young staffer from HHS and had also worked in the secretary's office and then with CMMI. Brendan coordinated all the working groups under Brad, making sure that deliverables were met and meetings were productive. He would later be essential for the development of the private retail partnerships that would scale to many thousands of testing sites. Rachel Baitel was a young staff member who came from USAID after working in the White House. She was only five years out of her undergraduate degree at Princeton but was able to find anyone we needed to talk to anywhere, obtain the relevant information, and form a plan of action. It was always "Yes, sir" from Rachel, and I had confidence in her from the very beginning.

Eric Hargarten was critical to the team as well and would remain so for the course of the pandemic. He was a former enlisted security specialist in the US Air Force who had subsequently graduated from Loyola University Chicago with a physics major and minors in finance and math. Brad had recruited Eric out of his venture capital analytics job to be Brad's right-hand man for innovative Medicare and Medicaid health-care delivery models. Eric started at HHS on March 1, not expecting to be thrown into the pandemic response. Eric was brilliant, quiet, disciplined, incredibly organized, and completely reliable. I have no idea what we would have done without him.

Jared and Adam had apparently already called and begun assembling several individuals from the private sector, including Nat Turner and several of his staff from Flatiron Health.

We were also going to need technical consultation and leadership from officers in the USPHS Commissioned Corps, so I called my principal deputy assistant secretary, R. Adm. Sylvia Trent-Adams, and the director of Commissioned Corps Headquarters, Rear Admiral Orsega. Both of these officers were already icons; nothing could really rattle them. They were veterans of Ebola in West Africa and the early fights against HIV. Rear Admiral Trent-Adams was a National Academy of Medicine member and had done pioneering work in developing and implementing the Ryan White HIV/AIDS Program. Rear Admiral Orsega and I had been deploying officers since early January and preparing for the US health system to be overrun.

The number of people on the White House COVID Testing Rapid Response Team was growing, and we could not work effectively in Brooke Rollins's small office in the basement of the West Wing. So on Saturday, March 14, we met in my office suite at HHS. We spread out, formed teams, had frequent group meetings and external teleconferences, and equally important, got pizza delivered. It was just like a start-up company—no question about it—except thousands of lives were at stake, and that fact permeated everything.

By Saturday, there were fifty-five people on the email list and many more who were on the team but not yet on the list. How they all got into the secure Humphrey Building, I am not exactly sure. But all got in—badges or not. Brad and I divided the overall team into working groups across all required functional areas.[4]

On Saturday morning, Brad and I led an overall team meeting, and then Brad led sync-up meetings with each of the work groups for about fifteen minutes every two to three hours, from 8 a.m. until 10 p.m. Each meeting detailed progress and impediments, and Brad changed plans and pivoted the organization frequently. There was a lot of change and redirection because we were starting from scratch and had to "kiss a lot of frogs" along the way.

Sometime in the first hours of planning, we decided to change the name from *drive-through testing sites* to *community-based testing sites* (CBTSs). This was important because we wanted these sites to be outside of the formal medical care system, which was already becoming overwhelmed with caring for the sick. We also wanted the flexibility to have walk-ups in places like Manhattan where people didn't actually drive. Later in the year, we actually had a person on horseback in Texas come through and get swabbed!

I loved working with Brad. He had skills that I didn't, and everybody's egos were left at the door. Like Brad, I had also graduated Harvard (except two decades earlier), but neither of us took that to mean we had all the answers. Brad's intellect combined with his common sense and operational acumen made him essential at many levels. We would fight many battles together over the next year—both external ones and internal ones within the White House. We often discussed the internal personnel conflicts and how to make them work or work around them when needed—including some that I had personally much later. Brad summed it up to the team in one of our first meetings: "We are going to build this ark, but it has already been raining an awfully long time . . ."

WHAT'S IN A TEST?

There was significant confusion, which remains today, about what a "test" means. In the Rose Garden as well as in communiqués from the CDC and the FDA, a test had been operationally defined as a kit that contained many (but not all) components needed to actually perform the diagnostic assay in a high-complexity laboratory.[5] Not a single item in these kits actually touched a patient.

When the CDC and the FDA told Azar and me that there were hundreds of thousands and soon millions of "tests" entering the market, the truth was that they were not complete. They had *some* components of the tests but not the whole end-to-end solution. For example, they had no swabs to obtain patient samples or tubes of media to transport the sample to the lab. They also did not supply certain scarce but required laboratory reagents needed to run the tests. I tried clarifying this distinction numerous times in the White House press room and on national media, most notably on April 20, 2020, when I spoke about the difference between a "test" and the "end-to-end solution." Simply put, the initial kits put together by the CDC and the subsequent commercial kits based on the CDC design did not include everything the laboratory needed to perform the test.[6] That was an enormous source of confusion in early March among the American people, the press, and even many subject matter experts.

The most famous missing components were swabs. Before a test could be run, a sample had to be collected using a swab, and in mid-March, the only swab recognized by the FDA was a nasopharyngeal (NP) swab that was inserted all the way up the back of the nose.[7] Once the swab sample was collected, it had to be placed in a specific test tube containing a solution called "viral transport medium." This assured that the patient sample was preserved during transport.

And, of course, nasopharyngeal swabs required collection by a health-care provider using an FDA-specified swab placed in an FDA-specified tube of transport medium. Once in the lab, the viral genetic material in the sample was extracted using an FDA-authorized method and tested using a specific kit that was authorized as a component of the entire aforementioned process. The health-care provider needed to be in full PPE including an N95 mask because a nasopharyngeal swab generally induced coughing or sneezing—which generated a highly infectious aerosol, exposing the health-care provider and everyone in the vicinity. PPE needed to be changed between patients to avoid accidentally infecting the next person through contaminated clothing.[8]

WHICH COMMUNITIES?

Even if our team could determine how to provide a full end-to-end testing solution, we would still only be able to establish a finite number of CBTSs in the short term. Where should they go? To me the answer was simple: we would establish sites where there was the greatest current need for testing and also where the need could soon explode.

I was concerned that if we involved too many people in this decision, it could get sidetracked by any number of considerations that were not the "greatest need," including politics and personalities. The CDC could provide this information, but we could not wait for days of internal debate and CDC bureaucracy. I had been dealing with Dr. Dan Jernigan, who was the CDC incident manager at that time and a solid guy. He was good to work with and responded to our needs even if it was not through proper CDC protocol. Dan would have a nervous laugh whenever I pushed him out of the CDC comfort zone; I was happy for this tell, which helped me understand the CDC's cultural boundaries and operational capabilities. So I told Dan, "I need your priority list of hot spots based on current or imminent need. And I need it in one hour." He provided it on time. I wrote the locations on a piece of paper, and someone transcribed them to a whiteboard (we had scoured HHS and collected as many whiteboards and flip charts as we could "borrow" from other divisions to support our weekend efforts).

That became our working list; there had been no politics or other considerations, just the CDC recommendations from Dr. Jernigan. I took a picture of the whiteboard not for a future book but so I would have on my phone a record of where we were planning to place testing sites. We were never pressured by Jared, Pence, or Trump to put testing sites anywhere except where there was the greatest need. I know that for a fact because I made the site decisions.

Getting from a targeted city to a specific address for a drive-through site was a very tedious process. Over the next forty-eight hours, Josh and his FEMA colleagues worked through the FEMA regional system to contact state and local officials and inform them of the evolving plan. CBTSs would follow the proven FEMA model, which was *federally supported, state managed, and locally executed*. Starting that Saturday, we contacted every FEMA regional representative individually and also had teleconferences where all regional representatives participated together. We called governors and state health officials. They wanted all the details, but we did not have them—at least not on Saturday. We were definitely "building the plane as we flew it."

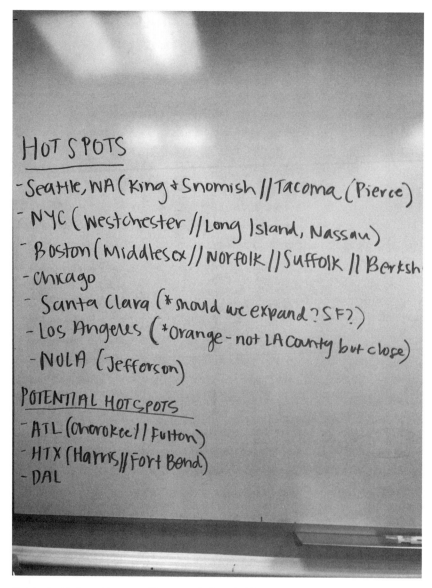

Original whiteboard listing of "hot spots" identified by the CDC as priorities for drive-through testing sites (personal photo).

The states needed to provide my team with specific locations with addresses. Midday Saturday, I made it clear that if we did not have addresses and a commitment by Monday at the latest, their state/county/city would have to wait for the next round of testing sites, and there was no guarantee when the next round would start. I was not being a heavy-handed jerk; it was just the reality of logistics and deployment. Remember, the emergency management framework is *federally supported, state managed, and locally executed*. We were following the playbook.

This operation should have been started two months earlier by the career officials at the CDC, but it wasn't. We only had forty-eight hours to begin shipping supplies and deploying officers.

SWABS

The testing team included many individuals from the Office of the ASPR and FEMA as well as volunteers from the private sector. The ASPR had already started working with contracting officers (who could sign federal contracts and commit federal government funding) and procurement specialists from the US Navy and US Army, which would soon include R. Adm. John Polow-czyk (Admiral P)—the logistics lead from the Joint Chiefs of Staff. Getting the Department of Defense involved in contracting was absolutely critical, since HHS had a long history of being remarkably terrible at contracting. Jared facilitated this personally—he wanted contracting on-site right next to the operators. If we needed something, he wanted a team right there to get it.

Admiral P began assisting the HHS-FEMA team on March 15 and then became the lead for the Supply Chain Task Force on March 18. He was one of the heroes in the national response, planning for the acquisition and distribution of supplies like PPE to every single nursing home and hospital in the United States. His team developed the overall strategy for a twenty-first-century SNS and implemented it on the fly. He and I became incredibly close colleagues over the next months. Admiral P, like most officers in the armed forces, had never heard of the USPHS Commissioned Corps. He later admitted to me that the first thing he thought when he saw us was, "Who are these people, and why are they wearing US Navy uniforms?"

On Friday night (March 13), I asked a very naive question, the answer to which actually made crystal clear the nation's unpreparedness for our testing initiative. That question was "How many swabs do we have in the SNS?" There was silence because there were none.

Diagnostics seemed to be an afterthought in the decades of planning leading up to the COVID-19 pandemic. Sure, BARDA had funded some new technologies for diagnosing influenza. But there were no supplies in the SNS—no swabs, no media, no laboratory reagents, no test tubes, "no nothing." We had no formal ties to the diagnostics industry, nor did we understand the supply chains even at a superficial level. No exercises had been conducted by any administration to help us understand the issues with distribution, uptake, and the long-standing biases and inflexibility among many laboratory elites ("lab snobs," we called them).

There was no national testing strategy beyond the CDC developing a test and providing those incomplete kits to public health labs. To further complicate matters as previously discussed, when the public health emergency was declared, the FDA tightened control over LDTs, which stopped local testing in its tracks for at least a month—the lost month of February.

Even the most recent FEMA-HHS federal leadership structure (dated March 13) had no task forces or working groups related to testing. This changed abruptly: by March 20, there was a task force dedicated to community-based testing and another task force focused on laboratory diagnostics, all reporting to the FEMA Unified Coordination Group (UCG). In the end, two of the six task forces were all about testing and staffed mainly by personnel from my office, OASH.

Since there were no swabs or transport media in the SNS, I asked Rachel Baitel and her volunteers to get on the phone, write emails, and do whatever else it took to find out where we could find a supply of swabs and transport media for our CBTSs. I did not know how many we needed, so I suggested one hundred thousand to start. Remember, one hundred thousand was about five times the number of tests that had been done to date cumulatively in the United States, so it was an aggressive ask. But on first look, there appeared to be at least a dozen suppliers of the exact swab that we needed, so I was cautiously optimistic. Later that week, Jared told me to get "one billion swabs"— and actually, by the end of our term, that turned out to be very close to the actual number we acquired.

On Saturday morning, Rachel had some bad news—awful, actually. All the so-called suppliers were really not suppliers at all but were repackagers of swabs made in one of two places: a company named Copan in Italy, which would soon be under national lockdown, with no supplies able to leave the country, or a small family-run business named Puritan in Maine that none of us had ever heard of. We needed to get to both of them ASAP.

To solve the immediate problem, Rachel and Eric had scoured all major health-care distributors for any available swabs and media that had already been procured and packaged from Copan or Puritan. They were able to source two hundred thousand swab kits (with media) from the company BD— amazing! They were also able to source additional swabs and media from Thermo Fisher. I was surprised that these supplies were available given what

I had been hearing about shortages throughout the country and from the CDC, but nonetheless, these supplies were indeed available. We bought all of them. *We literally bought everything we could get our hands on.*

But that was just the start—we were only going to get so far with the supplies from BD and Thermo Fisher. So Rachel was able to get me the phone number for Timothy Templet, the co-owner and executive vice president (EVP) at Puritan. He was alerted that I was going to give him a call, which I did on Saturday evening.

The EVP of a small family business in Maine was not generally accustomed to getting a call from an admiral in Washington, DC, stating that the United States was counting on his family business for its survival. I asked to purchase one hundred thousand swabs immediately and then a large percentage of his overall production indefinitely. He said that one hundred thousand was impossible, but we scheduled a follow-up call for Sunday morning. Between Saturday night and Sunday morning, Timothy found a way to make it happen, so we at least had one hundred thousand swabs from Puritan and a handshake for an unspecified future amount. Within a few months, we would invest nearly $300 million into Puritan to dramatically increase their production of several types of swabs, but that was much later in the story.

Honestly, I did not know anything about the Defense Production Act (DPA) at that point. It would have been possible, as I learned later, that after a few layers of approval by the White House, I could have instantaneously diverted Puritan's entire supply directly to our needs without their consent. But on March 14, everything was accomplished collaboratively with companies, including Puritan. The leaders of US industry were highly motivated to help—we did not need to force them. Their only reservation was a concern about losing their ordinary core customers to foreign manufacturers like those in China.

I understood that the nation still needed swabs to test people for strep throat and sexually transmitted diseases. But our team was not so concerned about these needs that weekend because the sky was falling. We knew what viral transmission and an exponentially growing number of cases looked like; we saw the future, and it was ugly. Another concern was that we did not want to parasitize the limited supply of swabs and media that was already destined for hospitals for COVID-19 testing—especially in hard-hit areas. CBTSs were never supposed to substitute for testing by the vast system of laboratories in hospitals and clinics; rather, they were meant to supplement and fill an acute need, especially for testing health-care workers, first responders, and the symptomatic elderly.

As for the only other supplier of swabs, Copan, thanks to Jared and the Department of Defense, I was also able to send a military airlift directly to Italy to rescue a shipment of swabs that might never have made it to the United States, since Italy was closing its borders. We took a percentage of that supply for the CBTSs but allowed the majority to flow through the US market for hospitals and public health agencies that were also in dire need of these supplies. We also ensured that Quest and LabCorp—our initial large laboratory commercial partners—had at least two hundred thousand swab-and-media packs to use to start up our CBTSs.

It was a good lesson for me—if I needed to send a US Air Force Boeing C-17 to Italy to pick up swabs, the Department of Defense would make that happen. There were no questions, weeks of deliberation, or advisory committees—just action. And that is what we needed: immediate *action*. That was not the way it happened in agencies like the CDC prior to this time. I thank God every day for our armed military (as well as the unarmed USPHS Commissioned Corps) and for the decades of investment that allowed uniformed services to do their jobs in times of crisis—whether eliminating terrorists, saving lives following hurricanes, or now getting supplies for us during COVID-19.

It would take us four more weeks to understand the status of every single swab in the United States, divert supplies from less important testing needs, invest in expansion, and ultimately be able to supply every state's request for swabs and media based on their projected needs. Yes, we did that, but you would never know it by watching the media or listening to political critics of the Trump administration.

LABORATORY TESTING FOR CBTSs

I had just met the CEOs of LabCorp and Quest one day earlier at the White House. For CBTSs to work, we could not rely on the CDC—because they did not have the scale required or the wraparound logistics and reporting that the large commercial labs had. We also could not rely on public health labs, which were generally small, focused on state priorities, and desperately in need of staffing and supplies. Moreover, we wanted the public health labs to focus on outbreaks in their own local areas, like at meat packing plants or nursing homes. We could not divert their resources to the CBTS program.

So I called the CEOs of Quest and LabCorp. Both labs were massive on a nationwide scale, with logistics (trucks and jets) and information systems that made the governmental public health infrastructure, including the CDC, pale in comparison. Both Quest and LabCorp were performing COVID tests following the recent FDA authorizations, and both labs were prepared to meet whatever scale we needed them to meet. With the recent EUAs for Roche and Thermo Fisher, there would be 1.9 million lab tests entering the market the following week. We knew LabCorp and Quest were going to be good for swabs and media (we just ordered those for them), so we directly allocated 200,000 of the 1.9 million tests to LabCorp and Quest as well. No DPA—just collaboration with the commercial sector.

We did not overthink easy decisions. For example, we decided that samples from half the CBTSs would be sent to LabCorp and half to Quest. If one lab had a failure or could not keep up with demand, we would pivot to the other lab or potentially add large commercial lab capacity as they came online. There was no time to nitpick and make everything perfect. My team had a good understanding of what was needed, and we had HHS lawyers in the office right next to the contracting officers to handle the legal questions. But to be sure, we made most of these initial arrangements through virtual "handshakes." The contractors trusted that we would eventually paper the deals and be fair to all involved. I certainly hoped we would not be the subject of a politically motivated witch hunt in the future, but that was a risk. The lawyers and contracting officers had a lot of cleaning up to do, but in the end, it did all work out. And I should note that *none* of the private-sector volunteers had anything to do with contracting or selecting our partners. Nobody crossed that line, to my knowledge, ever.

IT'S ALL ABOUT THE PATIENT

While finding sites and obtaining swabs were essential, the patient-facing side of CBTSs was for me the most important part of the process. It would also be the most visible to the public, and that was important to inspire confidence in the new system. From the start, I had two overriding questions and asked them constantly:

1. How do we keep staff and uninfected patients safe from becoming accidentally infected during a drive-through visit due to aerosols or infected waste?
2. What can we do to improve the patient experience and make it as stress-free and easy as possible given the circumstances?

There were a handful of drive-through test sites already popping up in a few states. However, these were low throughput and developed only for a specific local need. I applauded these efforts because there was no federal play-book, and local authorities and organizations were trying to improvise the best they could. Some states, like Utah, were really on the ball with a robust plan for the rapid expansion of sites.

At the time, South Korea was the obvious world leader. We reviewed everything we could related to their system—diagrams, news articles, web-sites, and so on—and I called several US representatives on station in Korea, including CDC staff assigned to the Korean CDC. South Korea had the idea for low-contact testing sites in late February and by the first week of March had a nationwide program. Many aspects of their sites were appropriate, and we adopted all the best practices, but we decided against many of their pro-cedures as well. For example, Korea placed one or two medical doctors at each site, which was not practical or needed in the United States, and the Korean sites were relatively low throughput, perhaps a hundred patients per day, compared to what we needed. Also, only a single patient could be in the car—which would not work for the United States, especially given our con-cern for the elderly and family units that might all be sick or exposed. Korea also had a web-based reservation system, and we knew that was not possible to have here in the short term.[9] Finally, South Korea had the geographic area of Indiana, with highly concentrated population centers, so the United States had a much larger scaling problem than Korea could ever imagine.

Fortunately, I believed (and still do) that I had the best resources on the planet to innovate a US drive-through model: the FEMA staff, who under-stood how to implement a POD concept, and USPHS Commissioned Corps officers—environmental health officers, doctors, nurses, nurse practitioners, engineers, and service access specialists—to get the science and medicine correct. Perhaps most importantly, I was able to call in the team that had recently returned from the *Diamond Princess* in Japan as well as teams previ-ously deployed to the repatriation sites at military bases. They could adapt the testing processes and personnel safety strategies from those missions to this new high-throughput testing scenario—and that is exactly what they did.

Among the USPHS leaders I brought to my office that weekend were Rear Admiral Trent-Adams, my principal deputy; Rear Admiral Schwartz, the deputy surgeon general of the United States; Rear Admiral Orsega, direc-tor of the Commissioned Corps Headquarters; and Capt. Cedrick Guyton (now Rear Admiral Guyton), the deputy director of HQ. Admirals Trent-Adams and Orsega immediately rostered the officers we needed and had them join our group, including Lt. Cmdr. Brian Czarnecki—definitely a go-to guy in the early process development. Czarnecki is an industrial hygienist and had been deployed in early February to Miramar Marine Corps Air Station in San Diego, where he received and assisted in the quarantining and testing of hundreds of Americans repatriated from Wuhan. Almost immediately after that mission, he deployed to Japan to assist in the testing and evacuation of the Americans on the *Diamond Princess* and also performed the swabbing of US responders on that mission.[10]

Major Tiffany Bilderback (now a lieutenant colonel) also deserves special mention. She was a US Army medical operations officer who was on detail from the US Army surgeon general to the ASPR. On her first day at the ASPR, she was assigned to assist Rear Admiral Schwartz, and so by the grace of God, we inherited her. Interestingly, she did not wear a uniform during her assignment because the ASPR believed that if people saw her with "only" the rank of major, she would not be taken as seriously as she needed to be taken. That would not have mattered in our very flat testing organization, but that is the way it was. I later learned that she had the call sign "MBA," which I thought was odd given the fact she did not have a "master of business administration." I later learned that MBA stood for "major badass," a nickname that she earned both on my team and from her earlier exploits in the war zone in Iraq.

Within the first day, the process team had outlined a feasible flow that could work under the principles of a FEMA POD system. The drive-through sites would have three primary stations:

1. Patient assessment and verification of eligibility for testing
2. Patient registration
3. Swabbing

The team developed specific procedures and roles for each station. For example, the swabbing station had five roles: a primary swabber, a decontamination staffer, a secondary swabber, a quality control staffer, and a runner.

Everything looked appropriate on paper, but we did not know if it would *actually* work. So we implemented a full-scale mock site in a parking lot in Maryland on Monday, just before we would "go live" at multiple sites throughout the country. We wanted to conduct this "under the radar" to avoid a media debacle, which was important for our effectiveness but also for the White House.

We fielded mock patients and injected as many problems as we could think of. We even had a drone fly over and monitor flow and safety, and the videotape was analyzed by our experts looking for ways to improve our processes even before we saw the first patient. We learned many lessons. For example, people flow could slow down dramatically if all the components were not working quickly and in sync, and there was a real risk of cross-contamination of patients and staff. So we added more personnel and additional layers of control to mitigate these risks. We also emphasized the importance of having a dedicated safety officer at each site, which we subsequently required as part of the program.

WE DON'T HAVE ENOUGH PPE
TO FULLY IMPLEMENT TESTING

Deciding what type of PPE to employ, who needed to wear it, and how frequently it would be changed was a very big decision at the time. The person leading this discussion and ultimate decision was R. Adm. Estella Jones, a veterinarian trained at Tuskegee and then Louisiana State University, who had been at the FDA for a decade. I had learned from Ebola in Texas and from the reports on the evacuation of Americans from China and Japan that the CDC was not reliable for operational matters—especially the appropriate use of PPE. I trusted Rear Admiral Jones, and she did not disappoint me.

She weighed the benefits and drawbacks of various protective layers of PPE, the use of powered air-purifying respirators (a system that uses a mechanical fan to deliver air in a hood), Tyvek suits (space suits), and other considerations. Eventually, she settled on a PPE regimen that included N95 masks for those in close contact with patients. Her team developed detailed protocols, and we designed swabbing and registration processes to minimize the number of people requiring PPE. For example, we would not have patients fill out their own forms because the pen and paper and clipboard would all be potentially contaminated and require even our administrative people to wear PPE.

The procedures and decisions were, in retrospect, exactly correct, but we had a very troubling realization on that Saturday. We were contemplating thirty to forty sites. Based on the calculated maximum throughput at these sites, *we would exhaust 80 percent of the strategic national stockpile (SNS) of PPE just on community-based testing within four weeks.* There was considerable interest by Dr. Birx in doing as much testing as possible and exhausting the stockpile if needed, but I decided that we would not take all the PPE from hospital personnel for the benefit of community testing sites. So we had to limit the testing done per day at each site, not because of a shortage of tests, but because of a shortage of PPE. A big part of the nation's "testing problem" was actually a PPE problem. Fortunately, an entire multiagency task force was focused on solving the nation's PPE issues, but it was going to take some time.

This was an example of the trade-offs that needed to be made given the extreme scarcity of resources at the time. There was no way to beat the shortages early in the pandemic, so we dealt with them the best way that we could in order to save the most lives and protect our health-care workers. Indeed, first responders, the elderly, and health-care workers were the only focus of our first drive-through sites. If our health-care workers got sick, there would be no one to care for everyone else—and that is a scenario that would have had profound and long-lasting implications for our nation.

NOT SO FAR UP THE NOSE . . .

As I stated many times in press conferences, on national media, and before Congress, we were never going *to test our way out of the pandemic.* That was clear early on and even clearer by the summer of 2020. COVID had been spreading silently in dozens of US cities long before the first patient was formally identified, and the asymptomatic spread made it impossible to do the type of contact tracing that would have been straightforward with a universally symptomatic illness like Ebola.

Nonetheless, we needed to expedite and expand testing—no question—even if it were only for symptomatic people and health-care workers. I was confident that there would be millions more lab kits, but the process for specimen collection and the labor and supplies that were needed were already becoming a rate-limiting step. It was obvious where we needed to go, but we did not have the data or the regulatory urgency to make it happen. It was my job to fix that.

The nasopharyngeal swab was uncomfortable for the patient. People described it as going halfway into your brain (which it doesn't but just feels that way), and even Trump remarked on how uncomfortable it was.[11] Using nasopharyngeal swabs imposed tremendous limitations on the system. First, collection by a health-care worker meant relatively low throughput at the sites, compared with a supervised self-collection process. But there was no way (and still isn't) for a patient to appropriately perform a nasopharyngeal swab. Second, collection by a health-care worker meant an unsustainable consumption of PPE because PPE needed to be completely changed after each swabbing by a provider. Third, nasopharyngeal swabs were so uncomfortable that the procedure could deter individuals from being tested. And finally, we were going to need all our trained health providers to care for people who were sick, not sticking swabs up people's noses in parking lots.

The solution was obvious—we needed a way for individuals to self-swab, which implied swabbing only the tip of the nose (anterior nares) and not performing nasopharyngeal swabs. But we did not have the data to know whether the anterior nares actually harbored the COVID-19 virus or as much virus as the nasopharynx did. So we immediately started collaborating with industry experts, the private sector, and academia to get the data we needed as soon as possible to support (or not) anterior nares collection. We scienced the hell out of this problem.

The FDA understood our needs immediately and let us know what they needed in order to authorize the use of self-collected tip-of-the-nose swabs. Companies like Roche and Thermo Fisher worked diligently to provide new data using anterior nasal swabs on their platforms. In the end, the data that were ultimately compelling to the FDA and to me were supplied by research-ers at the University of Washington and UnitedHealth Group, who provided their preliminary data to support FDA decision-making well in advance of publishing their work. I am eternally grateful to those teams for doing the work and collaborating with the FDA and me; their work changed the entire trajectory of testing for our nation.

On March 23, the push paid off. The FDA updated its guidance to state that for symptomatic patients, nasal swabs could be used that access just the front of the nose rather than the depth of the nasal cavity. This provided COVID-19 testing that was more comfortable for patients, allowed self-collection of spec-imens at sites (and eventually at home), and was performed with a simpler and more readily available swab.[12] This statement immediately changed the CBTS process only two weeks after the program had begun. It remained our process for the remainder of the pandemic and enabled innovations like home testing.

THE VICE PRESIDENT MAKES A VISIT

We were working furiously on Saturday to develop and implement a nation-wide system of CBTSs. I don't remember who delivered the message that Saturday morning, but I was told that Pence was coming to my office for a briefing. Say what? I knew that it was true because Secret Service agents started pouring into my office suite, which was already a train wreck from people working so feverishly, with papers posted on most of the walls and empty pizza boxes and Diet Coke cans pretty much everywhere. We spent a little time cleaning up, but not much.

I cannot tell you what a major event it is to have the vice president of the United States visit anywhere, much less the office of an assistant secretary on a Saturday afternoon, with about seventy-five of my new "closest friends" working on this project—many of them volunteers from the private sector who had just arrived from all over the country. In other circumstances, we might have been more worked up about the visit—but this was not ceremonial. It was a work visit. Pence needed information, but he did not want to interrupt our work by having us come to the White House; he knew that every minute mattered. So Pence came to us, and I would later understand the type of empathy and humility that was a defining characteristic of the vice president. He was very Midwestern in his courtesy and respect for others, and it didn't really matter to him that he was the second most powerful person on the planet.

The vice president was accompanied by Jared and Deb. Naturally, Azar and his deputy chief of staff, Paul Mango, were also in attendance, as were staff from White House Communications and Intergovernmental Affairs, who were also working closely with our team. Pence sat at the head of the table in my conference room, where I normally would have sat and led meetings with anyone else except the VP! The room was filled with USPHS officers, FEMA and ASPR operational staff, and private-sector volunteers—including my wife, who was also working around the clock with the communications team. She is a great writer and editor, and we needed to make sure the public-facing materials were crystal clear and understandable. There was no room for confusing technical phrases or CDC double-speak.

I led the briefing to Pence. I explained our strategy and approach, utilizing the FEMA regional network and integrating the FEMA POD concept with the USPHS practical pandemic experience. Brad talked about the operational challenges and the pace that was going to be required. Brad later stated that creating a nationwide CBTS program when there was nothing in place prior "turned out to be pretty hard." Yes, I agree with that!

We stated that we were going to have a mock site on Monday and that we could have at least "some" of the CBTSs up and running in a few days. There were many execution risks and substantial challenges in nearly every state—from concerns at the governor level to tactical concerns about traffic and security. But we were confident that these issues would be worked out. We did not have all the answers, but we felt increasingly confident that we were now asking the right questions.

Pence was pleased. The team was going to be able to provide, as he had promised for Sunday night, a way forward for testing—even if we did not have a website to provide internet-based screening or test results. We did not have a comprehensive national strategy yet, nor would CBTSs stop the pandemic in its tracks. But our sites would represent a significant contribution to the ongoing fight and make a meaningful impact on testing for health-care providers and the elderly.

More importantly, I felt like we were finally on the offensive against COVID-19, and the White House was providing the leadership and resources in a way that it had not done previously for COVID or honestly had ever done even for Ebola or H1N1 in previous administrations. It was hard to tell what Jared and Deb were thinking. Jared had that worried look on his face that he frequently had, but his "pickup game" of people who "get shit done" was working. The private-sector volunteers were smart, extremely driven, and highly effective. They were essential.

Jared was determined for our group to succeed, and therefore he committed to getting rid of any barriers that we would face—whatever they were. I believed him. And he did exactly that, even if in a nontraditional way. The media reported that Jared had a "shadow task force" that was not integrated with traditional government efforts and did not have any oversight; that was 100 percent wrong. All the volunteers working on testing directly reported to both Brad and me, and we had contracting officers and lawyers integrated into the efforts, literally in the same room. The attempt to imply this was some sort of sinister effort by Jared, I believe, was just another part of the ongoing

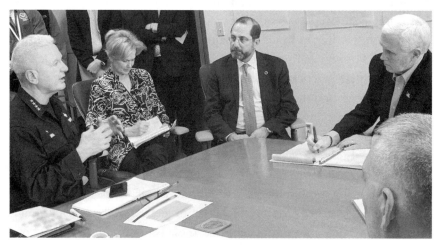

Impromptu Saturday visit by Vice President Pence to Admiral Giroir's office for briefing on drive-through testing sites, March 14, 2020 (personal photo).

media campaign to discredit anything to do with the Trump administration. For many weeks, Jared would call me sometimes multiple times per day to handle issues regarding ventilators or testing or really any need that had to be handled from a medical or scientific point of view. I am certain he did the same with Brad on the supply and operational side.

PUTTING IT ALL TOGETHER

March 15: 2,930 new cases, 21 new deaths.

Two days earlier, Pence told the American people that they would be able to go to a retailer near their homes to get tested, and also, he stated that there would be a website to provide information on whether a test was indicated and then direct people to a nearby testing site. At 5 p.m. on Sunday, we would be updating the American people on our progress. And clearly, the aspirational comments two days earlier were not going to be completely fulfilled that night—or any time soon. But we had made tremendous progress and would be operational within days, so there was some good news—and I hoped the president would agree.

On Sunday, we had an 8:15 a.m. check-in from all the teams, some of whom worked all night. Jill wrote down the first thing I said to the group, which was obvious but needed to be emphasized nonetheless: "This is the critical day."

We had a good start, but there were an infinite number of details to work out. Each working group had its own conference room in my suite, and we only needed to walk across a hallway to coordinate and plan with one another. At 11 a.m., we had a call with CEOs from the private sector, many of whom had been in the Rose Garden with me on the Friday before. And then at noon, Brad conducted another all-group check-in. Brad led these check-ins with remarkable clarity and efficiency. Tasks and deliverables were updated every two to four hours and sometimes more frequently. Having all the members of the "start-up" in the same suite enabled the continuous evolution of our approach to work around new barriers or challenges.

By working through the FEMA regional reps and the White House Office of Intergovernmental Affairs, we estimated that there were only about thirty operational drive-through sites throughout the country—mostly low volume and with variable criteria, popped up spontaneously by local health systems or public health departments. Our new federal plan aimed to add forty additional sites in multiple cities in the next week.

Each of the sites would have two process lanes servicing twelve cars per lane per hour for twelve hours a day and seven days a week. If there were more than one eligible patient in the car, we would direct them to the multiple-passengers lane and test all eligible passengers as long as they were sitting by a window so they were accessible to the medical personnel outside the vehicle. Having a multiple-passenger lane assured there would be no log jams in the other lanes. That would have completely wrecked throughput. We learned that from our mock site and the drone footage.

Initially, we planned to offer testing only to health-care workers and first responders (with a work badge required as proof) and those sixty-five years or older with a temperature of 99.6 degrees or greater. We made the temperature requirement lower than the CDC standard because the elderly don't generally mount high fevers. Why did the CDC not know that? If you ever worked in a hospital or with the elderly, this was a no-brainer.

States had the option of implementing sites *only* for health-care workers and first responders if that was an urgent local need. Again, within what was scientifically justified and capable given limited resources, we needed the states to tell us *their* priorities so we could help them meet their needs. Washington State was not New York, and neither was Texas or Louisiana. As it turned out, many states focused just on health-care workers for the first two to three days to assure continued staffing for their local hospitals and emergency rooms. Everyone meeting the criteria for CBTS screening was tested at no cost, regardless of whether they had health insurance coverage. I don't actually think we had the budget for that at the time, but we just did it and figured the financing out later.

We supplied each CBTS with the full array of PPE, swabs, and transport media, and we deployed a customized team of USPHS officers to provide leadership and ensure safety. For state-run sites, there would be three officers per site: a commanding officer, a safety officer, and an information technology / quality control officer. Retail sites, which required much more top-down organization and hand-holding at first, were fully staffed by USPHS officers until the retailers could learn the process. That meant fifteen to twenty officers per site. Each site had standard registration, process flow, shipping, and instructional materials for patients before and after testing. These materials were developed by the communications team working in my office and approved by me personally. I had a lot of patient care experience and reviewed every word on every document to make sure the information was clear and actionable for every segment of the US population.

We provided a handout with clear instructions to wear a mask if you were sick (that was the guideline from the CDC at the time—mask only the sick), to isolate the entire family if there was a positive test, and of when to seek (and not to seek) medical care, including when to call 911 for an emergency. We also emphasized that a *negative test* only meant that the person was not infected *at that time* but could have been exposed and test positive anytime thereafter, even one day later. How many times did I repeat that concept over the next eleven months?

After collecting, labeling, and bagging specimens at the test site, the site team express-mailed batches to either LabCorp or Quest. The labs would perform the test and transmit the results to the state public health lab within two to three days. The state public health lab would flow the results to the CDC through a preexisting but very clunky public health test result network. It was already in place, so we used it.

The issue remained, however, of how to get the results back to the patients. We would not have a website, that's for sure. Our volunteers were working on this problem. They contacted a major call center, Maxim Healthcare Services, which we ultimately contracted to directly call the patients and inform them of the test results. If there was no answer to the first call, the call center would call back twice more. We thought this was outstanding service and provided a patient experience as good as—or even better than—most private health systems. The call would also include scripted instructions about how to interpret the result and what to do if the patient was positive or negative. This worked out extremely well with few exceptions. Not bad for forty-eight hours of planning!

Maxim informed us that there would need to be an ordering physician so that they could legally provide the results back to the patient. This initially caused us real concern. How would we get local physicians to provide orders and be responsible for the test sites—and do this within forty-eight hours?

To take that issue off the table, I told the team that I would personally be the ordering physician. Rear Admiral Schwartz—a medical doctor, engineer, public health specialist, and lawyer—interrupted and said respectfully but in no uncertain terms, "Sir, I can't let you do that." I was the assistant secretary and might become more involved in the response at a political level in addition to the medical level. And we could not risk any confusion about patient care being influenced by politics. I agreed. So she volunteered to personally take the responsibility for the entire nation. Thus, Rear Admiral Schwartz became the physician responsible for ordering millions of tests across the country—undoubtedly the highest number of tests ordered by *any* single physician in the United States, if not the world.

For the sites already being operated by states but not formally part of the CBTS program, we decided to ship them PPE, swabs, and media. For CBTSs, there would be no flexibility in the materials, processes, or labs that were used. Flexibility would be fine at a later time, but not now. "Cookie cutter" was the quickest way forward to entail the least risk of failure—so that is how we proceeded.

The website was another issue. The idea of compiling a national database of testing sites was daunting—actually, it was impossible. In addition to CBTSs, there were state drive-through sites of different quality and with various eligibility criteria for testing. There were also health-care system sites, including walk-up sites, and testing in hospitals, emergency rooms, urgent care centers, and physician offices. But there was no source for this information! The CDC did not have it, nor did the CMS or anyone else. Without the information, updated daily, we could not inform patients where to go for a test and certainly could not schedule them at a national level.

In addition, I was personally concerned that we could inadvertently list sites with poor-quality testing or risky practices. If that happened, the federal government would be indirectly endorsing poor patient care. Furthermore, if people registered on the web, there would be privacy concerns since we would almost certainly not be compliant with health privacy regulations in the near term.

We had a great team trying to implement a website, but it was not going to happen, even though it had been promised by the president and vice president in the Rose Garden. I have no idea what Google said they were going to do because that interaction was directly handled by staff in the White House. Brad had a top team assigned to the digital front end, but it was an impossible task, and we dropped that work stream.

For me, I was certain that the information about testing sites would get out locally (as it clearly did) and that there was no urgent need for a US government national compilation of sites in a master federal database that would be outdated the moment it was created. Moreover, I was sure that even without a digital front end, we could double or triple national testing within a week. And that is what mattered. We were going to be limited by swabs and people, not electrons over the web.

We did have a way forward, though, for a screening tool to inform people whether they should be tested. Sumbul Desai, vice president of health at Apple, who had previously had a distinguished academic career at Stanford, called me on Saturday night to ask if Apple could help. That call was out of the blue and unexpected. Sumbul was a serious player and had the support of Jeff Williams, the Apple COO, who was also on that initial call.

For that first call, I invited Dr. Heidi Overton, a young surgical resident who was doing a stint as a White House fellow (an incredibly competitive position), to participate. She was working on various aspects of CBTSs, especially patient communications. On that call, in real time, the Apple team, Heidi, and I decided to codevelop a COVID-19 screening tool and place that tool on a cobranded website and in an Apple-developed app.

Heidi co-led the project with Sumbul, and we added two subject matter experts from the CDC who originally were hesitant but soon became enthusiastic. The tool walked users through a set of questions regarding symptoms, risk factors, and potential exposures and provided recommendations for the next steps, including if testing was recommended and whether to seek medical attention based on the input each user provided. Heidi, the CDC, and I developed the content for the algorithms, which I officially approved on behalf of the US government. Apple focused on the technical side, the user experience, and the details of every decision point. They were disciplined and acted rapidly.

We decided that the website would be cobranded by Apple, FEMA, the CDC, and the White House and that the underlying algorithm for decision-making would be made public—available for use by any other developers who wanted to copy our work. Apple did this for the greater good. They were unwilling to take any credit besides their logo on the site. The HHS-Apple team continued meeting every two weeks in order to update the algorithm and recommendations, which Apple translated into new versions of the website and app.

Remarkably, the testing decision tree and recommendations were developed and approved, and the website and app were launched on March 27, less than two weeks after our initial meeting. By July 12, 2020, fifteen weeks from the launch of the tool, the website had 7 million cumulative visits, and the iOS app had 2.5 million downloads.

Of historical note, Google apparently jettisoned the highly promoted website project immediately after Pence's March 13 announcement, but Google came back a few weeks later to develop a Google-built website on the White House coronavirus page. Google used the logic that the HHS-Apple team built and already implemented. Google never talked to me, not even once. Apple deserves great credit for their selfless efforts, and hopefully they got a thank-you card from Google that holiday season. Apple, like many US companies and individual citizens, wanted to do everything they could to support the national effort to combat the pandemic and save lives.

SUNDAY PRIME TIME

There are a few moments in my three years in Washington, DC, that I will never forget, and the Sunday press conference with Trump, Pence, and my uniformed colleagues was one of them. Pence wanted to recognize some of the officers who had actually done the work to create the program he had promised and to use them (us) to highlight the already important work of the USPHS officers in repatriating Americans, providing border screening, and caring for the elderly at the Kirkland Life Care Center in Washington State. Pence was always willing to recognize others and give them credit when they deserved it; even on this critical day, he was true to his character.

I was at Trump's immediate right; Deb was on his left. Eight of my fellow officers were also on stage, crowded on the podium, in ODUs. Those blue ODUs soon became familiar to most Americans and certainly to those who lived in the places where we were deployed, everywhere from Kirkland to the Javits Center and from Puerto Rico to Alaska. Secretaries Azar and Wolf were also on stage, as well as Tony Fauci and Adam Boehler.

The president opened with comments about the Federal Reserve and interest rates, which he had just learned about before taking the short walk from the Oval Office to the press room. In addition to controlling the virus, access to money was very important to Americans for good reason. He then made a brief remark about Google and frustratedly tossed a note in the air—I am still not sure what the note said or what had happened with Google. But there had clearly been some misunderstanding about what Google was doing. Alphabet, the parent company of Google, was indeed working on a project to assist in triaging people for testing, but this was in the very early stages and only intended for San Francisco. Someone put Trump and Pence out on a limb two days before, and that misunderstanding and overpromise dogged the White House for weeks.

Food security was also a major concern on that day—Trump had a call with the CEOs of major grocery chains and food suppliers earlier that afternoon, and the CEOs were committed to keeping their stores stocked and Americans fed. They would remain open for business, but perhaps with shorter hours in order to provide extra cleaning and sanitation. It was bad enough to have a pandemic virus on our shores, but Americans would not have handled empty shelves at the grocery store. We were very worried about panic, which would be counterproductive in every way. Trump urged Americans to buy what they *needed* but not *more than they needed*. This was a very good message, and I think it calmed down many worried families and communities that night.

Then the president of the United States thanked my USPHS officers for working around the clock and doing "an incredible job." Two years earlier, almost to the day, the OMB proposed to dissolve the USPHS Commissioned Corps after 130 years in uniform. At HHS, we fought this to the death—Azar, the surgeon general, myself, and many behind the scenes like Jen Moughalian, the chief financial officer at HHS. When the OMB realized they could not just eliminate us entirely, they decided to downsize us by half. We had no money for training, despite dozens of briefings to twenty-something-year-old OMB examiners. I personally briefed them and brought all my senior officers, including the surgeon general, but it didn't matter.

In just the two years I had been in uniform to that point, our officers deployed to several hurricanes, earthquakes, and wildfires. We deployed with DEA agents to communities across the country to assure that those patients dependent on opioids would receive appropriate addiction care after the DEA took down their "pill mills." We deployed to the southern border and solved a potentially disastrous spread of measles, influenza, and meningitis among unaccompanied children and family units. Then my officers led the mission to review every single record of every single immigrant child in order to reunite children who had been separated from their parents (or adults claiming to be their parents) by the Department of Justice. And now we were fully engaged in combatting the pandemic and on stage with the president of the United States. By the way, the OMB still would not give us a penny for training or equipping, even during the pandemic, and persisted in trying to dissolve us indirectly by requiring unachievable fiscal limitations on retirement. I don't blame the president, who was probably unaware of these facts, but I do blame many in the OMB, career and political, and a few individuals on the Domestic Policy Council who were the OMB puppet masters at the time.

At the press conference, Trump clearly acknowledged that COVID-19 was a very contagious virus and that elderly or chronically ill people were in significant danger. I was pleased that he said all the right things with an appropriate tone of concern. Then Trump left the stage to "make some calls" and turned it over to Pence. When Trump turned to leave the podium, the media went crazy yelling questions—but Trump left nonetheless.

Later in the pandemic, this is what the doctors on the task force wanted to happen at every press event. We advocated that Trump should make opening remarks and define major policy initiatives but then leave the podium so that questions could be directed to the VP, Birx, Fauci, myself, and any other significant figures on the day. Instead—and this was both an incredible virtue and a flaw—Trump rarely did that. He would remain on stage for an hour or more and answer whatever questions were asked by the media. He would also riff freely on whatever was briefed to him on that day—even a few minutes before—thus the comments (which were mostly misconstrued) about bleach and disinfectants, which the media immediately seized upon.

As I helped prepare Pence for his remarks at the press conference, it was very unclear to me whether he actually comprehended the public health messages we were telling him. His notepad looked like a multicolored treasure map from the latest adventure movie, with arrows and lines and scribbles all over. I remember thinking that the Sunday briefing would be a nightmare because there was no way that messy sheet of paper could translate into a cogent message. But it wasn't a disaster, and it would never be—at least from the Pence communication point of view. Pence heard everything we said, understood it, and simplified it to core take-home messages that the American people could grasp and hopefully believe and act on. He delivered the science as we briefed him, accurately and without stumbling on a single word. But his notes remained epic in their convolutions and color schemes! At least one should be in the National Archives.

That day, Pence was his typical serious, calm, and level-headed self. He emphasized the danger to the elderly and other vulnerable groups and urged everyone to heed the CDC and doctors' advice. He stated that the overall risk to the American people who were healthy was low—and that is exactly what all the medical experts told him, including Fauci and Redfield. He thanked the governors as well as the American people for their efforts. He did this repeatedly throughout the pandemic, and I always appreciated that. We didn't need to give Americans free beer or lottery tickets, or go door-to-door, or coerce them into performing government-prescribed behaviors. We believed we needed to give Americans the best information available, transparently, and trust them to make the best decisions for themselves and their families. It is the people's country, after all, not the federal government's country.

And then Pence began speaking about testing. He stated correctly that testing was now available in all fifty states, that there was an emerging partnership with the private sector, and that we recently authorized new tests from Roche and Thermo Fisher. He stated what Birx must have told him—that

Roche and Thermo Fisher would make it possible to open up testing at thousands of sites. That was theoretically possible because of the widespread availability of Thermo Fisher equipment—but there were many other barriers aside from lab kits and machines that were still rate limiting. We had spent the entire weekend tackling those rate-limiting steps and would continue to do so for many months. Thousands of sites, at least in the near future, were an overpromise, and I became worried all over again.

Pence then reviewed our prioritization for the testing of health-care workers and the elderly and the reasons for that prioritization. He also made the important point, again, that testing would be available for those *who needed it*—namely, the symptomatic or those whose health-care providers assessed might be infected with COVID-19. We were not able to provide testing to "anybody that wants a test."

On that night, we did not fully appreciate the importance of asymptomatic spread, nor did we have enough testing capability to even contemplate testing asymptomatic individuals. Our messages were right, given our knowledge on that day and the resources we had available, but it was not where we wanted to be or needed to be with testing. I knew that. And Birx really knew that.

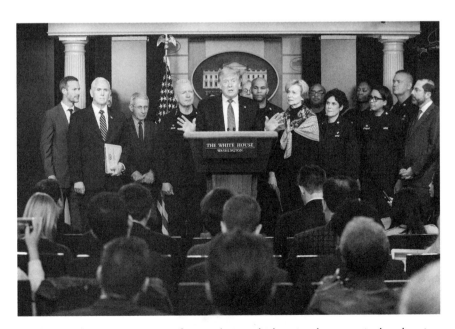

Sunday, March 15, 2020, press conference, during which national community-based testing sites program was announced and USPHS officers were acknowledged for their service (White House photo).

Pence thanked our team for our 24-7 work. He introduced me, and I thanked him. The brief notecard I wrote for myself started with principles that I wanted the American public to know. These were not written for me, nor were they talking points provided by White House communications. Both that night and throughout the pandemic, we doctors were able to write our own talking points and deliver them without prior editing or review. We typically wrote them in the few minutes we had to collect our thoughts after the task force meeting and briefing Trump, right before walking down that short hallway that led from the Oval Office to the press room.

The principles I outlined that evening were the following:

1. We were going to focus on the vulnerable as our priority for testing. This was important not only to preserve testing resources but also to again emphasize that the elderly and infirmed were at highest risk of severe illness and death.

2. Testing needed to be outside of the traditional health-care setting so as not to overrun emergency rooms with worried individuals and also to avoid the danger of bringing infected people into a setting where they could infect others who were vulnerable because of cancer or other diseases.

3. We needed to balance testing with other needs in the pandemic response. This was an indirect reference to our need to preserve PPE for doctors and nurses treating sick patients. I did not explain what dire straits we were in on the PPE front; perhaps I should have. But other teams were working on that issue.

I also emphasized, as I would do multiple times for the next months, that just having the lab kits was not enough. We needed mechanisms to collect samples (like community-based testing) as well as basic supplies like swabs, media, and extraction reagents.

We had indeed contacted all fifty states through FEMA. CBTSs would be able to screen two thousand to four thousand people per day per site. *Federally supported, state managed, and locally executed* was the mantra—many states needed everything; other states, like Texas, needed much less. Later in the pandemic, one state complained that we did not send them printers for their CBTSs—I let fly a few expletives, and that state figured out how to source printers for themselves.

Sites were scheduled to go live that week, and they did. I made the statement to the press, "This is not make-believe. This is not fantasy. We will have the capability of testing tens of thousands of people through the sites every week." Pence loved that line—I did not think it was that audacious, but given all the previous issues with CDC testing and the Google website that was not going to be available, I wanted Americans to believe me, and that phrase is what came out of my mouth spontaneously. We were shipping stuff in the morning around the country, and my officers were already deploying. Even Fauci said he was pleased and that we were entering a new phase of testing. But he reiterated, quite ominously but honestly, that the worst times remained ahead. And they certainly did.

Three days later, on March 18, the first CBTS opened; there were 6,114 new cases and 71 new deaths. An additional forty CBTSs opened within the next few days. On April 5, we changed the entire protocol from health-care worker nasopharyngeal swabbing to nasal self-swabbing under supervision. This expedited throughput, preserved precious PPE, and enabled the opening of entirely private-sector sites—as promised by Trump and Pence.

On April 5, we implemented our first CBTS 2.0 program, which was run entirely by retailers, under a flat-fee US government contract, with Rear Admiral Schwartz (the deputy surgeon general of the United States) still serving as the ordering physician. The 2.0 program would eventually expand to 2,800 testing sites in all fifty states, DC, and Puerto Rico, with two-thirds of these sites in zip codes of high social vulnerability. That meant we were reaching racial and ethnic minorities, immigrants, the homeless, and every other underserved group. We designed the system that way and were very proud that we executed it as planned. Perhaps we should have spoken more about our commitment to the underserved because the Biden administration has done nothing more than the Trump administration with regard to serving minorities and the underserved.

Two more versions of CBTSs (3.0 and 4.0) would follow the 2.0 implementation. Together with commercial partners, we did indeed develop and implement the most robust and advanced testing ecosystem anywhere in the world. You would never know that from listening to the media. After all, we were in the midst of a presidential campaign, and "anybody that wants a test" still could not get a test.

FEMA Full-Court Press

GETTING THE ORGANIZATION RIGHT

After President Trump's declaration of a national emergency on March 13, 2020, HHS continued to serve as the lead federal agency (LFA) according to the plan that existed for multiple administrations, including the Obama administration. But in retrospect, HHS did not have the scope, scale, command infrastructure, regional reach, experience, or operational processes to fight an escalating and lengthy war against this virus. The CDC had already demonstrated it had little actual operational capability or grasp of the overall national issues and trade-offs. The CDC's optimum role was to advise on narrow aspects of infection control, and even then, the CDC was challenged.

The Office of the ASPR was much more operationally minded, and Dr. Kadlec provided experienced and proactive leadership, but the organization within the Office of the ASPR was still relatively small and underresourced, and the staff—unlike their leader—tended to be insular. There was also substantial ongoing organizational tension between the CDC and the ASPR office, since the ASPR office recently assumed several traditional CDC functions including management of the SNS. And finally, although the Office of the ASPR was experienced in public health and medical services support (officially termed Emergency Service Function 8) during hurricanes and other temporary regional disasters, they were not built to lead a national emergency affecting every state, territory, and tribal nation simultaneously—especially one lasting for months or years.

In an unprecedented move and one of the most important decisions in the entire pandemic response, President Trump informed Pete Gaynor, the FEMA administrator, on March 18 that FEMA would be the LFA, and this decision was subsequently announced to the state governors and to the public on March 19. I am not sure if Trump made this decision or if Pence or members of the National Security Council advised him to. But it was made at the White House level—the only level such a decision could have been made.

On that same day, FEMA activated its NRCC (National Response Coordination Center) to Level 1 (the highest level of activation), and the UCG (Unified Coordination Group) was established on March 20 for the purpose of structured decision-making. Former DHS assistant secretary and then Harvard professor Juliette Kayyem nailed it in an interview that day when she remarked, "We have a saying in emergency management . . . go big or stay home."[1] And this move to FEMA was as big as the federal government could get. I personally breathed a big sigh of relief as soon as I understood what FEMA brought to the table—it was a true inflection point.

In retrospect, moving the lead to FEMA was 100 percent correct, but it was not completely obvious at the time. FEMA had never been the national lead for a public health emergency; that was always HHS's role. FEMA did not have the subject matter expertise inside its walls, nor had it ever led a mission of this magnitude that necessitated the national allocation of scarce resources and the overall coordination of global supply chains. FEMA was in the business of supplying whatever the states requested during an emergency—not adjudicating the legitimacy of those requests. But honestly, there was no other choice. FEMA had the NRCC, experienced incident managers like Josh Dozer, national scale, and known and well-rehearsed processes. Kadlec had the wisdom, in part gained from pandemic preparation exercises in 2019, to bring FEMA to the table in early February (and perhaps much earlier) as part of the interagency coordination strategy. As a result, representatives from FEMA had a good awareness of the situation and how it developed. And importantly, FEMA also had Pete Gaynor as its administrator.

Pete joined the US Marines after high school and then spent twenty-six years serving his country in uniform. He received his college and graduate education while in the US Marines and ultimately retired as a lieutenant colonel. He had various roles, including the head of Plans, Policy, and Operations at Headquarters Marine Corps during the September 11 attacks, and also experienced combat tours in the Middle East. Following his service in the US Marines, he returned to his home state of Rhode Island to assume various leadership roles in emergency management, ultimately serving as the director of the Rhode Island State Emergency Management Agency for three years. Pete was Senate confirmed as the deputy administrator of FEMA in October 2018 and became the acting administrator in March 2019 when his boss resigned. On January 14, 2020, Pete was officially confirmed by the Senate as the administrator and was sworn in two days later. I am sure he did not foresee the viral tsunami that he was walking into.

Although Pete was new in his role as the Senate-confirmed administrator, he did not show it. COVID-19 was a once-in-a-century event, but Pete had the skill set and, most of all, the frontline "chops" to lead the effort. We bonded immediately. Pete spoke with a heavy Rhode Island accent (which I learned to imitate almost perfectly) and had a naturally humble, friendly disposition. He knew what he knew and knew what he didn't know—he left his ego at the door. We needed that type of humility and service orientation at every level of the response and generally had it with few exceptions.

The UCG was the decision-making body at FEMA. Previously, a UCG was a structure implemented at the regional level after natural disasters; it included federal and state coordinating officials and other operational stakeholders. A UCG like this new one at FEMA, which included senior representatives from different cabinet departments, had never before been implemented but nonetheless still fit well into the National Incident Management System (the playbook for working together in an emergency). Everyone at the federal, state, and local levels knew this system, so we adapted what we knew, and it worked.

The Pandemic Crisis Action Plan (PanCAP) is the federal plan for pandemic responses—originally written in 2013, rewritten in 2018, and then revised again in the second week of March 2020. But the UCG and overall organization at FEMA evolved even more by the third week in March. Under the final structure, the UCG reported directly to the White House Coronavirus Task Force and was not separated by another administrative layer termed the Emergency Support Function Leadership Group as initially planned in the PanCAP. The final UCG not only consisted of CDC, ASPR, and FEMA leads but also included me as the assistant secretary for health (ASH). The task forces were realigned, and two new ones were added—the Laboratory Diagnostics Task Force and the Community-Based Testing Task Force, both led by my office (OASH) but composed of individuals from multiple agencies and technical backgrounds.

The CDC led only one task force, which dealt with community mitigation measures, making recommendations on issues like school attendance, masking, and social distancing. The Supply Chain Task Force was led by Admiral P and, under his leadership, developed all the tools necessary for end-to-end knowledge, growth, and management of the supply chain, including the use of the Defense Production Act. The Supply Chain Task Force formally included about 150 people, but these 150 were supplemented by another 100 or so acquisition professionals within the Department of Defense who rapidly wrote contracts and employed the Defense Production

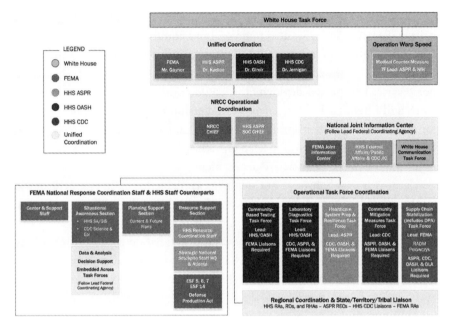

Organization of federal leadership for the COVID-19 response, March–July 2020: White House Coronavirus Task Force, FEMA Unified Coordination Group, and other task forces (figure from FEMA publication *Pandemic Response to Pandemic Coronavirus Disease 2019 (COVID-19): Initial Assessment Report*, January 2021).

Act. Each task force had experts from numerous departments and agencies, including the armed forces, FEMA, the CDC, the Office of the ASPR, the Defense Logistics Agency (DLA), the OASH, and others as necessary.

As testing coordinator, I drew on the resources I knew best—those within the USPHS Commissioned Corps and OASH. For the original development of the CBTSs during that long weekend in my office, I had tapped three outstanding leaders from the Commissioned Corps: Rear Admiral Trent-Adams, the principal deputy assistant secretary for health (PDASH); Rear Admiral Schwartz, the deputy surgeon general; and Rear Admiral Orsega, the director of Commissioned Corps Headquarters. Now I needed to designate one of these highly capable officers as the lead for the new FEMA task force responsible for scaling the fledgling community-based testing program.

I needed Rear Admiral Trent-Adams to lead OASH in my absence because I was officially deployed to the pandemic response, which was my only focus. Thus, I was forced to temporarily abandon my leadership role in programs that were also critical to public health, including Ending the HIV Epidemic in the US, the Dietary Guidelines for Americans, and numerous programs aimed at ending health disparities for racial and ethnic minorities.

Rear Admiral Orsega certainly could have led the CBTS program, and I believe she passionately wanted to do so, but I could not afford to let that happen to our officers. Orsega was the key to training and deploying the entire corps, and this pandemic was already the largest deployment in the history of our service. I suspected deployments would continue to increase in number, scale, and intensity. I also needed her leadership to provide support and care for our officers and their families, who were under tremendous stress, as well as force protection measures to keep our officers safe from COVID and all the other usual hazards of an active deployment.

Rear Admiral Schwartz not only was available for an assignment but in fact was the ideal person. Her impeccable leadership skills, brilliant mind, collegial nature, commitment to duty, and innate intellect were essential in this type of unprecedented national effort that depended on the smooth working collaboration among federal, state, local, and commercial stakeholders. She was a medical doctor with all the relevant expertise and training, a lawyer, and a public health specialist and had an undergraduate degree in engineering. Ultimately, I brought the three two-star rear admirals into a room and told them (as was later recounted to me by Rear Admiral Schwartz), "Heads up and pens down." Then I informed them how we were going to divide our workload to serve—and perhaps to save—the nation. Being the dedicated officers that they were, all three admirals took their marching orders and began carrying them out flawlessly.

The Laboratory Diagnostics Task Force did not yet have as clear of a mission as the CBTS Task Force. We were just getting started, and testing was still somewhat haphazard, but at least there was an early win with CBTSs implemented in cities across the country without any unforced errors. Trump critics said we had gone from an F to a C. I took that as a good sign.

Among the objectives we originally identified for the Laboratory Diagnostics Task Force were the identification, development, and securing of collection supplies and disposables (like pipette tips and test tubes), which had already posed huge challenges; incentivizing and allocating scarce laboratory diagnostic assays and eventually POC tests; filling in gaps in supplies, like extraction reagents; supporting and resupplying the public health laboratories, which had been left in a precarious position from FDA regulatory overreach and contaminated CDC tests; interfacing with large commercial and other diagnostic laboratories (thousands of them); collaborating with the FDA on the prioritization of test authorizations; communicating and dealing with requests from governors, mayors, state health officials, and other leaders; and responding to all the unforeseen challenges that would emerge as the pandemic evolved.

While I was personally accountable for high-consequence decisions and overall strategy, having an extraordinarily capable operational leader for this task force was "make or break" for the national testing program. Dr. Tammy Beckham was my choice. Tammy is a PhD scientist and a veterinarian. She started her career as a US Army officer, working in the high-level biocontainment laboratories at Fort Dietrich, and then became director of the Foreign Animal Disease Diagnostic Laboratory, a part of the US Department of Agriculture's Plum Island Animal Disease Center in New York.

I first met Tammy at Texas A&M, where she was director of animal infectious diseases and, more importantly, director of the Texas Veterinary Diagnostic Lab, where her team performed millions of tests on animals, many of which harbored diseases transmissible to humans (like avian influenza). During the Ebola outbreak in Texas, she assisted in the state response and personally cared for one of the victim's dogs that had been exposed to the Ebola virus. After Texas A&M, she moved on to be dean and professor in the Department of Diagnostic Medicine and Pathology at Kansas State College of Veterinary Medicine. She then wound up in the DC area leading the Cooperative Biological Engagement Program at the Defense Threat Reduction Agency (DTRA), meaning she was spending a lot of time supporting Central Command in dealing with chemical and biological weapons proliferation in the Middle East.

In 2018, to create synergies and eliminate silos, I planned to merge my National Vaccine Program Office with the Office of HIV/AIDS Policy, and I recruited Tammy to join OASH to make the merger happen. More importantly at the time, we were putting together the Ending the HIV Epidemic in the US initiative, later announced by President Trump during the 2019 State of the Union address, and I wanted her to lead it. Typical of the knee-jerk responses among Trump haters, I was criticized heavily by some individuals because I recruited a veterinarian to work on the problems of humans living with HIV—that sentiment faded rapidly as the HIV community came to know Tammy and understood our historic objectives.

Sure, Tammy had the technical skills as a true card-carrying laboratory professional who knew everything about zoonotic infections. She knew the instruments and the assays and could easily develop her own lab tests if she had to. But I wanted Tammy mostly because of her drive to achieve objectives and her absolute intolerance of mediocrity and indecision. She would butt heads many times with the CDC because of their slow responses and scattered decision-making and even more so with the OMB for their endless red tape and inexperienced staff, who regularly impeded nearly every request we made (at least until Russ Vought officially assumed the OMB leadership role in July 2020). I also knew that Tammy would take a bullet for me any day, but she knew I would never ask her to do that and that I had her back as well.

Everyone relocated to FEMA on March 19—and I do mean everyone, including all the members of HHS and the other agencies working on the response. Even though it was only two blocks away from HHS, I had no idea it was there until we relocated the operations. It was a short walk from my OASH office, past another HHS building and a McDonald's that always had several homeless people in front of the doors. I would frequently get coffee there in the morning and sometimes buy food for the homeless. They became pretty familiar with us during that daily walk to and from FEMA.

The task forces took up residence on different floors throughout the FEMA headquarters building, and the UCG members worked both on the floor assigned to their affiliated task forces and on the top floor near Administrator Gaynor's office. For the first couple of months, we were at FEMA at least eighteen hours a day, seven days a week. It was vital for us to be near one another and all the other task forces because there seemed to be a hundred new challenges every hour; we all needed to work together. It was also a little unnerving at times because we often had COVID cases on the floors, but none of us could go home to quarantine for fourteen days. So we just continued to work, and thankfully, to my knowledge, nobody was hospitalized or died.

The operational tempo at FEMA was full speed from moment one. Every day there was a national coordination meeting, organized by the NRCC chief (initially Josh Dozer) and attended in person by every agency involved in the response. The meeting would start with an update on the spread of the virus from the CDC so that everyone was grounded on the most current data. Each task force presented its ongoing deliverables and work plan and received direction as needed from the UCG. Then by video teleconference, each of the ten FEMA regional response coordination centers throughout the United States, in conjunction with HHS regional health administrators and ASPR regional leads, presented an update on their regions. Because these federal staffs were permanently located in the regions, they already had trusted relationships with state and local leadership. These relationships proved invaluable for implementing and coordinating the response, especially early on when resources were scarce.

The daily situational update at FEMA included ongoing challenges, new requests for supplies and personnel, and any hot-button items that needed attention. Next, there were updates from federal partners, including the Veterans Health Administration, the Department of Defense Northern Command (continental US, Puerto Rico, US Virgin Islands), the Indo-Pacific

Command (for US territories in the Pacific Ocean), the Defense Health Agency, the National Security Council at the White House, and the Joint Information Center (JIC) at FEMA (responsible for externally facing communications). This meeting typically lasted 1–1.5 hours and was our primary mechanism for overall communication and situational awareness. The FEMA region reports provided us with knowledge of what was *actually happening* on the ground, unfiltered and with brutal honesty. It wasn't always pleasant to hear, but we needed to hear it, and the FEMA guys and gals were never subtle. I really appreciated that.

Typically, there was also an additional daily meeting of the UCG, organized by a small number of senior staff, to make allocation decisions and to anticipate problems before they arose. I don't remember a single decision that was not unanimous among the four UCG members. If there was any disagreement, we worked it out rapidly, implemented the decision, and then reassessed our decisions on an ongoing basis. The UCG was also explicit about what decisions needed to be made at the White House level and what decisions should *not* be made at the White House level. The inclusion of Administrator Gaynor, Rear Admiral Polowczyk, and myself on the White House Coronavirus Task Force was, in retrospect, essential for consistent coordinated decision-making at

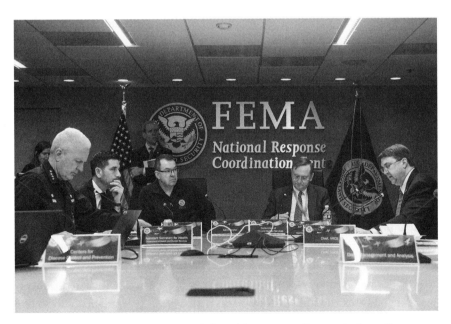

Senior leadership meeting at FEMA, including Administrator Gaynor, Assistant Secretary Kadlec, and Admiral Giroir (UCG members) and also Secretary of Veterans Affairs Robert Wilkie and Acting Secretary of Homeland Security Wolf (White House photo).

all levels. So to summarize the leadership of the early response, every day there was an NRCC update, a UCG meeting, and a White House Coronavirus Task Force meeting. Having a few of us participating at every level was critical for organizing and integrating the response and an important lesson learned for the next pandemic.

NEW YORK NEEDS FORTY THOUSAND VENTILATORS

No issue dominated the UCG's early decision-making more than the allocation of ventilators to states. As I have discussed, by training, I am an intensive care physician (for children). In the ICU, at least 75 percent of my patients were on ventilators at any given time in order to support their recovery from respiratory illnesses, surgery, or trauma. When oxygen and respiratory treatments are insufficient, putting an endotracheal tube in the patient's windpipe and placing him or her on a ventilator to maintain oxygen and remove carbon dioxide is a life-sustaining intervention. Ventilators don't "cure" the disease, but they do keep patients alive during their acute illness until the body's natural healing process kicks in (aided in the case of COVID-19 by drugs like remdesivir and monoclonal antibodies). If the natural healing process does not occur, the patient will develop organ failure and eventually die—ventilator or not.

During the fourth week in March, which was the first week in action for the FEMA UCG, we faced the prospect that potentially tens of thousands of Americans would need ventilators, which we did not have but without which the patients would die. Not only did that mean avoidable deaths and a collapse of the health-care system as we know it, but it also implied placing doctors and nurses in the horrific position of performing battlefield triage, essentially deciding who would live and who would die. We could not tolerate that situation in our nation—pandemic or not.

To understand the scale of the problem, HHS internal documents on March 14, 2020, indicated that there were 12,743 ventilators that could be deployed from the SNS. But between March 16 and March 31, the number of ventilators requested from the stockpile totaled 133,329. The most vocal of the requests came from Gov. Andrew Cuomo of New York, who stated publicly on March 24 that the state of New York needed 40,000 ventilators within two weeks, and at least 30,000 of them were needed from the federal government. Mayor Bill de Blasio had also requested 15,000 ventilators just for New York City, and it was initially unclear whether this was an additional request over

Cuomo's or already included in the Cuomo number. I immediately realized that I had better real-time communication with Cuomo and de Blasio than they apparently had with each other.

No matter what the exact number, providing forty thousand ventilators would have exhausted the SNS three times over and left nothing for other states. But if New York really needed that number of ventilators, would we let New Yorkers die with ventilators sitting in the stockpile unused just to cover for the possibility that other states might need ventilators in the future? That made no sense to me.

The first issue, and the most critical one, was whether New York actually *needed* the ventilators that they requested. In retrospect, they did not—not even close. But back in March, the UCG only knew how many ventilators we had sent to New York. We did not know how many ventilators were already in hospitals throughout the state, how many were being utilized, and how many were ordered from commercial sources independently by the state (or by individual hospitals) and when they would be delivered. Moreover, if we sent forty thousand ventilators, would New York have the trained staff to use them, monitors to adequately and safely employ them, and ICU bed space to put that many more critically ill patients on life support?

There was no mandatory reporting of ventilator usage and reserves, no information systems to automate the reporting, and no analytics to make predictions. It was a challenging situation, to say the least. How could this not have been planned for by the CDC or another HHS agency? Nonetheless, we had to deal with all these unknowns, and quickly.

During this critical time, Jared Kushner connected me to Jessica Tisch, the chief information officer for New York City. She was a Harvard graduate, a Harvard Law School graduate, and a Harvard Business School graduate. Jared had apparently met her in college and had kept in contact. Jared told me that she was maybe five feet tall and one of the toughest people on the planet, and she would not "bullshit" me in any way. I only learned while writing this book that she comes from a wealthy and benevolent New York City family—you would never know it by her affect and actions. She was an operator who enjoyed getting in a fight and dirtying her hands. My first call with her was late at night from my apartment. She had a number of public health officials with her. Over the next month, I spoke with her sometimes twice daily and the extended New York City team numerous times each week; their input was invaluable and saved countless lives both in their city and throughout the United States. Our information about New York was collected the old-fashioned way—human sources on the ground and via telephone.

The public hospitals in New York City were indeed in serious trouble. They were approaching the limits of their ventilator supply and PPE, especially masks, gowns, and gloves. Their staff were already exhausted and would need—really soon—alternate care sites and health-care staff reinforcements. The private hospitals appeared to be in better shape, with a reasonable supply of ventilators, PPE, and staff. Part of the problem, which New York City was ameliorating in real time, was the unequal sharing of COVID patients across the public and private health-care systems. It also became apparent that supplies provided to Cuomo at the state level, including ventilators, were not making their way to New York City and that the governor's office was saving many critical supplies for other areas of the state that might have an outbreak at some time in the future. So though Cuomo demanded that we *not* save ventilators for other parts of the country, he was at the same time saving ventilators urgently needed by New York City for other parts of his state. We should have put GPS trackers on every piece of equipment, and perhaps we will in the future, but we did not have that capability in March 2020. Jessica affirmed—with no subtleties or games—that New York City did in fact need several hundred ventilators as soon as they could be provided, or people were going to die. I believed her and also assessed that I could not rely on the governor to send New York City ventilators from his state stockpile.

The UCG took in as much information as we could on each request by every city and state, but at that time, our focus was on New York and New York City. When we decided to send four hundred ventilators to New York City, that decision was based on the information we had—and it was very good information. We sent those ventilators directly to New York City, not the state; that was the only way we knew that the ventilators would actually reach their intended target hospitals. By April 1, the total number of ventilators sent to New York State was 4,400, of which 2,400 were sent directly to New York City. I spoke to Governor Cuomo directly at least three times—and many more times to his immediate staff (in addition to frequent calls to New York City officials). That is why I found it so bizarre when Governor Cuomo went on his brother Chris Cuomo's CNN show on April 15 and stated that he did not know if I actually existed![2] Well, we had talked several times about ventilators, and I was on the podium with Trump and Pence regularly and on all the weekly governors' calls. What is true, however, is that Governor Cuomo never attended the governors' calls, or at least he never showed his face or asked a single question.

I believe that Cuomo had motives beyond merely securing ventilators and tests: he was making a public spectacle for the purpose of attacking the Trump administration and drawing attention to himself. The media was more than happy to give him a platform and praise nearly every word. The easy thing would have been to give in to Cuomo's demands and minimize the media criticism, but that was obviously not the right decision for the United States, so we never even considered conceding to his demands and bowing to the media onslaught. Unfortunately, being in government as a public servant, especially in uniform, it was inappropriate to counterpunch publicly despite my strong desire to do so.

DECISION-MAKING IN THE CONTEXT OF UNCERTAINTY

Cuomo was not alone in his request for ventilators, although he was unique in his adversarial approach to those of us actually trying to assist him. I had calls from numerous governors at all times of the day and night. On March 26, I had my first call with Governor Inslee at 8 p.m. Although Inslee was brutal to Trump and his administration, his dealings with me were polite and professional. He also knew that we had officers on the ground at the Kirkland Life Care Center nursing facility, and he was very appreciative of their efforts. He was square with me, and I never had any issues working with him operationally.

In general, Cuomo and most other governors were not making requests based on need; they were making requests based on "projected need" for the future. And the projected need was ten times what was available for ventilators and nearly everything else. Making decisions on how to allocate lifesaving resources kept all of us awake at night, especially me, because I knew everything there is to know about ICU care and what would happen to patients without ventilators.

In truth, there was one thing we needed more than anything, and that was better information and analytics to support our decision-making about the allocation of scarce resources. To improve our information and situational awareness, we decided on a three-pronged approach: (1) objective data gathering through FEMA channels, (2) modeling and prediction, and (3) boots-on-the-ground intelligence through a "secret weapon."

DATA

At FEMA, we instituted a formal process to allocate ventilators (and all other supplies). That formal process started on March 21, within forty-eight hours after FEMA was named the LFA. By March 31, it was highly evolved, savvy to games being played by some requestors, and fully functional. The new FEMA Data and Analytics Task Force tracked state ventilator supply and needs. Ventilator requests needed to be substantiated by data demonstrating the number of ICU patients in that state, the number of patients on ventilators, and the overall supply of ventilators available. Some states were doing this in the course of their own incident response. Kudos here to Gov. John Bel Edwards of Louisiana and his staff, who provided detailed spreadsheets, daily, of their utilization and needs broken down by regions and even by individual hospitals. Each request for resources was fully vetted by subject matter experts from multiple agencies, all stationed at FEMA. Every single ventilator request went to the UCG for adjudication. All other requests—for example, PPE—were typically handled at the level of the NRCC chief, but because of the life-and-death nature of ventilators and their allocation, the UCG needed to shoulder that responsibility—and we did.

There have been numerous accusations that politics entered into the allocation of federal resources and that blue states were shorted while red states were supplied generously. I can absolutely refute that. There were no politics involved in ventilator allocation or the distribution of any other resources. I can say this definitively because the UCG was the allocation authority, and I was a member of the UCG. Sometimes the requests did go directly to Jared Kushner or Pence or other senior White House officials. In those cases, requesters were instructed to formalize their ask through the FEMA web-based portal. This was a very familiar process for states—done in every disaster—and we used it for the tracking and analysis of ventilators and all other supplies. The allocation of ventilators was reported at the task force level to the vice president and occasionally directly to the president, and future needs and projections were discussed. No one in the White House ever tipped the scales of our allocation decisions—that would have crossed the line for me, and I am certain for my fellow colleagues on the UCG.

While we were allocating the ventilators already present in the stockpile, the Supply Chain Task Force—working closely with the White House—began using all national authorities, including large bulk purchases and the Defense Production Act (DPA), to secure more ventilators. By mid-April, the number of available ventilators was expected to double and then expand dramatically month by month. Until that time, we were going to be tight, at best. As a result, the surgeon general and I issued guidance on March 31 entitled "Optimizing Ventilator Use during the COVID-19 Pandemic."[3] This guidance was the result of intense work by Jerome and me personally, since we were both subject matter experts in mechanical ventilation, but also the result of the committed efforts of medical societies, including the Society of Critical Care Medicine, whose president (Dr. Lewis Kaplan) personally flew to DC and spent several days at FEMA working on this and numerous other health-care initiatives. His contributions were enormous and exactly what we needed from his professional society.

Our ventilator guidance included recommendations to cancel elective surgery, reallocate resources within regions, and use nontraditional ventilators such as anesthesia machines, transport ventilators, and home ventilators. We also provided as much information as we could about coventilating two patients on a single ventilator; that information included statements allowing for the acceptability of such a practice by the FDA and the CDC as well as protocols from prominent academic institutions for coventilating patients. We also included a joint statement from multiple medical societies that *objected* to coventilation as a practice in order to provide balanced information to health-care providers and systems. It was a tough call, but Jerome and I understood that if the last ventilator was used, coventilation might be the only alternative, and many institutions were indeed planning for that eventuality. Coventilation would have been unprecedented in our country but much better than handing out a death sentence to a patient in need.

Very rapidly, we were gaining real-time situational awareness of the utilization of ventilators and other supplies. In retrospect, the type of system developed by Rear Admiral P and his team at FEMA should have been planned for and invested in by relevant HHS agencies such as the CDC and the Office of the ASPR over the course of multiple administrations. It could have been initiated by the White House or Congress a decade earlier, but it wasn't. So Rear Admiral P and his Supply Chain Task Force at FEMA built it quickly, on the fly, and it was remarkably effective.

MODELING

Knowing the situation at every moment of every day was necessary but not sufficient. What we really needed was an estimate of future demand, especially for ventilators, so we could better plan the allocation strategy. I also needed to know how likely it was that we were going to need battlefield triage to prepare federal guidance for that tragic potential contingency.

The lack of predictive models was a source of enormous frustration at the time. The modelers at the CDC, now integrated into a team at FEMA, simply could not—and would not—provide us with models to inform our decisions about the allocation of scarce resources. Of course, they did not have enough data to be certain that their models were correct, but we weren't requiring certainty. We needed to know the range of possibilities. I was personally both very involved and very frustrated by the situation. I wrote down a note on March 31 that we were still waiting on the CDC to provide us with utilization projections!

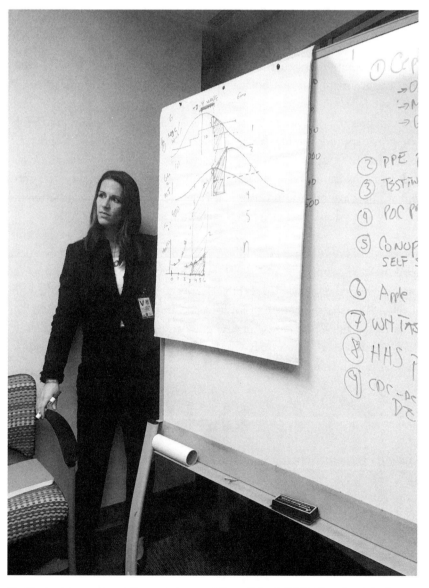

Dr. Blythe Adamson providing real-time modeling of the COVID-19 outbreak in the United States from the HHS headquarters building, March 2020 (personal photo).

So instead of relying on the CDC, we utilized the best models that were available at the time—and those were models generated by the Institute for Health Metrics and Evaluation (IHME), an independent health research center at the University of Washington, and by Blythe Adamson, PhD, MPH, an infectious disease epidemiologist who was one of the "volunteers" from Flatiron Health. Blythe dropped everything—and even left her two children—and came to DC to join the fight. When at FEMA, she detailed epidemiologic models on a whiteboard in real time so we could ensure that she was using the right assumptions as a foundation for her estimates.

Even when alone in her hotel, she apparently drew models on the window, which led to the picture below, which she sent me. I don't understand the math, but I didn't need to because she understood it, and more importantly, she could explain the implications to me and the FEMA teams. I told Blythe she was like our very own Greek goddess of epidemiology descending from Mount Olympus right when the nation needed her; she said she would add that to her business card in the future!

Both the IHME model and the Blythe model had several common conclusions, which increased my confidence in their accuracy. Both were based

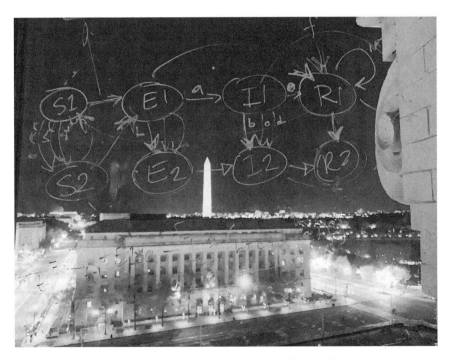

Disease modeling by Dr. Blythe Adamson on the window of her hotel room overlooking US Treasury Building (photo courtesy of Dr. Adamson).

on the empirically observed death curves and then correlated hospital service needs to those death curves. This was a critical strategy and one that I strongly supported because we had no idea what the true case numbers were because of asymptomatic spread and inadequate testing. Both models used lessons from China and Europe but adjusted them for various factors, including the ages of those infected in the United States and the age-specific mortality—critical for our projections given our elderly population. And finally, both models assumed that there would be emergency mitigation measures adopted by states, including nonessential business closures and stay-at-home recommendations.

We did not rely exclusively on these models, but they were tremendously informative. I noted on March 29 that the models predicted that peak ventilator use would occur in the last week of April or the first week of May. The model also indicated that an estimated 19,500 additional ventilators would be needed from the federal stockpile to meet the national need. Of concern, however, was that the range of possibilities spanned from a minimum of 10,000 ventilators up to a maximum of 40,000 ventilators nationally—19,500 was just the best single estimate. With ventilator orders soon arriving, we knew we could handle shipping 19,500 ventilators from the stockpile, but there was no way we could even come close to meeting a requirement for 40,000 ventilators within that short time frame. So the fact that we were in such a precarious position made it essential to recommend community mitigation measures to "slow the spread" in March. If we did not flatten the curve, Americans might die by the thousands because hospitals lacked ventilators.

Based on these considerations, including the IHME and Blythe models, my actual media talking points, taken directly from my notes on March 29, were the following:

- In some parts of the United States, the availability of precious medical resources, including ventilators, may be limited because of the number of patients suffering from COVID-19.

- The American people have heard many predictions about potential shortages, but please understand that most of these are guesses or alarmist overestimates.

- The best available data show that ventilator supply will indeed be very tight, but we can—and will—meet the demand if we all work together.

- Most importantly, the best projections—including the recent ones provided by the Institute for Health Metrics and Evaluation at the University of Washington, suggest that if everyone follows

  ○ strategies to slow the spread,

  ○ guidelines to optimize the use of current ventilators (which are being posted in a simplified form so everyone can follow), and

  ○ the judicious, data-driven use of the federal ventilator stockpile,

  then everyone who needs respiratory support should be able to receive mechanical ventilation, even at the peak of the crisis.

Our confidence in the models was increasing because federal predictions at the macro level were starting to match predictions at the local level. On March 30, I had one of my numerous New York City status calls, that time with Jessica Tisch, Dr. Mitchel Katz (CEO of NYC Health + Hospitals), and Raul Perea-Henze, deputy mayor for health and human services. They reported that NYC had 3,900 ventilators and that 2,400 of the 4,400 sent to New York State were indeed shipped to NYC, as negotiated; another 1,000 had been sent to other centers in the state; and 1,000 were being held in reserve by the governor. NYC's own model predicted that peak utilization would occur in the first week of May (just like IHME and Blythe predicted), with a range of needs between 7,705 and 15,142 ventilators. The IHME model predicted that 8,855 ventilators would be needed for NYC. In general, this was good news because given the expected arrival of new ventilators, we would be able to meet NYC's needs. Based on these predictions, we also prepared another 1,000 ventilators to be sent to NYC if they requested them. I knew I could trust the New York City officials, and they knew if they made a request, ventilators would be on their way within two hours.

We were still waiting for CDC models about the trajectory of the pandemic and the future requirements for specialized supplies like ventilators. Waiting . . . waiting. CDC modelers complained vociferously about our use of the IHME and Blythe models, but the CDC offered no alternatives. The IHME and Blythe models turned out to be pretty damned close to what eventually happened, and as such, they were invaluable as we pieced together the information needed to effectively run the response.

My interactions with New York City were superb in all regards. NYC officials were smart, knowledgeable, and focused only on solving the problems they faced. There was excellent communication, as illustrated by the

March 30 call I just recounted. I rarely spoke with Mayor de Blasio, who was obviously on the opposite side of the political spectrum from Trump. But when I did speak to him, he was uniformly polite, positive, supportive of his professional staff, and genuinely appreciative of our efforts. I would probably never vote for Mayor de Blasio for anything, but I would be happy to buy him a beer.

NORTH, SOUTH, WEST, AND EASTMAN

The last and perhaps most important part of our situational awareness strategy was to have "boots on the ground" we trusted. Certainly, the FEMA regional representatives were doing an exemplary job, but they could not perform the kind of technical medical assessment and command coordination that we needed. The CDC was uniformly helpful for issues of infection control, but in terms of operational savvy and problem-solving, they were not at all useful. What I needed was someone who could travel to all the hot spots, provide technical assistance and operational recommendations, and give me (and the UCG) an unfiltered and unbiased assessment of the ground truth.

Dr. Alex Eastman and I went pretty far back. He is a trauma surgeon and former director of the Parkland Trauma Center in Dallas, one of the meccas for trauma care and research, initially made famous by providing care to the mortally wounded Pres. John F. Kennedy. Alex was also a lieutenant and lead medical officer for the Dallas Police Department who regularly deployed with the Dallas Police Swat Team, got shot at by bad guys, and even performed emergency surgical procedures on downed officers while under fire. I knew Alex from the Ebola days in Texas, when he was in charge of the Parkland Ebola response unit.

Since September 2018, Alex was also the senior medical advisor for operations in the DHS, which meant he worked on everything from defense against weapons of mass destruction to protecting the health of immigrants in Customs and Border Protection (CBP) custody on the southern border of the United States. Alex and I worked intensely on the border issues with unaccompanied children and family units in 2019. Aside from being a trauma surgeon with a badge and a gun (usually two guns, if I recall correctly), Alex had unique charisma and charm. He was the kind of person whom people immediately liked and trusted. He was not afraid to say the truth to anyone about any situation—which I imagine kept him on the hot seat at the DHS, especially with their revolving door of leadership. If things were effed up, he would tell us that in no uncertain terms but then have a plan to "un-eff" the situation and get things working.

I called Alex on March 21. He was with his wife and kids at home in Dallas. I asked him to pack his bags, get to DC as soon as possible, and not buy a round-trip ticket back home. Get whatever clearance he needed through DHS, but we needed him to go to hot spots and do what he does best—assess and adapt, provide feedback and guidance, and give us the skinny. I told him that I did not know where he would go or what exactly he would do, just to get his ass to DC and we would make it up from there. I don't know the conversation he had with his wife, or trauma service, or the Dallas Police Department, but he was in DC within forty-eight hours, and on March 26, he provided his first of sixty-one sitreps, this one from New York City—the epicenter of the outbreak and where we needed additional ground-truth information to supplement our daily communication with New York City health officials.

In New York City, Alex worked with numerous officials, including on day 1 with the Office of Emergency Management commissioner Deanne Criswell (now the FEMA administrator in the Biden administration), who was "great, committed and just wants to make things better. Was a great

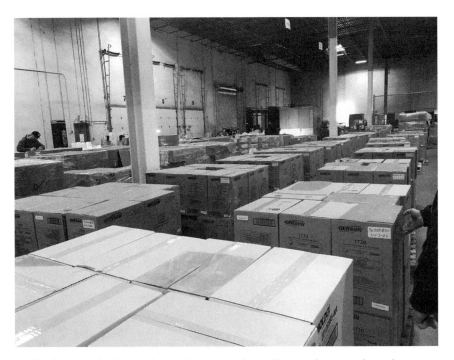

Cache of New York City supplies, including ventilators discovered in a warehouse by Dr. Alex Eastman (personal photo).

partner all day."[4] The commissioner communicated her priorities, and these were relayed back to me and subsequently the UCG, and we acted upon them immediately. Alex also quite famously showed up at an NYC warehouse operated by a contractor in Edison, New Jersey, and provided me with this unexpected update:

> Found literally tons of supplies (see pics below) including the SNS ventilators, N95s, face shields, and much more.
>
> Note: Some of the SNS ventilators were still being unloaded.
>
> In short, figured out a flawed strategy by NYC Department of Health and Mental Hygiene to hold onto supplies based on unpredictability of inbound replacement supplies.
>
> Worked side by side with NYC OEM Commissioner Deanne Criswell to correct.

After two full days in New York City, Alex started his cross-country travel—going to places that I identified as needing coordination, technical assistance, trust building, and ground truth back to FEMA. At most sites,

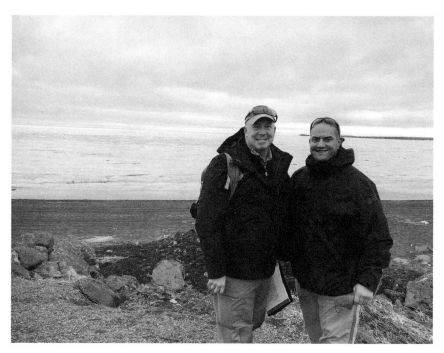

Dr. Alex Eastman (right) with his chief of staff, Jeff Birks (left), standing near the Arctic Ocean on their site visit and assistance visit to Alaska (personal photo).

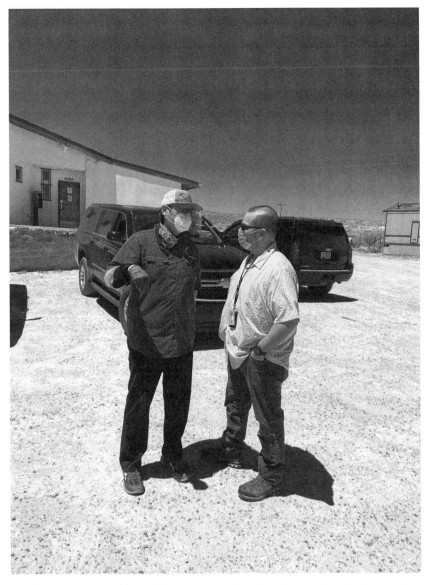

Dr. Alex Eastman with Navajo Nation president Jonathan Nez at a food distribution in the Navajo Nation near Window Rock, Arizona (personal photo).

he met with state leadership, including the governor and state health officials, as well as federal representatives in the region. After New York City, his coordination activities included site visits everywhere from Florida to Alaska, Louisiana, Illinois, and the Navajo Nation. The information he provided was essential for those of us in DC to understand what was really happening throughout the nation and to then provide rapid solutions without delay or bureaucracy. Summaries of his daily sitreps can be reviewed in the appendix to this chapter.

None of us could ever adequately thank Alex for his arduous and honestly dangerous journey across the United States. He saved countless lives and made our job at FEMA manageable. But I did thank him—he is like a brother to me. Before the end of my term in office, I awarded him the highest decoration from the US Public Health Service to a person not in the military—the assistant secretary for health's Exceptional Service Medallion. He deserved it and much more.

BACK TO HHS

The organization and daily operations remained at FEMA until June 15, when the task forces were turned into "working groups" and the center of operations transitioned back to HHS. The reason for this shift was multifactorial. First, the three months with FEMA as the lead agency established the processes and battle rhythms that were needed, built the multidisciplinary teams (including the armed forces) necessary to bolster the capabilities of HHS, established the information systems, and expanded supply chains for products like ventilators and PPE. Second, FEMA was preparing for a forecasted severe hurricane and wildfire season, which in and of itself might demand most or all of FEMA resources. Third, OWS (Operation Warp Speed) had been announced one month earlier, and it was clear that its success or failure would be the defining event for the administration and the only way to end the pandemic without millions of US deaths. OWS was squarely in the sweet spot of HHS and especially Secretary Azar.

The FEMA UCG as a leadership body ended, and a new UCG at HHS was formed consisting of Secretary Azar, Deborah Birx, and Pete Gaynor. My time at the UCG was over. Pete was kept fully in the loop in case the response needed to jump back to FEMA, which was a distinct possibility if there was another surge.

Every morning, Secretary Azar led (and attended in person) a sync call that included leadership from all relevant HHS divisions, including myself, the CDC, the FDA, the Office of the ASPR, the CMS, the NIH, and others. Also included was the JIC, now organized under HHS, to focus on communication to the public and media messaging.

The surgeon general was almost always traveling, bringing messages directly to states and localities, but he typically called into the meeting to provide boots-on-the-ground feedback. He was also working intensely with Francis Collins to increase minority enrollment in the vaccine clinical trials. We did not want a situation in which too few minorities were enrolled to be able to draw firm conclusions about the safety and efficacy of vaccines in minority populations. Jerome worked tirelessly through all the channels he knew—many he was part of—and he was extraordinarily successful. To my knowledge, this was the largest and most fruitful effort ever undertaken by the federal government to assure adequate racial and ethnic participation in clinical trials. I always attended the secretary's daily sync call, reported on all issues related to testing, and also functioned as a technical subject matter expert to coordinate policy and assist in the development of overall guidelines.

AND THEN THERE WAS THE MEDIA . . .

Before COVID-19, I had only a modest media presence, mostly regarding specific national policy initiatives led by my office, such as the Physical Activity Guidelines for Americans and the Ending the HIV Epidemic in the US. But that all changed on March 15, 2020, when I first appeared behind the White House podium with the president and vice president. It was clear that the primary way we were going to communicate with the American public was through the media, so there was no choice but to fully engage with the press. As such, for many weeks, I frequently led segments of the official White House press conferences and then also appeared regularly on multiple networks, morning and evening, and of course on the often contentious Sunday morning news shows.

I initially received almost no coaching or support from the official HHS communications team in the Office of the Assistant Secretary for Public Affairs—they were there for Secretary Azar and, with rare exception, did not meaningfully engage me or my issues. Similarly, the White House communications team did not prepare me for appearances, except for their routine late evening group preparations with all those appearing on the Sunday morning shows. I was certainly holding my own, sticking to straightforward and transparent messages, being as honest and humble as I could while portraying confidence, and using all the communications skills I learned as a public speaker and bedside ICU physician. But I definitely needed help.

I relied on my small communications team in OASH, which had been carrying a very heavy load ever since that long weekend after I became testing czar. It was not built for this type of challenge, but they rose to the occasion under great duress. Fortunately, in June 2019, Mia Heck joined my team as director of external affairs. While Mia was not a "coms person" specifically, she was a highly seasoned professional who knew how to interact with external groups and the media. She was serious, dedicated, and loyal and had a very high emotional intelligence; I trusted her completely. Before joining my office, Mia had served as a senior advisor to the HHS Department of Intergovernmental and External Affairs and before that as a senior advisor to Seema Verma in the CMS. Perhaps more importantly, after her brief time at HHS in the George W. Bush administration, she gained significant professional experience in the National Incident Management System and had several certifications in emergency response. These diverse experiences made her invaluable once the pandemic hit.

Mia led a small but talented group of career communications staff in OASH. Critical to this team was a seasoned USPHS officer, Cmdr. Kate Grabill, who led public affairs for the Commissioned Corps and the Office of the Surgeon General. We had worked together for a year carefully crafting messages about modernizing the Commissioned Corps. She could withstand any challenge and keep her cool. Finally, Patricia Haigwood, whom I first worked with at DARPA and then later at Texas A&M, was a tireless worker and did everything from communications to data mining; she was actually the primary source for many of the analyses and charts Pence and I used from the White House podium.

In March and April 2020, my communications staff went to the mat for me. They had my back. They identified issues, including making sure I was aware of combative partisan reporters before I went on live national TV. The team even held Sunday afternoon meetings, where they predicted and outlined the most important public health messages for the week and then modified and supplemented these messages with daily updates for me in a written "nightly" communications report. My team did everything they could without much outside help from the assistant secretary for public affairs (ASPA) or the White House, but we were barely keeping all the balls in the air. And increasingly, headlines were becoming more about the few times I was perceived to contradict Trump and less about the critical public health messages we were trying to convey.

Then, all of a sudden in late April 2020, Michael Caputo arrived as the new ASPA. Certainly a book could and should be written about him, but here I only want to emphasize that the situation immediately changed for the better. Instead of his office ignoring my needs and neglecting my communications staff, he reached out immediately and stated he was there for us, not just the secretary. He brought in an incredibly skilled and savvy communications strategist and Republican consultant named Gordon Hensley, who worked with us daily to help me prepare for the media and for the public. His advice about clear messaging, and especially his nearly clairvoyant anticipation of "gotcha" questions, positively transformed my ability to provide clear communication to the American people.

Caputo also provided top cover, which I had never had previously from the media and communications standpoint. Beginning in late April, it was becoming very difficult to get clearance from the White House (which was required) for national media appearances, including network and cable morning and evening shows. There was so much going on that I think my appearances frequently never made it to decision-makers, or they were focused on Trump and Pence, and the opportunity "timed out." This was incredibly frustrating because fighting the pandemic was heavily dependent on providing factual information over the airwaves so the public could make potentially lifesaving decisions for their families.

Caputo immediately changed the dynamic and ended the stalemate because he felt the doctors in his HHS purview (particularly Surgeon Gen. Jerome Adams and I) were the ones who really needed to be on TV, not the politicians and administrators. So when the White House did not clear appearances in a timely fashion, Caputo "cleared them" on behalf of the president. If he weren't there to do that, I would not have been able to talk sensibly to the American people as often as I did.

Gordon and Mia also decided to be proactive. They knew that outside of the press room at the White House, many reporters were just hungry for accurate information—data, statistics, a deeper level of understanding, and information about what was going to happen. They were also scared for themselves and their families. When not on camera, reporters are people with problems just like the rest of us—elderly parents, kids home from school, and perhaps family struggles with depression or addiction.

So with Caputo's blessing, Gordon and Mia arranged a weekly media call starting in early May. Eighty to one hundred reporters from print and broadcast media routinely attended the call. I always opened with about fifteen minutes of remarks—these were always my topics and my remarks but were honed by Gordon and Mia. That was followed by about forty-five minutes of Q and A. Not only did this provide reporters with the background

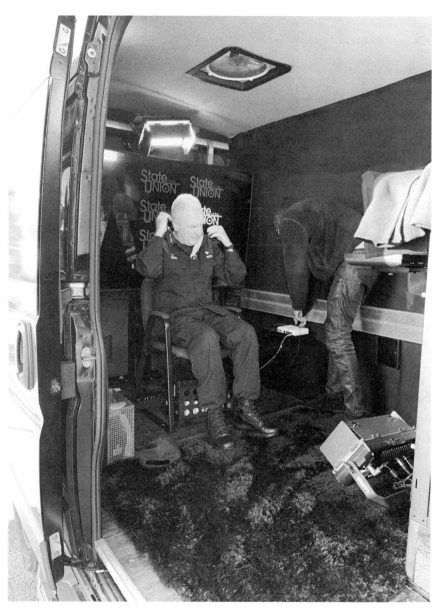

Admiral Giroir in mobile media studio ("studio van") preparing for Sunday morning show *State of the Union* with Jake Tapper. During the pandemic, live studio appearances ceased. Instead, appearances were done remotely, often in studio vans that pulled up outside his apartment. Needless to say, the complexities of a live national interview were often compounded by poor audio feed, cramped and constrained quarters, and frequently freezing temperatures (personal photo).

information they needed to understand and cover the pandemic, but it also enhanced the trust they had in me and my team. The few times when a reporter tried to be aggressive or political on the calls, Patricia and Mia would hold up a small sign with a fish hook on it—"Don't take the bait!"

I kept this weekly call until the end of the administration, and to this day, I feel very good about those interactions with reporters. Those who attended these calls were from the *Washington Post*, the *New York Times*, Politico, ABC, CNN, and other news outlets, and many still call me today about issues— sometimes on the record but mostly just for background and understanding. We still need a clear message, and as the Biden administration has discovered, it is not all that easy, even with a favorable and forgiving media, something we never had during the Trump administration.

APPENDIX

Selected Situational Report Summaries from Dr. Alex Eastman to the FEMA UCG

- New Jersey: Focused on supporting hospital capacity issues, providing additional ventilators and PPE. Assisted in coordination of beds in the Veterans Health Administration for nonveterans and deployment of federal personnel. Site visit to PNC Bank CBTS confirmed it was "performing well. Exquisitely well set up and organized. No issues noted."

- New Orleans and Baton Rouge: Coordinated with hospital systems, provided technical assistance on implementing Morial Convention Center Alternative Care Site, worked to alleviate PPE shortages, requested enhanced federal assistance for critical care staffing, worked to enhance mortuary facilities, submitted request for Mortuary Assistance Team from FEMA, and corrected problems with reporting of CBTS results from major lab partners.

- Dallas: Conducted technical assistance visit to the Kay Bailey Hutchison Convention Center alternative care facility.

- Detroit/Lansing: Provided technical assistance to Detroit Police Department command staff on specific protocol to protect officers from COVID and handling of officers if they become sick or exposed, identified and remedied significant PPE shortages for EMS, identified issues and resolved them at TCF Center alternative care site. Sourced drugs needed for critically ill patients. Assessed and improved ICS [incident command system]. Coordinated with and provided technical assistance to Michigan State Police.

- Chicago: Provided coordination and technical assistance on the design and staffing of the McCormick Place Alternate Care Site with numerous local and federal partners, worked to resolve excessive requirements of Department of Defense in order to staff McCormick Place, observed and provided assistance to staff undergoing scenario-based training, solidified planning with Illinois Department of Health for inmates in correctional facilities. Met with Mayor Lightfoot and Gov. J. B. Pritzker and senior staff. "Recognized local leadership for assembling a cohesive, interdisciplinary ACS [alternate care site] leadership team. A national best practice from what we've seen thus far."

- Philadelphia: Met with multiple health system leaders. Main issues revolved around long-term care facility outbreaks, but there remained substantial hospital capacity within the city and region. Received feedback about the lack of coordination between hospital systems (as opposed to within hospital systems), and then in response held a coordination meeting among systems to improve sharing of patients. Identified needs and began solving for increased mortuary services and more medical input at the EOC.

- Miami: Conducted technical assistance visit—Miami Beach Convention Center Alternate Care Facility; "improvements from 'early' model ACSs make this the most capable facility yet." Conducted technical assistance visit with Jackson Memorial Healthcare Division of Disaster and Emergency Preparedness and Dr. Abdul Memon, system chief medical officer for disaster and emergency preparedness, who is "a Florida legend of sorts." Identified and communicated main regional concerns: long-term care facilities with very limited testing, including group homes and shelters; jails and their inability to cohort and isolate; and the potential marked effects of asymptomatic transmission on the pandemic when the state reopens.

- Topeka, Kansas: Worked with state officials, meat processing centers, unions, and federal partners, and coordinated with Dr. Tammy Beckham at HHS who is an expert in animal health and food processing. Four counties in western Kansas are home to three large beef production facilities; combined they produce 25 percent of the nation's beef, and COVID is a real threat to the nation's food supply due to labor shortages because of sick workers. Identified poor living conditions of employees (low income, multiple families living in same household, poor sanitation). Performed site visits to meat processing facilities and provided technical assistance; personally participated in butchering of carcasses with a massive chain saw to fully understand work-related potential exposure risks and requirements to perform job functions with such equipment. Coordinated with the CDC team for comprehensive solutions to assure the US food supply.

- Navajo Nation: Reviewed specific plans and needs for four locations of concern—Gallup, Chinle, Crownpoint, and Shiprock—because inpatient COVID cases were doubling within twenty-four hours. Identified lapse in communication such that the federal data significantly underestimated burden of disease—a truly critically important finding. Provided technical assistance to facilities and staff. Participated in Navajo Nation daily operational briefing; built and improved relationships with Navajo Nation president Jonathan Nez and his cabinet directly; solved critical credentialing issues necessary to utilize deployed federal health-care staff in Indian health services facilities; identified food insecurity as a major concern and driver of new infections; assisted in loading three hundred personal cars of tribal citizens with food and water, side by side with President Nez, to ameliorate food insecurity issues.

- San Diego and El Centro: San Diego hospital system was found to have good reserve capacity at that time; met with the mayor, public health leaders, and hospital leadership; collaborated with San Diego mayor on complex issues related to the border: ~250,000 US citizens live across border and return to the United States if they get sick. Also, San Diego health-care staff critically dependent on many workers who cross the border daily; identified urgent needs in Imperial County and assisted in filing FEMA requests; social issues, including food insecurity and poverty, worsened overall situation with pandemic.

- Alaska: Performed critical coordination with outstanding state health official—Dr. Anne Zink—who was working intensely with Admiral Giroir on providing massive surge testing to support the Alaskan fishing season. Provided coordination and technical assistance visits for Anchorage hospital systems and reviewed plans for alternate care sites; communicated with UCG concerning the logistics challenges of distance and weather; met with governor to understand dual concerns of protection from virus and keeping the economy going in Alaska and participated in press briefing; conducted technical assistance calls with Juneau and Fairbanks city leaders; visited US Coast Guard Station in Kodiak; performed site visits to numerous seafood processing facilities, including Trident and Ocean City, which together process four million pounds of seafood each day; conducted technical assistance visit to alternate care site in Kodiak and Cordova as well as health centers; met with tribal leaders in Dillingham to understand their devastation from 1918 flu pandemic and concerns over COVID repeating history; performed site visits in Dillingham to health-care facilities and seafood canneries; performed community outreach visit and consultation to Egegik Tribal Council, and visited seafood facility; performed technical assistance and community outreach visits to city of King Salmon and Naknek; coordinated implementation and troubleshot problems with implementation of Cepheid testing devices sent from HHS to support on-site testing.

9

Anybody That Wants a Test . . .

Twenty-six minutes and twenty-three seconds into his March 6 press conference at the CDC, President Trump made a statement that would dog him, the administration, and certainly me for the remainder of his presidency: "Anybody that wants a test can get a test. That's what the bottom line is."[1] Fifty-two seconds later, likely realizing his mistake, the president stated what I think he intended to say in the first place: "But I think, importantly, anybody right now and yesterday, anybody that needs a test gets a test. They're there." In fact, over the course of the next sixty seconds, Trump used the "needs a test" phrase three more times, as if he instinctively knew what he said would lead to a public relations nightmare and perhaps even a crisis for his reelection campaign. On March 15, during the Sunday press conference with me and my fellow officers in the White House press room, the vice president also emphasized that we could not provide tests for everyone who wanted a test but that "tests would be available for everyone who needed a test." I went even further in my remarks from the podium that evening to clarify that we actually would be defining specifically who "needed a test" because we had to prioritize testing capacity for the elderly and other vulnerable groups. Bottom line, we clearly did not have enough tests to perform widespread community testing or complete contact tracing in March 2020, and we were not able to fix that situation until late in the summer of 2020.

But the horse was already out of the barn twenty-six minutes and twenty-three seconds into Trump's CDC remarks on March 6. The media and the Democratic Party leadership seized upon the "wants a test" as the required national performance standard—which, of course, was medically unjustified (what kind of medical test is ever done whenever a patient wants one?) and practically unachievable for many more months.

Who "needed" a test depended heavily on a number of interrelated factors, including the status of the outbreak, the effectiveness of mitigation measures like masking, the specific goals for testing at that time and in that place, the willingness of individuals to quarantine after close exposure, and the number and types of tests that were available. That complexity was real but hard to communicate, especially when the naive simple standard of "anybody that wants a test" accomplished the political goal of reliably discrediting the Trump administration's efforts.

It didn't help that on May 11, 2020, for some unknown reason and contrary to everything Pence and I had been saying, Trump reiterated the phrase "If somebody wants to be tested right now, they'll be able to be tested." Later in that same press conference, I tried to respectfully correct the president (always an uncomfortable thing to do) by clarifying that we could test "everybody who needs a test." I explained that we were still focusing on people who had respiratory symptoms or who needed a test because they were exposed to the virus by contact. Nevertheless, the media pounced.

Other popular narratives were that the Trump administration never had a national testing strategy and that we pushed all the burden of testing to the states. Not only were these narratives false, but they were also the exact opposite of the truth.

Our administration developed a detailed strategy and implementation plan, rolled it out sequentially with increasing sophistication, and only relied on states to do their part after they received from the federal government requested supplies, personnel support, authorities, technical assistance, direction, and all other resources that they needed. At least that was the situation beginning in late March. Nonetheless, these false narratives were continually repeated by Democrat leaders like Senator Patty Murray, who obsessively pummeled us with those mischaracterizations. Senator Murray—at least in my experience—could never engage in meaningful debate or discussion of any issues because she just could not see past her disdain for President Trump. Aside from Senator Mitt Romney and perhaps Senator Bernie Sanders, I don't think I would put any other senators in that category—most were great to work with and gave important input to the overall efforts, especially when the cameras were off.

The truth is that there had been no previous plan for testing at a national scale during a pandemic—not even for known viruses like influenza, much less a novel virus like SARS-CoV-2. There were no tests, swabs, or collection tubes in the stockpile; we didn't even have a description of the industrial base or phone numbers to call. Our initial resources were Google and many phone calls to large medical distributors, like Henry Schein, who helped us understand where the supplies actually came from and how to potentially get them. The much-referred-to "Obama pandemic playbook" rarely mentioned diagnostic testing in its sixty-nine pages, and when testing is mentioned, it is part of unactionable statements like the following: "FDA can provide assistance by working closely with manufacturers and US government partners to expedite the development and availability of biologics (including vaccines), drugs, and devices (including diagnostic tests and personal protective equipment)."[2] That is hardly a fully fleshed-out plan of attack for me—or anyone—to follow. I don't blame the Obama team because Democrat and Republican administrations had the same blind spot. That tunnel vision perhaps reflected the relatively inbred processes for pandemic planning that did not include enough private-sector or academic partners or public health labs, or perhaps the blind spot occurred because the focus was on pandemic influenza, which has its own set of challenges, but testing is not one of them.

There is no doubt that the CDC fumbled testing early and that the FDA imposed artificial barriers that prevented academic and some large commercial labs from developing their own LDTs. In retrospect, one of the legitimate criticisms of the Trump administration's response—at least early on—was that the senior leadership put their faith in, and relied too heavily upon, government bureaucracies like the CDC and the FDA, which did not recognize that they were failing. The White House did not exert control (nor empower Secretary Azar to do so) in January or February. Taking early control at the White House level would have helped the nation better prepare for March and April, when the crisis really hit. Quite opposite from the accusation that Trump exerted too much control over the health agencies, it was the exact opposite.

To be clear, at the "tree level," HHS agencies performed well, even exemplary. Who can argue that over three hundred EUAs for diagnostics by January 20, 2021, is not a kick-ass effort by the FDA? Or that the CDC did not perform well, if not brilliantly, on local disease investigations, for example, during outbreaks affecting our food supply in the Midwest?

But at the macro level, the "forest level" of national policy and strategy, the agencies could not perform without significant integration and direction from Senate-confirmed HHS leaders like me or from the White House Coronavirus Task Force. In retrospect, that is not surprising given the silos in federal departments and the narrow specialties of their career leaders who may be, for example, the top people in vaccine discovery but have no idea about the overall public health consequences of a lockdown or loss of employment and a financial crash. No matter how many technologies and whiz-bang gizmos we have, if we don't get the organization right, we will never have an adequate response for the next pandemic.

In relation to testing, from the moment that the White House took control (specifically, when I became testing lead after Jared busted into my meeting with the secretary), we did indeed develop and implement the most robust and comprehensive testing program in the history of modern public health. The numbers speak for themselves. By January 13, 2021 (the last day I analyzed the data), within a ten-month period of time and from a near-standing start, we accomplished the following:

- We completed 264 million tests in the United States, as reported to HHS through the official public health reporting systems. This number was likely underestimated by at least 30–50 percent because very few of the >180 million rapid BinaxNOW tests we distributed were ever reported to public health authorities. But even with these underestimates, the United States conducted more tests than any other country and more tests per capita than any other country with a population over ten million.[3]

- The United States had the full end-to-end capacity to perform 170 million tests in the month of January 2021, not including pooling,[4] which could have increased that number by at least twofold. Although HHS under the Biden administration no longer provides supply projections to the public as I did, nonprofit groups estimated the number of tests available within the United States in September 2021 at 417 million tests, again not including pooling.[5] If Biden would have continued to support testing and not lost a critical eight months between January and September, we projected that the nation would have had one billion tests fully available *per month* in the winter of 2021. And those increases are entirely based on the programs of the Trump administration or programs we initiated but had not yet contracted by January 20, 2021.

- Through the use of the DPA and other authorities, we controlled essentially 100 percent of the major POC markets and supplied 5.3 million rapid tests (and associated reader devices when required) to all 15,300 nursing homes in the United States in order to protect their residents, who had the highest risk of mortality in our country.

- We purchased and distributed to governors, tribal nations, and vulnerable groups, including nursing homes and other populations, the first 180 million BinaxNOW rapid POC antigen tests in the fall and winter of 2020; this redefined the testing ecosystem in the United States. In January 2021 before the change in administration, I announced funding for the purchase of another sixty million rapid antigen tests as continued support for states, nursing homes, and other vulnerable populations.

- The Trump administration built the capacity for, purchased, and distributed free of charge to states 191 million swabs, 221 million tubes of transport media, and 4.3 million Abbott IDNOW POC molecular tests. We also directed the distribution of test kits in the commercial market, even when the federal government did not buy them outright. Beginning in late March 2020, we developed complete visibility and situational awareness of the testing market. The part of the free market we allowed to operate was done intentionally because those parts of the market worked well with only a soft touch by my team—meaning supplies were allocated according to our recommendations to the areas of high need (without directly purchasing them or using the DPA).

- We established over 9,500 federal or federally enabled testing sites, including 7,700 retail and community sites, 1,300 federally qualified health centers, and 658 surge-testing sites in twenty-three states. We guaranteed that a majority of these sites were located in communities of moderate or high social vulnerability, as defined by the CDC, meaning they reached racial and ethnic minorities, migrants, homeless people, those in poverty, and other disadvantaged groups.

- We established six K–12 school pilot testing programs in collaboration with the Rockefeller Foundation and the Duke Margolis Center for Health Policy (120,000 tests) and an additional pilot strategic surveillance program with the CDC in six states, the Department of Veterans Affairs, and several tribal nations (1.8 million tests).

- Just for testing, we used the DPA thirteen times and conducted forty-two airbridge flights (jumbo jets or military equivalents) to assure the expedited availability of testing supplies like swabs, pipette tips, and other commodities.

- We spent over $6 billion to support testing through the task forces that I led, and that does not include the billions of dollars spent on research and development through programs at the NIH and BARDA.

- Through funding appropriated by Congress and signed by the president, we supplied >$30 billion to states, territories, and tribes solely for the purpose of supporting testing and related activities, like contact tracing. Most of that money remained unspent by the time the administration changed.

After President Biden took office, testing fell dramatically. By July 2021, testing was less than half of what it was in January, despite the Delta variant raging across the nation. Even though testing rebounded in August and September, by my estimates, only 10–20 percent of the national testing capacity was being utilized at that time.

But you rarely heard about testing in the media in mid-2021. Biden's initial testing czar was rarely on camera. In contrast, I did a comprehensive media briefing every Monday or Tuesday to between sixty and one hundred members of print and broadcast media, during which I specifically detailed the status of testing as well as the overall key issues in the pandemic response for that week. This is in addition to my national TV appearances on multiple networks each week.

President Biden has rarely ever been asked a question about testing, nor has Dr. Fauci, Dr. Walensky, or Mr. Zients (the first White House COVID coordinator), at least at national-level briefings and press conferences. There were no longer outcries by Ashish Jha and other political operatives for massive increases in testing, perhaps even testing daily for every single person in the country, as was demanded from the Trump administration.

The majority of media outlets did not report the fact that the US industrial base for testing cratered in the spring and summer of 2021 because of a lack of continued federal investment and leadership. Because of this federal neglect, the CDC was forced to publish a laboratory advisory to warn of POC testing shortages in September 2021.[6] To put a finer point on this, although the United States was continuing to invest in certain types of testing capacity expansion, the Biden team did not sustain the testing industrial base through government orders. That almost killed the industry even while the pandemic was worsening with new variants.

Finally, what happened to the National Pandemic Testing Board, highlighted in Biden's initial pandemic plan and executive order on Inauguration Day? To my knowledge, as of early 2022, we are still waiting for it to have any impact or even preliminary recommendations; in fact, we don't even know who the members are or the nature of the charter. In contrast, my team laid the groundwork for public-private collaboration by implementing the National COVID-19 Testing Forum, which began in July 2020.[7] This type of public-private-academic partnership needs to be further developed—not relegated to a political talking point—if we are going to keep the United States biosafe, and I will detail this concept in the last chapter of this book.

It is clear that testing was a blunt-force object against the Trump administration, and that fact is even clearer now by its near disappearance from the media early in the Biden administration, until it could no longer be ignored during the Delta and Omicron variant surges. What is tragic, however, is that although I still maintain that we can't test our way out of this pandemic, we have already started to forget how incredibly useful and important testing can be once we achieved a minimum threshold of capacity. During the Delta outbreak, while we correctly pushed for vaccinations, the Biden team could have sent rapid tests to every single household in outbreak areas multiple times per week. Why didn't they do that? Why isn't testing more available for workplaces or schools? More importantly, instead of sending tests to anyone who signed up on a website (which Biden eventually implemented), tests should have been allocated to those at high risk (elderly and/or those with chronic health conditions) for whom a positive test meant they were eligible for the new, highly effective pills against COVID-19 (Lagevrio and Paxlovid). Those pills have dramatic positive effects on preventing hospitalizations and deaths.

Bottom line, I am worried that the nation's rapid transition from "testing obsession" to "testing oblivion" will doom us to repeat the mistakes of our recent past. Our federal testing apathy is also sending clear warning signals to the US industrial base that financial decisions to rapidly expand capacity and personnel during the next crisis will not be sustained by the federal government, and that signal will translate into risk aversion and inaction among our industrial partners. We had no industry reluctance during the early days of COVID-19, but that could change dramatically in the future if the Biden administration does not commit to long-term sustainable solutions.

THE NATIONAL TESTING STRATEGY

My team developed and implemented a national strategy long before the first official announcement of the national strategy on April 27, 2020, when the White House released the *Testing Overview*[8] and the *Testing Blueprint*[9] and before I personally documented our detailed plan in an eighty-one-page report to Congress entitled *COVID-19 Strategic Testing Plan*.[10]

That official plan was supplemented by an *Addendum to the Testing Strategy*[11] from the White House in June and then supplementary reports updating the national strategy to Congress in August and November 2020. Moreover, the testing guidelines from the CDC and the Center for Medicare and Medicaid Services, which were coordinated with my team, provided additional specific recommendations that further implemented the national strategy.

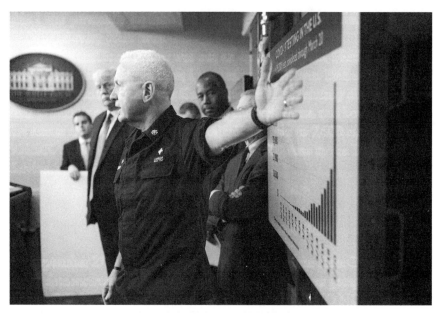

Admiral Giroir briefs the White House press corps on early progress of testing and national testing strategy, March 2020. President Trump, Secretary Carson in background (White House photo).

In March and early April 2020, we needed to build capacity and a variety of test types, including lab-based testing and POC testing. By late April, we had the beginnings of a toolbox to achieve our objectives. These objectives would not change for the remainder of our term, but our capacity to achieve them and the tactics involved would evolve as we developed new tests and addressed different stages of the pandemic, region by region, population group by population group.

Our overall specific national testing objectives were the following:

- *Identify emerging local and regional outbreaks*

     We achieved this objective by maintaining sufficient baseline testing to detect early changes in percent positivity (the percentage of overall tests that were positive). A rise in percent positivity was the key leading indicator—and a very reliable one—that would precede a rise in actual clinical cases, which would inexorably be followed by an increase in hospitalizations and deaths.

     We monitored the percent positivity down to the county level daily and used this information to prioritize our responses and also inform state and local officials in our weekly official written guidance (and frequently daily verbal recommendations).

- *Support isolation and contact tracing*

The Achilles' heel for COVID-19 contact tracing is the large amount of disease spread by asymptomatic individuals. If everyone were symptomatic, like with Ebola or even MERS, then isolation and contact tracing would be very effective tools to snuff out the disease. With COVID-19, the virus is spread efficiently by those who are not sick, and the majority of individuals have no idea where they became infected or who infected them. So unless everyone in a population is tested at least twice per week (as was done in nursing homes but is still unrealistic on a nationwide scale in late 2022), it is impossible to isolate all those who are spreading the infection.

I was very specific about the importance of masking in indoor crowded spaces and physical distancing when appropriate (prior to vaccinations) but also that it was beneficial in areas of outbreaks to identify as many asymptomatic spreaders as possible through testing. This was particularly the case for young people who lived in multigenerational households, for example, and for other groups where asymptomatic transmission could be of high consequence.

We achieved this objective by having sufficient baseline testing but also by emergency surge testing in areas that had increasing numbers of cases or were predicted to do so (by percent positivity). In total, we implemented federal surge-testing sites in 658 locations in twenty-three states beginning in July 2020. We also guaranteed that >90 percent of federally qualified health centers (FQHCs) had testing capacity. This was important because FQHCs care for one of every three people in poverty in the United States, and those in poverty often did not have the luxury of physically distancing or teleworking.

- *Diagnose COVID-19 rapidly in hospitalized patients and, later in the pandemic, in those who were eligible for antibody therapy*

We achieved this by prioritizing testing for these groups, including instructing the ACLA labs (Quest and LabCorp) that hospitalized patients needed to have results in twenty-four hours or less. This was accomplished by a simple coding on the test paperwork indicating the fact that the patient was hospitalized. Later in the pandemic, most hospitals were doing their own COVID testing, and there was widespread availability of simple POC tests.

- *Protect the vulnerable*

In the early stages of the pandemic, 40 percent of pandemic deaths occurred among nursing home residents. And even through the summer of 2020, >80 percent of all the deaths occurred in those over sixty-five years of age.[12] In addition to the elderly, racial and ethnic minorities were disproportionately affected, with their hospitalizations being four or five times the rate of nonminorities.

We went all in to protect nursing homes by providing POC testing (results on the spot in fifteen minutes), as soon as it was available, to every single nursing home in the country. To protect minorities and the poor, we established free testing at FQHCs and mandated that at least two-thirds of our CBTSs be located in areas of moderate or high social vulnerability.

- *Support the safe operation of schools and businesses*

The Trump administration *never advised closing schools*, and indeed, we warned against the consequences of doing so. That being said, we understood that until vaccines became widely available, routine surveillance testing (regardless of symptoms or known exposures) of specific populations could be useful to provide another layer of protection. This strategy worked extremely well at a number of universities, which provided weekly or twice-weekly testing for students and kept the case counts reasonably low without Draconian measures.

But in order to do this on a national scale, we needed rapid POC antigen testing (which could have taken years to develop under normal circumstances). The authorization of the Abbott BinaxNOW antigen card on August 26, 2020, opened the door. I had been working with Abbott for months in anticipation of this breakthrough, and the FDA was primed to prioritize their review of this test. Following authorization, we immediately purchased the entire national supply for months and sponsored pilot testing programs in schools so that communities could learn and make their own decision about whether intermittent surveillance testing was right for them.

- *Enable state testing plans*

  The states were no more "left on their own" with testing than they now are related to COVID-19 vaccines. Each state testing plan was developed after direct and comprehensive technical guidance by my federal multiagency team, employing evidence-based criteria and transparent objectives. We enabled the state plans by directly shipping test materials according to the states' requests and their testing goals. We provided $10.25 billion in May 2020 (and more to follow) to fully fund state testing plans. By the end of our term, states had spent less than $3 billion of this initial $10.25 billion in funding but were provided with even more funding ($19 billion more) by Congress in the 2021 supplemental appropriation.

When Senator Murray, the media, and the occasional academic spectator stated that there was no testing strategy, they either were intentionally misleading the public for political reasons or had not read the plans that we submitted to Congress and made public. Irrespective of the facts, media like the *New York Times* misrepresented the strategy and underplayed the support by the federal government to states—even making analogies to government-led "hunger games."[13] Schumer and Pelosi stated that the Trump administration was not taking responsibility for ramping up supplies when in point of fact, that is what we did 24-7 as outlined in this chapter. In retrospect, my assessment is that support for the states was far greater during the Trump administration than during the Biden administration in terms of both specific guidance and actual supplies distributed. Facts should matter, except the only thing that mattered to most Democrats and media was to defeat Trump.

I regularly called, in good faith, any public commentator, including detractors and political opponents, and asked for suggestions and for them to participate in finding solutions. With rare exceptions, there were no specific suggestions and, in general, a complete lack of willingness to actually grapple with the issues or assist me or anyone else in the administration. I remember calling Ashish Jha from the Roosevelt Room of the White House after one of his highly critical media commentaries. I asked for his specific suggestions and participation, which we would welcome. He was condescending and dismissive and actually had nothing to contribute. Now that Jha has joined the White House team in the Biden administration, which might have been his goal all along, he will finally be accountable for his commentaries and unrealistic demands.

Jha was in sharp contrast to other academics, like Professor Michael Mina from Harvard, who was frequently an outspoken critic of the Trump testing program and specifically the FDA but who provided useful recommendations and commentary at every stage to me personally. His assistance was extremely helpful, and I took many steps (and tried to get agencies to take many more) as a result of his scholarship and recommendations.

There were many individuals like Mina for whom I will forever be appreciative, and the nation should be as well. They critiqued loudly, but they also contributed. Even the Rockefeller Foundation—not at all ideologically aligned with the Trump administration—was a straight-up player in their interactions with me. They discussed their reports and recommendations with me *before* they were published, acknowledged our successes when appropriate, and then actively participated in (and led) pilot efforts for surveillance testing in schools for which we supplied free state-of-the-art testing supplies. Unfortunately, a few trade associations also fell into the Jha category; surprising to me was the AAMC (Association of American Medical Colleges), an organization that I had previously felt positive about. Even though I invited them to participate in the national testing forum and informally called their leadership many times. It seemed that their president, David Skorton, was much more interested in press coverage generated by issuing "surprise reports" to the media than actually discussing their recommendations at an operational level so we might implement them.

I learned a lot about politics and conflicts of interest at every level and at every stage of the response. There were many heroes, but there were also many self-interested or ideological zealots who made my job a lot harder than it needed to be. They contributed to the misinformation campaign that ultimately caused distrust and division among Americans who were just trying to figure out how to best care for their families.

STRATEGY: IN THE BEGINNING . . .

Before the formal strategy was presented to the nation in April, my team began executing a comprehensive testing plan during those initial "seven days in March." It was pretty obvious *what* we needed to do but not *exactly how* to do it. At every part of the response, there was a complex and dynamic relationship among what we knew about the virus, the stage of the pandemic, the available testing technologies and supplies, and the regulatory position of the FDA. It does no good to opine on television that we need to test everyone in the country twice a week when we have no capacity to do so. If I had a magic wand, I would have waved it because we all aspired to have billions of low-cost, highly accurate tests as soon as possible, and we did everything in our power to do so.

But I want to be clear: in late March and the first weeks of April, we were just trying to solve the acute hemorrhage; we did not have the capacity to put Band-Aids on flesh wounds. To summarize, our initial *tactics* in late March 2020 were the following:

- *Rapidly expand the CBTS from the initial drive-through federal sites to federally enabled retail sites in the commercial sector (CVS, Walgreens, others).*

CBTSs were never meant to be the major collection sites—but they would be critical to supplement the traditional health-care system, especially in areas of high social vulnerability because people in these areas were bearing the brunt of the pandemic and had the least access.

- *Immediately increase reagent capacity (meaning test kits—for example, from Hologic, Cepheid, and others) and supplies (swabs, media) as quickly and as massively as possible.*

These materials were critical for the clinical laboratories in hospitals, public health labs, ACLA labs, and academic institutions—nearly everyone. Playing off of a comment that Jared Kushner made, our strategy was to go as fast and hard as we could, but if "we got to a billion of anything," according to Jared Kushner, we could reassess and see if we could back off. While we certainly needed long-term investments, immediate expansion came primarily from technical breakthroughs and FDA regulatory flexibility—and that is where we pushed.

- *Provide rapid testing to hard-hit communities.*

In the beginning, there were no rapid POC tests whatsoever. In late March, an extremely limited supply of POC molecular tests (ID Now, Abbott) became available, but this unique and essential resource would be squandered if not allocated strategically. Jess Roach, a young public health professional who recently joined our office, worked way above her pay grade for months to implement our allocation decisions and later the combined recommendations of the FEMA allocation team that flowed through the UCG.

- *Keep US infrastructure intact and national leadership functioning.*

It became crystal clear beginning in March 2020 that my team would have special responsibilities to keep several key parts of the US domestic infrastructure operating—like the White House and the national electric power grid, as two examples. I personally fielded the calls and discussed the issues and then made some difficult decisions about who would get resources and who would not. The pressure and consequences were very high, but there was no ducking the decision-making. There were plenty of people to ask for recommendations and assessments, and I took advantage of those whom I trusted.

TESTING FOR DUMMIES

Actually, understanding the types of tests, their advantages and drawbacks, and the right way to employ them befuddled even experienced public health professionals and laboratory scientists throughout the pandemic. There are still problems in understanding the full range of testing options, and many arguments remain based more on culture and bias than actual data. So if readers are interested in gaining a fairly sophisticated understanding of the types of tests and their advantages and limitations, please refer to the appendix to this chapter. The explanations are as simple as possible but not simpler.

EXPANDING COMMUNITY TESTING THROUGH THE CBTS PROGRAM

During those eventful seven days in March, we began the CBTS program at forty-one sites under the leadership of USPHS officers. The sites were chosen because they were in areas of significant community spread or where significant spread was likely. My team was given the task to design and implement a national drive-through strategy on March 13. The first site opened on March 18, with another dozen opening that week. By April 2, all forty-one sites were fully operational. In my briefing to the vice president on May 31, 2020, I reported that these forty-one initial sites had tested over 230,000 individuals, with a positivity rate of 13.9 percent. That meant we were testing the right people, but it also meant that testing needed to continue to expand dramatically to achieve a goal of less than 10 percent positives—which at that time was the generally accepted global metric to demonstrate sufficient testing.

The forty-one initial sites were a great success but only a drop in the bucket of what would be necessary. Moreover, because they were run according to a single "cookie-cutter" plan, there was minimal flexibility for states aside from specifying the population to be tested (health-care workers, elderly, etc.). The federal government supplied all materials. Rear Admiral Schwartz was the ordering physician of record. The labs were contracted and paid for by the federal government. It worked but could not scale effectively. We clearly needed to leverage existing infrastructure but infrastructure that was outside of the typical testing landscape of doctors' offices and hospitals.

When Trump announced the public-private partnerships in the Rose Garden on March 13, the announcement was correct in a sense but a couple of weeks premature. Certainly, the retail giants wanted to help, but they would need to do much more than just offer up their parking lots. Similar to what was later done with vaccination, once the testing procedures were worked out in the forty-one initial sites, we wanted the private-sector retailers to contribute not only their parking lots but their staff, logistics, and informatics as well. So my team designed what we termed CBTS 2.0. This was launched live on April 5, the same day that the nasal self-swab was authorized, eliminating the need for a health-care provider to perform nasopharyngeal swabs. This was not a coincidence. It would have been impossible to scale testing to CBTS 2.0 without supervised self-swabbing because of both throughput issues and lack of PPE and everything else involved in provider swabbing. Looking back, the fact that it only took twenty-one days to launch 2.0 after the initial Rose Garden vision was pretty amazing. Brendan Fulmer—an advisor within the Office of the Secretary assigned to Rear Admiral Schwartz's task force—led this implementation effort with big assists from the White House team, especially Adam Boehler.

Under CBTS 2.0, the federal government paid retailers a flat fee for performing tests, and the fee was somewhat generous but still much less than the CBTS 1.0 program's overall cost per test. We were not looking for bulk discounts—we wanted something that would work and be a win-win for everyone. The retailers were responsible for all aspects of testing—supplies, contracts, scheduling, patient result reporting, and so on. This was well within the wheelhouse of retailers like CVS and Walmart if they could get paid fairly and were guaranteed a supply of testing materials. We decided on the flat fee from the federal government because, at that time, it was unclear who could get reimbursed for testing and how that would happen.

Under most rules, reimbursement (both private insurance and federal programs) required an ordering physician, and aside from CVS, which had a structure in place to do so, the other pharmacy chains did not. Testing uninsured people would eventually be reimbursed by the HRSA but required a layer of paperwork that would slow the process. So a flat fee, paid by the federal government, irrespective of whether there was an ordering physician or the person was insured, made the most sense—and most of all worked for the retailers and the American public. It was all going to come out of one federal pocket or another, so we implemented what worked best for our partners. We hit the "easy button."

The retailers generally had contracts with LabCorp or Quest, but some made arrangements with local laboratories. A few had POC testing in their stores. Our administration had requirements for the retailers to be reimbursed; for example, two-thirds of the sites had to be focused on vulnerable populations. Fortunately, the CDC publishes their Social Vulnerability Index (SVI), which takes into account race, poverty, language barriers, disability, and a number of other factors by zip code. So it was easy to ensure that CBTS 2.0 locations were in areas of moderate to high social vulnerability by checking that the zip codes matched the moderate to high SVI areas.

Also, the retailers were required to use criteria for testing that were aligned with guidance from their local public health authorities. This ensured that the available tests were being used appropriately to meet local needs. We provided federal/CDC guidelines for testing if there were no local standards, but the default was to the local recommendations—and local officials based their decisions on the outbreak status and needs within their communities. Local officials could get technical assistance from my team—or me personally—at any time they needed it, and they often did.

Retailers were also required to report results to state public health authorities and to HHS. Every day, I reviewed a dashboard sent to me by Rear Admiral Schwartz reporting the number of tests performed, the positivity rate, and very importantly, the turnaround time. I reviewed this daily by state, by retailer, and by zip code. It was the type of information we needed for the entire country but did not have the systems to collect. My final dashboard report on January 20, 2021, indicated that there were 3,027 live CBTS 2.0 locations on that day and 6.44 million tests had been accomplished, with an overall positivity rate of 10.17 percent. In January 2021, the turnaround times ranged from 1.87 days to 2.89 days, and we were very pleased about that.

CBTS 3.0 was intended to be the final evolutionary step in the program. For 3.0, retailers transitioned to an insurance-based model in which billing and reimbursement were through the traditional mechanisms of private insurance, Medicaid, Medicare, and HRSA funds for testing the uninsured. CVS was completely ready for this type of model and began transitioning in the summer of 2020. Other retailers could not transition without significant effort because their underlying organizational structure did not employ physicians or nurse practitioners. However, there was one retailer that could have transitioned but resisted doing so because it was just too easy to get a flat rate from the government. That retailer complained to members of Congress about the Trump administration pushing them to transition to this model and how it would deny testing to the needy when it was really about keeping high profit margins with the least amount of effort expended. But in general, the retailers were great partners throughout the administration.

Between CBTS 2.0 and 3.0 models, we implemented over 7,700 retail testing locations, all stemming from the initial public-private partnership announced in the Rose Garden. Again, there was no playbook, no models for contracting or engagement, and no pandemic exercises that ever contemplated such actions. The work on testing laid the foundation for the OWS vaccination program that similarly leveraged all the major pharmacy chains to get shots in arms.

All the CBTS 1.0 locations either closed or transitioned to state control by July 31, 2020, having tested over 400,000 individuals. Many localities wanted to transition to local control early on, and for good reason, and they did just that. Local control meant they could send tests to local labs, improving responsiveness and turnaround times. They could also manage registration and reporting results in ways that were more appropriate for that specific area at that specific time. But several sites wanted everything the way it was, seemingly forever, even though retail sites were fully implemented in their areas. This led to all sorts of false rhetoric, which the media was happy to exaggerate, about the federal government closing down sites in areas of high need—which was totally wrong. But some local politicians wanted to mischaracterize the situation for political advantage against the Trump administration. Rear Admiral Schwartz and I bent over backward to transition this program—and finally, we were able to do so by the end of July.

We did not anticipate a CBTS version 4.0, but we developed it because of the need and launched it on July 7, 2020. If you remember, the nation was right in the upswing of the post–Memorial Day surge. And aside from masking and "lockdowns," the only tool in our toolbox was to increase testing to identify infectious people and encourage them to isolate until they were no longer infectious. So CBTS 4.0 became our federal surge-testing program, available literally to any city, town, or county that requested a surge site.

We learned some lessons from CBTS 1.0 and 2.0. First, we wanted an end-to-end solution, preferably through the private sector. We absolutely needed to engage all of the United States in order to achieve the scale we needed, and the private sector had to be a big part of the answer. And, of course, I am a believer that with appropriate metrics for success and oversight, capitalism works. The private sector will innovate and be flexible; it will always perform better than a system of central government control. Second, we would limit surge sites to a specific number of weeks or number of tests so we would not create the expectation of an endless entitlement that would be used against us for political advantage when we tried to move to a new outbreak area. We implemented this by signing an agreement with the local authorities so there would be no misunderstanding or back-end mistruths. That being the case, we often extended the time period if it was justified—that was no issue at all. Third, we needed the flexibility to meet the needs of surge testing in various locations. Central drive-through sites could be helpful, but we also wanted mobile testing in hard-hit areas. We wanted to test special populations, whether that be multigenerational homes in Miami or public housing in Houston.

Rear Admiral Schwartz was doing market research on what companies could potentially meet the rather complex requirements for surge testing. She was struck by a company named eTrueNorth, a relatively young firm dedicated to bringing more health-care services to people through their local pharmacies. eTrueNorth had already been teaming with some of the major retailers—namely, Walmart, Health Mart, and Kroger—on their CBTS 2.0 testing. They were functioning as a system integrator, as we might have said at DARPA or in engineering circles. They would understand the need and the objectives and then put together the pieces (integrate them) to get the job done. Earlier in the pandemic, when turnaround times were getting very long at Quest, eTrueNorth came in with their partner labs and tailored solutions. It worked for huge customers like Walmart and Health Mart. I had not dealt previously with eTrueNorth. Rear Admiral Schwartz made the call, and it was vital.

To us, Coral May (eTrueNorth cofounder and CEO) was as close to a "force of nature" as I saw during the response from the private sector. In our initial conversations with Coral, Rear Admiral Schwartz and I asked if eTrueNorth could surge to any site anywhere in the United States (including Hawaii) where we directed them. Coral said, "Yes, just give us about three days' notice."

We asked if they could do multiple sites, some of them mobile, and focus on at-risk communities, like multigenerational households, going door-to-door as needed. Coral said, "Sure, no problem." We asked if they could pilot POC testing for surge sites. Coral said, "We would love to do so." We later asked if they could pioneer saliva testing at surge sites and compare that to traditional anterior nares testing, and Coral said, "Yes, we can do that too."

In DC, talk is really cheap. But Coral and eTrueNorth delivered. We told them where to go, how many tests they were to perform at each site, and the populations we needed to reach, and they did every task to our specifications and to perfection. We made surge-testing sites available to any governor who wanted them; we never said no to any request. By January 20, 2021, the CBTS 4.0 program had done surge testing in 658 different sites in twenty-three states. This resulted in approximately 900,000 tests being administered, with an overall positivity of 7.28 percent. The overall turnaround time was 1.84 days, and during the peak need for testing in January 2021, it had dropped to 0.75 days (yes, under 1 day).

DID THE CBTS PROGRAMS REALLY MATTER TO THE RESPONSE?

The CBTS program made several important contributions. First, it was the major innovation engine for testing by developing and implementing safe, efficient, and scalable models that were used throughout the nation. The needs of the program also drove the rapid adoption and FDA authorization of anterior nasal swabs, which changed the entire scope of testing in the United States. Sure, that would have eventually happened, but it was accelerated by at least four to six weeks because of the urgent needs of the CBTS program and its prioritization by my office. Second, especially early on, CBTS was the primary mechanism for hard-hit communities to keep their health-care personnel and first responders on the job while minimizing the risk to others. Later in the response, it was our assurance to socially vulnerable communities that the administration cared about them; we were testing in their communities. Third, the program was the physical means through which the public-private partnership operated. Giving a motivational speech in the Rose Garden is one thing, but actually making the program work and expanding it to thousands of sites is another thing altogether.

There were so many people on my team that made this program a success. But I cannot overstate the amount of credit that is deserved to Rear Admiral

Schwartz, Major Bilderback (Major Badass), Brendan Fulmer, and all the people working with them (night and day) to keep pushing this program to its eventual massive scale. The CBTS program also laid the groundwork for the more than forty thousand pharmacies that were enrolled to provide shots in arms for OWS. The transition from testing to vaccination was a natural progression, building on the foundation, structure, and trust engendered by the CBTS program.

ABBOTT ID NOW: THE FIRST POINT OF CARE

March 27, 2020, was a critically important day that provided us with an early break the nation needed. On that day, the FDA authorized the Abbott ID NOW POC test. Instead of collecting a sample, putting it in transport media, sending it to a high-complexity lab, and waiting days for the result, the Abbott ID NOW test used a sophisticated amplification technique in a toaster-sized instrument, with results available in five to thirteen minutes. In fact, there were already over eighteen thousand of these instruments available throughout the United States in clinics and physician offices testing for flu and other common illnesses; they were just waiting for the COVID-19 test to be FDA authorized and delivered. The main drawback was that only one test could be done at a time in each machine, making it only able to test four to six samples per hour per machine. The other consideration was that it was less sensitive than lab-based molecular tests, but in retrospect, it was likely to be positive if the person had enough virus to be infectious to others. And that is really what we needed to know.

Abbott told my team that they would rapidly achieve a production of three hundred thousand tests each week, which seems like a large quantity but is not really given the United States' seemingly infinite demand for rapid testing. I knew that there would be such an overwhelming demand for these tests that this precious resource could be squandered if not managed carefully. And so started my relationship with Robert Ford, CEO of Abbott. Over the next ten months, we would speak several times per week, first about ID NOW and much later about the BinaxNOW rapid antigen tests. Robert was a matter-of-fact type of guy, a little crusty, brutally honest, and always clear that he had all the resources necessary to do the research and maximally scale production. At least he thought so early on. He was straight up when he disagreed with me, but those instances were rare, and we worked through our disagreements as colleagues.

Like me, Robert realized that ID NOW was a precious resource. I asked him to work with me on getting the most out of this resource that we could, and he agreed immediately. In March 2020, I had not heard of DPA, nor had the president yet invoked it for any supplies, not even ventilators or N95 masks. But even if I had known about the DPA, I would not have invoked it with Abbott. The DPA was not a magic wand—it could not create matter out of nothing or violate the laws of physics. The pandemic was going to be a long haul, and it seemed better for me to work collaboratively and transparently without the heavy hand of the DPA—unless, of course, it was absolutely necessary. Robert was going to work with me, and I trusted him. So we proceeded. My trust was well founded.

As a priority, we wanted to ensure that every public health lab had both instruments and tests every week. The public health labs could use these for outbreak investigations—like in nursing homes or critical industries like food processing. Because of the size and portability of the instrument, it could be brought right to the spot of the outbreak, and tests could be done on-site with results in minutes. It would be a godsend to test a nursing home worker during an outbreak and be able to tell immediately if he or she were positive. If negative, they would continue to mask and stay in the workforce to provide care to the elderly residents. The same thing is true for critical infrastructure workers. So the public health labs were at the top of my list. We also wanted to fully supply underserved populations, especially where expansive geographies and overall lack of medical access were insurmountable barriers. There were special needs—some of which we could fix, but not all. These were very hard decisions, but I needed to make them.

I don't recall the specific date, but I was in my office when Attorney General Barr called me about the Federal Bureau of Prisons. I had not spent much time with him before; in fact, the only interactions I had with him were in the Oval Office briefing the president about fentanyl and methamphetamine trafficking across the southern border. On the phone, the attorney general was very soft spoken and deliberate with every word. He talked to me about the horrible COVID outbreaks in the federal prisons and that we as a country and he personally had a special obligation to care for those in our custody. He was very sincere, and I believed he was personally troubled by the situation. Of course, we would supply rapid tests per his request, and as he probably knew, my officers in the USPHS Commissioned Corps supplied a substantial amount of the health care in those same federal prisons. So I knew the tests would be used wisely for this vulnerable population.

Abbott ID NOW was authorized by the FDA on March 27. Beginning April 3, my team took charge. We bought every available instrument in the Abbott warehouse and sent fifteen of these to at least one public health lab in every state. For Alaska, I sent fifty instruments because of their vast geographies and the inability to transport samples due to distance or weather. The Indian Health Service received 250 instruments for similar reasons. And we also sent instruments to the US Pacific Islands—since they were thousands of miles away from the nearest commercial labs. After the initial order, we committed to buying between fifty to one hundred instruments each week—which turned out to be a good investment because needs always arose, and we were able to meet those needs without completely disrupting the commercial supply to traditional health-care institutions.

Along with the instruments, we needed to purchase tests and allocate them. My team, together with Abbott, did some rough calculations on the numbers we wanted. Part of the decision was how much of the supply we would take out of the commercial market because all tests would have been used for COVID purposes—whether bought by the federal government or the private sector. It was a zero-sum game. I decided that the federal government would procure one hundred thousand of the available three hundred thousand tests per week. And that is what we did, with the option to increase the number if needed. And so every week between April 3, 2020, and January 2, 2021, sixty thousand tests went to the state public health labs, twenty thousand were allocated to the Indian Health Service, and ten thousand were sent to the federal prisons. Smaller states by population got proportionally more tests per capita because the smaller population states (like Montana) had challenges of rural geographies and a lack of laboratory infrastructure. Major academic medical centers like those in Boston did not really need a handout from us to support testing, but Massachusetts still got a small share of the POC tests because they needed them for special circumstances just like everyone else.

In addition to the one hundred thousand we purchased directly each week, Robert Ford and his head of diagnostics agreed to allocate the remaining two hundred thousand tests to states in rough proportion to the number of cases reported. And thus my team received and approved every week how many tests were ordered and were going to be sent to states—down to the specific laboratory, urgent care, or doctor's office. We rarely heard of any needs beyond what we were sending, but when we did, we always had a small reserve of machines and tests in the stockpile to send on short notice.

In retrospect, the most important aspect of this program was an assurance of the supply to the recipients. All kinds of strange things happen when the supply is uncertain, like New York City storing masks and gowns in the warehouse waiting for the system to crash before resupplying their hospitals. The public health labs, state health officers, the Indian Health Service, and federal prisons could use all their tests each week because they knew there would be resupply from my team the following week.

If you do the math, there were about ten thousand tests per week unaccounted for by the allocation I indicated above. For those ten thousand, I felt like I was judge and jury because there were requests from so many places, and it truly was a zero-sum game. But there were needs that rose above the others. The Department of Defense needed rapid tests—and I understood that from my time at DARPA and other Defense Department touchpoints. It would have been really bad to launch one of our ballistic nuclear submarines from port—needed perhaps more than ever to deter the Russians and Chinese during a time of potential US vulnerability—but have to scrap the mission because of a COVID outbreak on the submarine. Similarly, the United States could not afford to deploy Special Forces or US Navy SEALs with an infected and infectious member. So the Defense Department always received their requested allocations—how they used them specifically, I did not have a need to know and never asked.

The Department of Veterans Affairs also had special needs. I was committed to supplying the armed forces and veterans, as the vice president rightfully insisted—and so we did. We also supplied tests to the Secret Service, the DHS, and a very select group of technical specialists organized by the Department of Energy (about a thousand of them) that literally kept the US power grid operating. We also supplied, for a time, FedEx and UPS. The Chinese (after being the origin of the pandemic and then failing to be transparent about it) were imposing strict testing requirements and potential incarceration on US pilots flying into and out of China. FedEx and UPS were essential components of our airbridges to obtain supplies we sourced in China, and so my team supplied instruments and tests so that the pilots and crew could continue their vital airlifts of PPE and other supplies from Asia.

Last but certainly not least, the White House needed tests in order to screen people meeting the president or the vice president. I made sure that the White House was fully supplied but always urged that testing be only one component of protection, not the entire strategy. Tests could be falsely negative, even very good tests, meaning that infected people could get through the screening process, and even if truly negative, that person is only negative for that moment in time and could turn positive in eight to twenty-four hours.

But the White House, in general, thought that *testing negative* was a golden ticket. And until Trump tested positive on October 2, 2020, there was almost no mask wearing or physical distancing in the White House. Most of the task force doctors were surprised by that situation, and we wore masks whenever we could—especially in the narrow hallways of the West Wing. But the average age of White House staffers was probably thirty years old, and there was rarely a mask to be seen, even in the tight quarters near the Oval Office. When the Trump family tested positive, masking habits generally changed at the White House. And for the first time, there was also physical distancing practiced at the White House Coronavirus Task Force meetings, meaning that attendance was virtual except for those actually needed around the main conference table in the Situation Room.

I make it a point in this book to talk about the people involved on my teams because they were really the ones who made the response happen and deserve a great deal of the credit. Jess Roach was one of those people who worked on many major initiatives in the response, but one of her most important contributions was leading the Abbott ID NOW testing planning and allocation. Jess was a 2008 graduate from the University of Michigan who later received her master of public health from George Washington University in Washington, DC. She was quite successful as a global health officer in the Office of Global Affairs at HHS. I met her when she was my lead staffer during the World Health Assembly of the WHO in 2018, when for several days, I was the lead US representative, since the secretary was detained in DC. At the WHO meetings, Jess was meticulous and detail oriented and provided me with not only what I needed to know but everything I should know about every issue, the history of every US policy position, and even every minister I met from dozens of other countries. She was a talent, and I wanted her in my OASH office. I actually tried to recruit her to be my deputy chief of staff, but she turned me down!

But in October 2019, she finally accepted a position as the senior policy advisor in the OASH Office of HIV and Infectious Disease Policy—to work on the Ending the HIV Epidemic in the US initiative under Tammy Beckham (then director of that office). When COVID hit and Tammy assumed leadership of the Laboratory Diagnostics Task Force, I knew Tammy could use assistance from Jess. Therefore, Jess became the deputy director for policy and communications for that task force—basically Tammy's right-hand person. Jess was incredibly capable but young and not accustomed to daily being subjected to the stress of the century or dealing with demanding and often desperate individuals from every segment of our nation. She came to me one day and said that she "just wasn't built for this," but I reassured her that not only was she indeed *built for this* but she was uniquely capable because of her expertise, her integrity, and her dedication to service. Jess did her job under great duress and little sleep, working seven days per week for months. She is a great example of one of the highly dedicated career public servants who live only for public health and the greater good of every person on the planet. She represents—and to some degree epitomizes—many of the career officials throughout the government who regularly go above and beyond and serve as the "glue" keeping things running between administrations.

CEPHEID GENEXPERT

A week before Abbott ID NOW's EUA by the FDA, another very important EUA was issued, this time for the Cepheid GeneXpert—a truly unique diagnostics system with which I was very familiar. Cepheid advertised their system as a "point of care," which is partly true and partly not. The Cepheid device is a true PCR system but one that is highly automated so that the many steps involved are done micromechanically inside a sophisticated cartridge. The technician literally pipettes the sample from the test tube into the cartridge and puts the cartridge into the device (about thirty-five pounds for the small version of the device), and the result is available within forty-five minutes. Depending on the instrument, four, eight, sixteen, or even thirty-two samples can be done simultaneously.

Seeing Cepheid rise to the challenge early in the pandemic was very satisfying to me. Twenty-plus years earlier, Cepheid had been a DARPA-funded project supporting the cutting-edge microfluidics needed to automate a testing system. DARPA's goal was to take sophisticated PCR technology and have it available in a suitcase system that a US Army corporal could use on the battlefield to detect biological weapons like anthrax. The program was a complete success, and Cepheid revolutionized PCR testing. Dr. Birx told me that for PEPFAR, Cepheid devices were in vans traveling all over Africa to diagnose HIV and tuberculosis. DARPA had again silently made an incredible impact on the world, but DARPA's role was basically forgotten.

There were already over eight thousand GeneXpert systems in the United States doing testing, and that was good news. Similar to Africa, the systems were being used primarily for HIV and tuberculosis testing but also for many other infectious diseases. Cepheid would be able to produce about one million tests in April 2020 by shifting production from other tests like HIV, but they would only be able to ramp up to 1.5 million tests per month by the late fall. It was not a matter of money or supplies that slowed Cepheid—they had all the money and resources they needed. The paradox was this: the sophistication of the platform made it easy to use but very hard to manufacture at scale. The systems inside included numerous microfluidic pumps, mixing chambers, a sonic device to disrupt the viruses, and so on. The cartridge was highly sophisticated and even had a very exacting design with multiple chambers and microfluidic channels. I would have purchased twenty million per month if I could, but that was physically impossible. So Cepheid was going to occupy a critical niche in the ecosystem, but it would never dominate US testing.

By late April, Brad Smith's team at the White House located and mapped every single testing device in the United States that could possibly run COVID tests (from every manufacturer). This was a monumental advance in our knowledge and was critical for us to best allocate testing resources. Brad's team determined that many small metropolitan service areas were at least 50 percent dependent on Cepheid for their testing needs. There were many rural areas that were actually 100 percent dependent on Cepheid. That made sense—it was a very accurate system, highly sensitive, extremely easy to use, relatively inexpensive, but not high throughput. This was perfect for small rural hospitals and medium-sized towns that needed accuracy but did not have high numerical demand nor high-complexity labs or abundant trained staff.

We decided that these Cepheid-dependent areas would receive a much higher proportion of Cepheid cartridges per capita every month than other areas. And when there were regional outbreaks in areas that were highly dependent on Cepheid, we surged Cepheid tests to those areas preferentially. We sent a dozen Cepheid devices and tens of thousands of tests to Alaska during the salmon fishing season, during which some sixty thousand fishermen and processing plant workers would descend upon that state (and their very vulnerable Native Alaskan population) from all parts of the world and congregate in extremely close quarters for months.

"THE STATES WERE LEFT ON THEIR OWN FOR TESTING"

Aside from the false claim that there was no national testing strategy, the most egregious mischaracterization of the federal response was the disingenuous allegation that "states were left on their own" for testing and diagnostics. Certainly, the states had an essential role in implementing testing, just like they had in the OWS vaccination program. For both testing and vaccination, there was extensive collaborative planning between the states and the federal government, with supplies provided federally and scale provided through federal contracts with commercial retailers. In addition to the federal leadership and coordination of testing, the White House Coronavirus Task Force provided detailed recommendations for everything from testing to masking and antiviral treatment down to the county level to each governor every week—and I will discuss that in chapter 11.

But specifically related to testing and the states, the federal government established and supported over 7,700 CBTS locations (not counting surge sites) as well as testing in 1,200+ community health centers in many thousands of locations. We also provided surge testing to every city/county/state in which there was even a hint of an emerging outbreak. From my first week as the testing czar, we also supplied the state public health labs with reagents and supplies like swabs and media. We assured that public health labs had the latest in point-of-care technology—namely, Abbott ID NOW tests beginning in late March. As soon as FEMA was named the lead agency, we received requests for materials and responded to them via the FEMA process to the degree that we could. I spent incredible amounts of phone time with governors and state health officers personally trying to understand the true need and intended uses—because *yes*, everything was in short supply. We would not have enough tests for everyone in the country to be tested—not even close. Everybody that wanted a test could not get a test. We needed to focus on the most urgent needs, which was frustrating to everyone, but that was the reality. No magic wands were available on Amazon!

In mid-April, we ramped up national testing to a different level. By that time, we had fully engaged every single manufacturer of assays, swabs, and media within the United States or with ties to the United States (including Copan in Italy). We knew exactly what diagnostic assays were going to be available at what time and from which manufacturer and where they were going to be shipped. In fact, beginning in April, we knew there would be more diagnostic tests available on the market than would be used, and this surplus would become larger and larger every month of our administration.

The real issue was that *not every lab would be able to get the exact test system that they wanted and were most familiar with*. Most large labs wanted Roche or Hologic, but there were not enough of those tests to go around. We needed labs to have flexibility in their choices (take a Ford versus a Ferrari: both will get you where you want to go, but there are a lot more Fords available, and sometimes Ford wins the race anyway!).

We had many bases covered by mid-April—or perhaps "pieced together" is a more accurate description than "covered." The large commercial labs would continue to scale rapidly and consistently supply about half the nation's testing. The public health labs would do about 10 percent of testing, which was their maximum given their small footprints and regional missions.

Thanks to Deb Birx, who was a laboratory scientist in addition to being a clinician, we knew where every PCR machine was throughout the United States and geolocated them on maps. Finally, the last important piece was funding for the states. The Paycheck Protection Program and Health Care Enhancement Act (Public Law No. 116-139), signed on April 24, 2020, by Trump, provided $11 billion to state, local, territory, and tribal organizations to develop, purchase, administer, process, and analyze COVID-19 tests, scale-up laboratory capacity, trace contacts, and support employer testing.

Just like the CDC "microplanned" COVID vaccinations for OWS, we engaged in coordinated planning with every state and territory. The logistics burden was carried primarily by a young political appointee working in the White House, Quellie Moorhead, who began in February 2017 as a research analyst in the Office of American Innovation and in May 2019 became special assistant to the president and director of the Office of Policy Coordination. It did not matter what her duties had been previously because she ran into the "burning building" of COVID when the pandemic hit. Quellie was unflappable, ultraorganized, and determined to achieve the mission. She worked closely with Brad, and together they were essential to the next phase of testing.

On April 20, each state received the specific location of every piece of major diagnostic equipment that could be used for COVID testing in their state. On April 21, a multidisciplinary federal team with experts from the OASH, FEMA, the CDC, and other agencies held a technical assistance overview call with 304 individuals in leadership roles from every state and territory. In general, the state participants included a representative from the Office of the Governor, the state public health laboratory, the state health official, and the state epidemiologist—or their equivalents.

The multidisciplinary federal team then held a series of individual, personalized technical assistance calls with each and every state, DC, and Puerto Rico beginning on April 23. On April 29, we began a second round of technical assistance calls individually with each state. The outcomes of these calls were the testing goals for each state for May and June and detailed plans to maximize testing capacity.

The overall testing goals were set by considering multiple factors, including the rate of new cases, plans for mitigation, percent positivity, and other factors. The federal team would guarantee all the swabs and tubes of media each state needed and would deliver these supplies weekly to a central state cache to be further distributed according to the state testing plan. The federal team also instructed each state on how to obtain additional diagnostic testing by using the ACLA labs and other testing resources. Specifically, we told each state which specific tests it could expect to receive, like Hologic, and how it could make up any deficits by switching to other available platforms like Thermo Fisher or PerkinElmer, which were in overabundant supply and could be scaled almost infinitely.

At that time, we projected twenty-eight to thirty-two million end-to-end tests would be available in May 2020. There was more than enough actual capacity to supply the projected state needs as long as individual laboratories exercised some flexibility in their choice of tests (Ford versus Ferrari). The federal team provided states with contacts at companies and facilitated the distribution of tests as requested. Each state was also given the name and contact information of a dedicated federal point of contact (their personal federal "concierge" whom they could call at any time for any issue related to testing). This is the opposite of states being on their own!

We in the federal government did not mandate a specific amount of testing be done in each state. We did not know the right answer and also did not have the authority or means to mandate anything in that regard. However, we did provide specific technical assistance and "required" each state to have a minimum goal of testing 2 percent of its population within that month, but we encouraged much more than that. The 2 percent number was empiric, based on our observations that 2 percent was minimally sufficient to detect a change in the percent positivity, which inexorably foreshadowed an increase in cases, hospitalizations, and deaths. Once changes in positivity were seen, we could surge the entire panoply of resources to that region, including testing and hospital personnel, and provide specific advice to the governors, which we did weekly.

Indeed, many states had goals around the 2 percent level for those first months, including Georgia, Nebraska, Kansas, and Oregon. Several states had more aggressive targets, including New York at 7.7 percent, Massachusetts at 10 percent, and Rhode Island at nearly 15 percent for the month of May. The overall testing goal for the states and territories was 12.9 million in May, and we could support that number—twice that, actually, with the materials we projected.

The state testing goals and plans would be formalized by each state submitting its comprehensive plan to HHS by May 30, 2020, as a condition of receiving the $11 billion allocated from the Paycheck Protection Program. Congress had actually *not given HHS any authority* to mandate that states meet specific requirements in order to receive the money, but we acted as if we had the authority anyway so that we could ensure every state would have an acceptable plan.

Tammy and I developed a specific template that we "required" the states to complete. After submission, each plan underwent peer review by a multidisciplinary federal team of subject matter experts, including members of the CDC as well as the Testing and Diagnostics Task Force and the White House. States then received feedback about the quality and sufficiency of their plans across every parameter in the template. And, of course, this was not an "exam" that they would "fail." The federal team was there to help and was available throughout the process to work on any aspects of the state plan in a collaborative fashion. The plan was submitted in two parts: The first was due in May for May and June. There would be a second submission, which was an expansion of the first plan, due at the end of June to cover the period from July through December 2020.

Our template "required" the state plans to be comprehensive and robust. The template included planning sections for contact tracing and surveillance of asymptomatic persons to determine community spread; a section to ensure that the state could surge testing if needed using POC instruments; plans for testing at nontraditional sites, including community centers and retail sites; special provisions for testing at-risk and vulnerable populations, including the elderly, the disabled, those in congregate living facilities such as prisons, and racial and ethnic minorities and other similar groups; testing of individuals working in critical infrastructure sectors; and plans for partnerships with academic, commercial, and hospital laboratories to successfully meet testing demands.

The review panel was chaired by me personally and included experts from the Diagnostics Task Force, the NIH, the CDC, and other agencies. Every plan received specific feedback in writing and verbally. A great majority of the plans were very good or outstanding, but a few were woefully lacking and needed major revisions. By the second plan submission, essentially all of the state plans were excellent and had been specifically tailored for their states' needs. In the interest of transparency, on August 10, HHS published all the state plans.[14] Congress was about to demand these be disclosed to them, and I am sure the "Senator Murrays" within Congress would have used (abused) them for political purposes, so we just published all of them on an HHS website to get ahead of any political games. I never received *a single comment or criticism* from any media expert or pundit regarding the state plans or the process for their development. And that is because the plans were well thought out and appropriate for that phase of the pandemic.

Beginning in May, we sent states every swab and tube of media they requested according to their plans (totaling 191 million swabs and 229 million tubes of media by January 2021). We advised on the distribution of lab assays to meet state needs, even if the lab assays were not always the first choice (Ford versus Ferrari).

In May, the materials we sent were a mix of whatever we could procure, including multiple different swab and media types—all FDA authorized but not always the typical product labs were familiar with. In fact, in May, we had to piece together fifteen different suppliers of swabs and media, who all sent their materials to FEMA for repackaging and shipping. It was crazy logistics. In May, we got two weeks behind schedule and needed to make that up later in the month. We also had to use materials in formats that were unfamiliar to test sites. For example, instead of individually wrapped swabs, we supplemented individually wrapped swabs with sterile bulk packages of swabs, accompanied by specific instructions on how to use them without contamination. Such bulk packaging was specifically OK'd by the FDA, especially for use in large testing sites, but a few officials in states only wanted individually wrapped swabs and balked at the bulk swabs. In May, though, there just were not that many options. We needed flexibility, and the lack of flexibility among some was incredibly frustrating and actually quite narrow-minded. It was a pandemic of unprecedented scale, and we needed everyone to use what was authorized and available.

One of the most publicized and politicized episodes was when we had to send some swabs in packages that were not reflective of the package content. Specifically, we had to send some spun polyester swabs (which were FDA authorized for PCR) in baby Q-tip packages because that is the only package that the manufacturer had at the time. We had calls with all states informing them of the packaging issue before they were sent. We sent letters to all the states. And we put instructions and documentation with the actual supply that was shipped, again detailing what was actually in the packages. So everyone knew about the packaging issue, but some political hacks nevertheless took the opportunity to make a media spectacle and try to embarrass the administration.

I made the decision not to delay sending materials by a month because the packaging wasn't correct—my decision. Perhaps I should have delayed it to avoid the politics and the media spectacle. But our actions were not driven by politics or the media—they were driven by trying to get testing to the right people at the right time. That being said, all packaging and labeling were perfect by the beginning of June, with shipments delivered on time as requested by the states. The program went off with few additional hitches.

CUOMO AT THE WHITE HOUSE

There was obviously a lot of tension between President Trump and Governor Cuomo. I had never personally heard Trump speak badly about Cuomo, which was unusual, since the president spoke freely about many people and issues with members of the task force. His dislike for certain governors and congressional members was clear and not hidden from the media, but I had not heard a single negative comment about Cuomo in any meeting with the president. And if anything, despite not immediately sending New York forty thousand ventilators (which they did not need and we did not have), Trump and Jared responded to New York's needs attentively. There was no reasonable request by New York that went unfulfilled. If anything, New York was prioritized because it was hit hard early, and the president empathized with the plight of the people there. It was his home turf.

After a couple of weeks of back and forth in the media and according to press reports on calls between Trump and Cuomo, the two leaders decided to have a meeting on April 21 privately, mano a mano, at the White House. The main issue was that Cuomo wanted to double testing to forty thousand tests per day and felt that the US government was not supplying his state with the reagents and supplies he needed. He also needed additional clarifications about the roles and responsibilities of the state versus the federal government—not only for testing but for reopening. Cuomo believed that he should have the authority as governor to determine when to reopen instead of Trump. In general, I actually was in full agreement with Cuomo's position, since I supported our federal system—for better or worse.

I was not going to be in the meeting with Trump and Cuomo. But Jared Kushner had arranged a meeting for Cuomo with Brad Smith, myself, and a select few members of the White House team in the Roosevelt Room—immediately before the meeting between Cuomo and Trump. Our team was seated for a few minutes before the governor arrived. He entered from a hallway near the entrance to the Oval Office, so he had obviously been meeting with someone else (likely Jared) before our meeting.

I think both the governor and our team were prepared for a long, confrontational, and unfulfilling meeting. I did not look forward to it. But the governor was professional and cordial. He had never been very collegial on my previous phone calls with him during the first week at FEMA, but he was professional and polished that day at the White House. He stated how he absolutely needed to double the testing in New York, and that meant doubling federal support for supplies: swabs, media, and most importantly diagnostic assays. Probably more advanced than any other governor at the time, Cuomo had already figured out how to create state testing centers by bringing PCR machines together in a cluster and using them to expand the traditional health-care system. He stated that fact in the meeting. These clusters could supplement the already advanced and capable New York health-care infrastructure, combined with our CBTSs and the large commercial labs that serviced the area. Cuomo was actually doing exactly what we wanted him and every other governor to do.

It was perhaps the shortest meeting in history. Cuomo came into the room and stated he needed to double supplies in order to double testing. If we could do that, New York could do the rest. Brad and I both responded, "Yes, sir. No problem. Done." Cuomo said something like "Really?" We confirmed the response. We had surplus PCR capability from Thermo Fisher (which actually could expand to almost any level we needed), and the governor said that platform would work fine for his state, since New York had hundreds of instruments that were perfect to run those assays. The governor was happy, and so were we. Whatever else Cuomo did or did not do effectively during the pandemic, he was on top of testing and understood clearly how to work together with the feds in a collaborative fashion.

I don't know what was said between Trump and Cuomo, but Cuomo's press conferences after the White House meetings indicated that he was very satisfied and received the commitments he sought. Even the *New York Times* had nothing negative to report about the meeting.[15] Within the next week, our one-on-one coordination meetings with New York actually set a goal for fifty thousand tests per day, more than the original commitment Brad and I made to the governor. We were happy to increase the number and then continue to expand from there.

Everyone who wanted a test still could not get one, but we were increasingly confident in our ability to ensure that everyone who "needed a test" could find one conveniently and quickly and with highly reliable results.

APPENDIX

A Primer for COVID Testing

RT-PCR Tests

The initial CDC tests, the WHO-sponsored tests, and the South Korean tests were all tests based on RT-PCR, which involves copying the viral RNA onto a DNA template and subsequently amplifying that template through the repeated heating and cooling of the sample over dozens of cycles. With PCR, two copies of the viral targets turn into 1,090,000,000,000 copies (over one trillion) in about four hours! PCR is not a new technique—it is used daily in labs across the world for detecting viruses like the HIV or hepatitis C viruses. With one exception (Cepheid), all RT-PCR tests were initially done in high-complexity laboratories at major health-care systems, public health labs, or commercial referral labs.

For COVID-19 RT-PCR, first a sample by a swab must be collected and then placed into a tube with transport media or saline. Then the sample is transported to the lab (which could be next door or across the country), where the actual test is performed inside a PCR device (which takes several hours once the samples are sufficiently batched). The results are subsequently reported back to the patient and the state health authorities. When the process is working smoothly and there is no backlog, results are returned in twenty-four to forty-eight hours. But during the early stages of the pandemic and extending into the late summer of 2020, because of several rate-limiting steps at the level of the laboratories themselves, results took three to five days and often longer to return. There were times when results took seven days and on rare occasions even longer, depending on the location of the patient and the prioritization we gave that specific test (e.g., tests needed for hospitalized patients versus those for people traveling to another state). I followed turnaround times on a daily basis from all major commercial labs, and decreasing these was a constant focus of my team's efforts.

The advantages of RT-PCR tests were their familiarity among all laboratories and the fact that the basic RT-PCR procedure could be easily adapted to SARS-CoV-2 by large labs and even small academic ones (as was done by South Korea, the WHO, and even the CDC if it were not for contamination and a slow fix). The other apparent advantage, which also turned out to be its greatest and most misunderstood weakness, is that RT-PCR is very sensitive (remember, two copies are amplified to one trillion copies). That means that if there is even any small remnant of viral RNA present, the RT-PCR test will likely be positive. Much later on in the pandemic, we understood that a person could be positive even weeks after no longer being capable of transmitting the virus to another individual. So being positive according to an RT-PCR test does not equate to being actively infected with the live virus or being able to transmit the virus to other people. This fact was operationalized when the CDC recommended the release from quarantine based on the amount of time since the first symptoms, not a negative test.

Whoever says that RT-PCR is the "gold standard" is speaking from a very narrow clinical diagnostics point of view. Yes, PCR was certainly the *first* standard and a valuable one, but knowing when and when not to rely on it—and for what specific conclusions—has remained a heated debate throughout the pandemic, even to this day. We affectionately called these people who, despite data and the important public health implications at a population level, would only recognize nasopharyngeal swabs analyzed by RT-PCR as an acceptable test "lab snobs." These snobs resulted in great harm to the overall mission of testing, and I believe that resulted in lives lost.

Nucleic Acid Testing Not *Using RT-PCR*

There are a number of methods that amplify the genetic material of the virus but do not do it by sequentially raising and lowering the temperature. Since the temperature does not change, these methods are generally characterized as "isothermal amplification." Avoiding the rapid changes in temperature allows amplification to be done more quickly and in a much smaller instrument. For example, the Abbott ID NOW COVID-19 assay uses isothermal amplification technology in a "toaster-sized" instrument that is extremely easy to use, relatively inexpensive, and employed in thousands of emergency rooms, urgent care clinics, and physicians' offices every day to diagnose infections like influenza and strep throat. For ID NOW, only one test can be run at a time, and it has to be run at the point of collection (not transported in media to another location). But results are available in fifteen minutes or less. And sometimes that speed really matters.

Early isothermal technologies like Abbott ID NOW were generally considered less sensitive than RT-PCR but also more sensitive than antigen tests. These were also on average about half the price of RT-PCR tests (with exceptions) but more expensive than antigen tests.

Antigen Tests

Antigen tests do not detect the presence of viral genetic material after amplifying it. Rather, antigen tests use antibodies (like the ones people develop after recovering from an infection or getting vaccinated) to identify specific protein components of the virus. Antigen tests are very commonly used in clinical medicine. For example, they are by far the most common tests for strep throat and influenza, employed widely in doctors' offices and school clinics. Although there are multiple new variations that were developed later in the pandemic, antigen tests on the market before COVID-19 generally came in two varieties: one that required a very inexpensive instrument (a "reader") to determine whether the test was negative or positive and a second in which the health-care provider (or the person being tested) physically observes a change in the test (like the common pregnancy test) to indicate whether the test was positive or negative.

Antigen tests (most types are lateral flow tests, or LFTs) are also rapid, with results within fifteen minutes or less. A health-care provider can also easily daisy-chain multiple tests at the same time, so it is possible to do fifteen to twenty tests within an hour. This can be done in any laboratory that is "a laboratory" by CLIA (Clinical Laboratory Improvement Amendments) standards, and some can even be performed at home. They are the least expensive of all tests. To make a long story short—and the evidence is now very clear—antigen tests are very likely to detect the virus (become positive) when the person is actually *infectious* but less likely than RT-PCR at detecting remnants of the virus in people who are no longer infectious to others. Antigen tests might also fail to detect small amounts of the virus when a person has just become infected, so repeat testing a few days later takes care of the problem of people with very early infections.

So in summary, RT-PCR is much more likely to identify a person as positive but much worse at differentiating if that person can actually spread the disease. As a public health leader, I really wanted something that was rapid and cheap and could tell me who was capable of infecting others. And that was Professor Mina's continued (and continuing) point. This is why antigen tests, if deployed correctly and as part of an ordered testing ecosystem, should be the foundation of a national public health testing strategy for COVID-19 and any other pandemic we may face in the future.

False Positives

All tests, no matter what type, are highly *specific*, meaning that if you are positive on the test, you are actually positive for what the test is looking for (viral RNA or antigens). However, since RT-PCR is so sensitive to even a few molecules of genetic material, there is always the possibility of a contaminant getting into the mix—in which case the test will perform correctly (detect the RNA or DNA that is truly there) but be falsely positive about the actual patient because the test is picking up contaminating genetic material that does not belong to the patient. Although this happens rarely with modern laboratory techniques, it did happen on numerous occasions during COVID, including the initial contaminated CDC tests. Most notably, in August 2020, there were seventy-seven false positive RT-PCR tests among NFL football players from the same reference laboratory. If not for the fact that these were high-profile athletes and the results were shocking to the NFL, these false positives might have gone unnoticed and uncorrected. Those seventy-seven might have believed they were infected but actually were not.

10

Rapid Antigen Tests Finally Arrive

THE NURSING HOME IMPERATIVE

Nothing in the nation's early pandemic response incited more emotion and visceral reaction than the issue of nursing homes (also known as skilled nursing facilities or SNFs, pronounced "sniffs"). From the initial viral onslaught that ravaged the Life Care Center of Kirkland, Washington, in February and March 2020 to the catastrophic governor's mandate in New York that nursing homes must accept patients who are still infected and contagious, it was clear that nursing homes were ground zero. Indeed, in the first months of the pandemic, 40 percent of deaths occurred among nursing home residents. These people were vulnerable not only because of their advanced age and chronic health conditions but also because they lived in a congregate setting for which staffing was generally insufficient and inadequately trained. Infection control for a respiratory-transmitted virus like COVID-19 was extraordinarily challenging, if not impossible. Even with imperfect information, we understood the urgency for decisive actions. Over 1.4 million people lived in 15,500 nursing homes in the United States, and every minute delay would cost lives.

Within the federal government, the Center for Medicare and Medicaid Services (CMS) has the responsibility to oversee and regulate nursing homes and shares with state agencies the responsibility for ensuring that nursing homes meet federal requirements for quality and safety. Even before the pandemic hit, Seema Verma, the CMS administrator, took this responsibility seriously and was proactive about issuing guidance and regulations to improve quality and patient safety. In November 2018, Seema enhanced CMS oversight to ensure adequate staffing. In March 2019, together with the CDC, the CMS offered free online training to improve infection control practices in nursing homes (prescient, to say the least). In July 2019, Seema eliminated the burden of unnecessary regulations in nursing homes through her "patients before paperwork" initiative. There were many other steps to improve quality and transparency before COVID attacked our elderly. With the arrival of COVID-19, the CMS frequently updated guidelines for nursing homes, including PPE recommendations, infection control, visitation, and every other aspect of patient safety.

Prior to the pandemic, I had many interactions with the CMS concerning opioid-prescribing policies, but Seema had a potential conflict of interest and thus recused herself from any interactions with me on that topic. As a result, I had not worked much with Seema and did not know her personally. But once COVID escalated, I began collaborating with her on a daily basis at the White House Coronavirus Task Force level and also individually on many challenges. Seema had a bad reputation among many at HHS, and her rivalry with the secretary was widely reported in the media—but I had no firsthand knowledge of that. Personally, I found Seema to be one of my best colleagues in the response. She deferred medical and science issues to the doctors, but when a recommendation was clear, she was fearless about implementing it. Seema felt personally responsible for the welfare of nursing home residents and to a large degree the quality of the US hospital system. She preferred to use carrots, but if she needed a stick, there was no one in the United States who wielded a bigger one than Seema. Losing Medicare participation was the biggest of all sticks, and she controlled that. Everyone in the health-care industry knew it. I also believe they trusted and respected her in addition to obviously fearing her.

We immediately thought testing could become an important tool to mitigate the horrific mortality rate among nursing home residents. During my first week as testing czar in March 2020, we prioritized symptomatic nursing home patients and the elderly, only behind hospitalized patients and symptomatic health-care workers. Symptomatic health-care workers included nursing home staff (nurses, aides, food handlers, etc.) because we needed to diagnose them and remove them from the workplace before they infected their vulnerable residents.

In March 2020, we focused on those who were symptomatic because we did not understand—nor could we have predicted based on previous coronaviruses—that asymptomatic spread would be nearly as important as symptomatic spread. But even if we had appreciated this fact, we did not have the national testing capacity to routinely screen asymptomatic people. To do so would literally mean testing everyone who was elderly or connected in some way to health care because everyone in health care was potentially exposed to COVID-19—from the doctors and nurses to the dining room and janitorial staff. We were intent on building the capacity for asymptomatic screening as quickly as possible and targeting that capacity first to nursing homes. But we could not do that early on.

In addition, the entire task force felt it was a compelling physical and mental health priority and also one of basic human compassion to restart visitation by family members to nursing home residents as soon as possible. How awful that our seniors were confined, isolated, and lonesome! The effects on both residents and families were becoming devastating, and we knew it. We heard it daily. And we felt the pain personally and deeply. But reopening visitation needed to be done safely to avoid another fatal catastrophe like what had happened in several East Coast states early in the pandemic. So with significant input from the CDC and White House Coronavirus Task Force members, Seema issued the "Nursing Home Reopening Recommendations for State and Local Officials" on May 18, 2020.[1]

The recommendations included several considerations for reopening visitation such as the incidence of COVID cases in the community and in that specific nursing home, the ability to isolate and provide adequate infection control within the facility, the availability of and the training to correctly use PPE, and the capacity to provide routine testing for staff and residents. Specifically, the CMS recommended that "nursing homes should have a comprehensive plan for testing. *All residents* should receive a single baseline test for COVID-19. Also, all residents should be tested upon identification of an individual with symptoms consistent with COVID-19 or if an employee or staff member tested positive for COVID-19." In addition, "*all staff* should receive a baseline test, and continue to be tested weekly."[2] These new recommendations reflected our evolving understanding of the importance of asymptomatic and presymptomatic spread. The testing of the staff was even more important than the testing of residents because we knew that COVID was being brought into SNFs from an external environment, and that meant it came from SNF staff who brought it in from the community.

Seema provided flexibility regarding exactly how those recommendations could be implemented because she (and I) recognized the limitations and constraints faced in many communities. This was an unprecedented crisis. To jump-start the ability of SNFs to implement these recommendations, their publication was followed within seventy-two hours by the announcement that SNFs would receive a $4.9 billion payment from the Provider Relief Fund. This provided the resources necessary to implement the new CMS recommendations, including testing. Indeed, by the end of our administration, SNFs would receive a total of more than $20 billion in supplemental funds to support quality care and patient safety.

But there were still many impediments to implementing the testing rec-ommendations, as we expected there would be. Maggie Flynn was an excellent young reporter for the website Skilled Nursing News, and she very accurately and fairly portrayed the situation on the day of the recommendations.[3] Test-ing was substantially better than it had been even one month before, but most SNFs relied on lab-based PCR testing, which was expensive—generally $125 per test—and SNFs could not afford that. The additional $4.9 billion in funding mitigated that concern. But even with adequate funding, we knew there would be additional challenges for SNFs. There were more than enough tests available (over thirty million per month), but there were throughput issues in many regions. The commercial labs were also variable in their turn-around times—often within four days but sometimes up to six days or longer. We asked for Quest and LabCorp to prioritize testing from SNFs, which they did, right behind the priority given to hospitalized patients, but the demand overwhelmed the system, and any major expansion relied on states enhanc-ing their testing capacity (through direct federal resources and guidance, as Governor Cuomo was doing) or on the federal testing program pioneering a technical breakthrough to bump the system to a new level of capability.

TURNAROUND TIMES

Turnaround times (TATs) are an important factor in the effectiveness of test-ing but are difficult to precisely measure. For many labs, turnaround times were defined as how long it took to report a result once the specimen was obtained in the laboratory. For me as a clinician, that was not the right defi-nition. What was relevant is the end-to-end turnaround time, including the time it takes to transport the specimen. For example, it may only take a lab twelve hours to perform an assay and provide results once the specimen is received, but it could take thirty-six hours to collect and transport the sample to the laboratory. Therefore, we defined a TAT as the time from when the physician ordered the test until the time the result was returned to the patient.

Short TATs are a goal for all testing, with the ultimate one being POC testing with fifteen-minute results. But short TATs are very important for some tests and less relevant for others—especially in a resource-constrained environment. For example, it is critical to immediately diagnose anyone admitted to a hospital and anyone else who could potentially benefit from outpatient treatment like monoclonal antibodies or more recently oral anti-viral drugs. Delays in diagnosis mean delays in therapy, and delays in therapy could mean death. It is also essential to test exposed health-care workers and first responders immediately with fast TATs. If they are positive, they need to stay home (and receive treatment if eligible). But since early in the pandemic, employers had the option (and generally exercised it) for critical infrastructure workers to remain on the job, even after a close exposure, if they remained asymptomatic and had a negative test. This is truly the only way it could have worked, or else by April, there would have been no doctors or nurses or SNF staff, since they would all have been on fourteen-day quarantines.

For a person in the general public who had close contact (within six feet for fifteen minutes or more without proper masking) with a person diagnosed with COVID, the CDC recommendations at the time were to stay home for fourteen days in quarantine. Even if you had a negative test on day three or five or seven, the requirement for fourteen days of quarantine did not change. So it is arguable (and we did argue a lot internally about this) whether those exposed actually needed a test at all, since the outcome would be the same either way, at least for that person. In December 2020, the CDC guidance included an option for local public health authorities to end quarantine at seven days if there was a negative test within forty-eight hours prior to ending quarantine. But until that time, there was no such option.

Turnaround times for SNFs were an entirely different issue on two levels. First, if a resident was newly admitted or symptomatic, that person would need to be isolated until the SNF proved that the person did *not* have COVID. There were still many reasons an elderly person might have a fever and fatigue, like a urinary tract infection or a decubitus ulcer (bed sore), and not need respiratory isolation. COVID isolation took significant staff time and bed space, and burned PPE—all of which were critical for SNFs.

The second level where TATs mattered for SNFs was even more important, and that was the routine screening of SNF staff and the screening of all residents when there was a case. For staff, even though masking and appropriate PPE were required, these measures were imperfect, especially when utilized by undertrained staff. Therefore, it was vital to get any staff member who might have COVID out of the workforce immediately. This was even more important because many SNF staff actually worked at multiple nursing homes, enabling a massive spread across multiple facilities from even a single case. And although less likely to spread the disease compared to staff, individual residents still interacted with one another and could spread the infection, so we needed to know as soon as possible if any resident turned positive as well.

Given these factors, prolonged turnaround times for SNFs were a big deal, at least in my mind. Yes, we surged supplies when requested. Yes, we prioritized SNF testing at commercial labs. Yes, we recommended states do the same at their public health laboratories and use their POC Abbott ID NOW instruments and tests for this purpose. Yes, we encouraged innovative solutions like using Cepheid instruments as they did in Africa: putting them in a van and driving them to SNFs for testing. Florida and a few other states were actually doing that. And all of this was partially effective. But it was not a comprehensive solution for the 15,500 SNFs of variable sizes and resources scattered throughout the country.

At that time, I was able to track turnaround times for large commercial labs like LabCorp and Quest, and that was a great asset, since they did half the testing in the United States and the majority of testing at SNFs. For the large commercial labs—including LabCorp, Quest, and a dozen others—I received daily reports for the nation and for each state on standard deviations and ranges of TATs, the percentage completed in three days or fewer and five days or fewer, and the specific TATs for hospitalized patients. The bottom line was that TATs for hospitalized patients were excellent. TATs for the general population were often in the range of four to six days in the early summer of 2020, which, although not ideal (and we constantly strove to decrease them), would work for those exposed, without symptoms, and in quarantine—because there would be no change in the plan either way. They were advised to remain in quarantine for fourteen days even if the test was negative. But four- to six-day delays posed enormous problems for SNFs. Catastrophic problems. We needed a different plan, or else deaths among nursing home residents would continue and perhaps escalate, despite the aggressive actions of Seema and her CMS team.

IS POC TESTING A SOLUTION FOR NURSING HOMES?

My maternal grandparents lived just across the yard from my childhood home in Marrero, Louisiana. My grandmother, with whom I was very close and spent a lot of time on a swing under the big family oak tree, developed Alzheimer's at a relatively young age. At that time, she was diagnosed with "hardening of the arteries," but it was clearly Alzheimer's in retrospect.

My grandfather and mother cared for her as long as they could at home, but it soon became impossible. What they accomplished at home would never even be considered by today's standards. There were no home-care nurses at that time, no "visiting angels"; my family did everything. But after a couple of years at home and for my grandfather's health and mental status, our family decided to put my grandmother in a nearby nursing home. My mother and grandfather were there with her every single day. And although I was in elementary school, I visited her multiple times per week. Even as a child, I was deeply affected by what I saw.

Although many families visited often and some even participated in care, many elderly residents were put in the nursing home and forgotten. Even those with dementia could feel pain and express emotions, as my grandmother did. The staff at this home seemed generally well meaning although not well trained. So although I did not do geriatric medicine (in fact, just the opposite), I was always very sensitive about nursing home residents and their families. That sentiment permeated my family as well. From a very young age, my older daughter, Jacqueline, sang and played music at nursing homes to entertain the residents and staff. And my younger daughter, Madeline, advocates for elderly-accessible parks and recreation activities.

Maybe because of my childhood experiences or maybe it was just my upbringing to care for the elderly, the nursing home situation during COVID-19 haunted me—especially because testing could potentially make a big difference. The protection of the elderly was also always extraordinarily high on the vice president's priorities. He felt this commitment deeply, and it was a frequent topic of discussion at the White House Coronavirus Task Force meetings. I am not sure if it was his sense of duty, his religious principles, or some other personal reason, but I knew Pence would back any program I would devise to protect the elderly.

The size of the problem was pretty large. We had approximately 1.2 million SNF residents and another 1.2–1.5 million SNF staff who would require testing at variable frequencies. And to adequately do surveillance, we needed tests that would have the shortest turnaround times—and by definition, the best TAT is achieved by POC tests. Although we did not have POC technology available in those numbers early in the pandemic, there were some emerging opportunities—and those opportunities were in the domain of antigen testing.

BinaxNOW, the simple $5 card-based antigen test, would not be authorized by the FDA until August 26, 2020, but of course in May, we could not predict that authorization. Another antigen test from Quidel, which required a specific instrument to read the results, was authorized on May 8. The Quidel Sofia 2 was widely used in physician's offices and clinics throughout the United States; in fact, there were over twenty thousand of these instruments already in the US health-care system. The test used a nasal swab that, after collection, is swished in a test tube (provided) for a minute and then transferred by a pipette (provided) to a detection cassette. After fifteen minutes, the cassette is placed into an instrument, and the result (positive or negative) is displayed. We knew this could be a solution for nursing homes because it was simple, rapid, and about one-quarter the cost of lab-based PCR tests. But there was a big problem: there were not even close to the number of tests available that we needed for a nursing home program. There were only six hundred thousand tests available in the first month, which would supply only about 15 percent of the SNF needs. This test supply was projected to ramp up somewhat in July and August but would never be sufficient to even begin to fulfill the SNF needs.

Because we worked daily within the industry, I knew that the dominant player in this market segment was BD Life Sciences. Their similar instrument to Quidel, the BD Veritor, was already utilized in over twenty-five thousand US sites, and their company had the capability to significantly ramp up production of both instruments and tests. If BD could develop a COVID-19 test and the FDA authorized it, we imagined that the combination of BD and Quidel could be just the ticket for SNFs.

This strategy led to another very important collaboration. Every week, my team and I held a virtual meeting with the president of BD Life Sciences (Dave Hickey) as well as the company's senior scientific and regulatory teams. Dave was very collaborative, as was his team, and he was completely transparent with me about their status and potential obstacles to both authorization and ramp-up. They wanted to help, and I could sense that they had pressured their internal system to the max—so I only need a light touch to nudge BD in the right direction. Together we reviewed their trial designs, data, production schedules, and interactions with the FDA. We facilitated their supply chains, some of which were in Asia; we shook them loose through the White House and State Department.

I emphasized to BD leadership the importance of their BD Veritor platform to our national strategy. I never interfered with the FDA review, but I did emphasize the importance of the BD Veritor to the overall national response. With literally hundreds of EUAs pending at the FDA, FDA staff had a good idea of what they needed to prioritize, even without my urging, and BD was at the top of the list at that time. BD eventually received their EUA on July 2, 2020, which gave us the opportunity to begin the implementation of a plan to enable nursing homes to test their residents and staff comprehensively and meet the guidance from the CMS.

ARE ANTIGEN TESTS "GOOD ENOUGH"?

With the authorization of Quidel and the expected authorization of BD and their low costs and ability to scale up, the question remained whether rapid antigen tests were appropriate for use in nursing homes as an alternative to PCR tests. While this was specifically a nursing home issue at the time, it exemplified the overall tension between the *importance of screening tests for public health* versus the *precision needed for diagnostic tests for individual patients.*

Later in the pandemic, it became fairly clear (even if still not universally accepted) that rapid tests like BinaxNOW or BD Veritor may not detect every remnant of the virus (like PCR does), but rapid antigen tests are likely to detect those individuals who are infectious and pose a risk to others. At the time of the nursing home decision, we did not have exact metrics, but we rightly assumed that Quidel and BD would be less sensitive than PCR (meaning that some people who were positive would not be picked up by these tests). As an estimate based on the data we had, we assumed that PCR was 95 percent sensitive in actual practice and that both BD and Quidel were in the range of 85 percent sensitive. What that meant is that for every one hundred people who were really positive for COVID-19, the antigen tests would pick up only eighty-five of them. Balancing that, however, was the fact that PCR tests were too expensive for many SNFs to obtain, and if they could obtain them, results were typically returned with a delay of four to six days due to the overwhelming demand at the commercial labs.

I needed assistance and decision support, so I requested that the CDC modeling group help me by predicting the real-world effectiveness of PCR testing versus antigen testing in nursing homes, taking into account sensitivity and TATs when combined with other infection control and prevention activities. I avoided typical CDC bureaucracy and processes and directly contacted Lt. Cmdr. Rachel Slayton, a young USPHS officer whose "day job" was as a modeling unit lead for the Division of Healthcare Quality Promotion at the CDC.[4] Lieutenant Commander Slayton was truly a "modeler," which meant she was very comfortable with complex math and statistics but had a little problem relating the complexity of her models to us "normal human beings." But she was great throughout the pandemic from my earliest visits to the CDC, and I had confidence in her analyses—if I could provide her with exactly the right question. There was no way I was going to tell her how important the analysis was until it was completed. As an officer in the corps, I knew she would provide me, her admiral, the highest quality work, whatever the stakes.

Within a few days, Lieutenant Commander Slayton provided me with the following slide, and I include it because of its historical significance. I was floored by the results. Slayton and the CDC team assumed that masking in nursing homes was approximately 75 percent effective and PPE was 50 percent effective. These were good assumptions. Then they used the known sensitivities of PCR and antigen testing and also the fact that turnaround times for PCR tests from nursing homes were four to six days at that time. They also modeled testing twice weekly (every three days), once weekly, and once every two weeks.

The results were compelling. Hands down, whatever the frequency of testing (every three days, seven days, or fourteen days), the less sensitive antigen tests (the fourth bar in each group) beat PCR for reducing infections in nursing homes. Twice-a-week testing (every three days) was much more effective than once-a-week testing or testing once every two weeks. And surprisingly, increasing the sensitivity of a POC antigen test to 95 percent (the fifth bar in each group) only minimally improved the effectiveness! *What this meant was that the predominant factor was the frequency of testing and turnaround time, not the sensitivity!* As such, there was no reason to put billions of dollars into trying to improve the sensitivity of antigen tests. I reviewed the

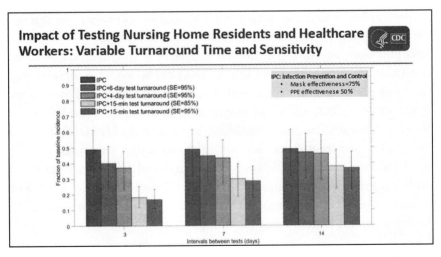

Original slide from CDC indicating the superiority of frequent rapid tests compared to PCR tests with slow turnaround (personal files). IPC = infection prevention and control measures (masking, gowning). SE = test sensitivity. "Fraction of baseline incidence" means only indicated fraction of cases would occur with IPC plus testing regimen. For example, IPC alone prevents about 50 percent of predicted cases. IPC and a fifteen-minute turnaround test with an SE of 85 percent prevent more than 80 percent of cases.

model in detail with the CDC and questioned all of their assumptions. The model appeared to be solid, and I believed it and so did my colleagues on the Testing and Diagnostics Task Force.

The path forward was clear: provide POC antigen testing to the nursing homes in high-risk communities. But while we had solved the technical hurdle of developing POC tests at scale, there remained major barriers to implementing the program, even though it was obviously the right thing to do.

First and foremost, the FDA had not authorized antigen tests for use in asymptomatic individuals (only symptomatic ones), but testing asymptomatic nursing home staff was exactly what was required based on the modeling. This was a *huge* impediment, although a self-imposed one. Second, CMS standards required all labs to only use tests in a manner for which they were authorized. Third, many states had regulations that prohibited the use of tests outside their FDA authorization; state experts might not have understood the importance of screening antigen tests (yes, the testing snobs we spoke about earlier could not get their heads around this). And if we could solve those issues, we actually needed to obtain instruments (thousands) and tests (millions) in the quantities that we needed—and that was not going to be easy under any circumstances. Finally, we had to train nursing home staff on how to use these new testing resources.

First, the FDA . . . I worked obsessively to convince the FDA that they needed to make a statement about using authorized tests in a manner that was not explicitly authorized. To the FDA, this seemed unnecessary and obvious, since physicians use off-label medications all the time. But in this public health emergency, the precise limits of FDA authorization became the governing doctrine about how tests were used. Without permission from the FDA, very few if any nursing homes would use antigen tests for asymptomatic staff because they feared the absolute power, including the fact that the FDA (and the CMS) can enforce their regulations with criminal penalties and hefty fines.

I had multiple conversations with Jeff Shuren and Tim Stenzel (the career leaders at the FDA who regulated tests) over this issue, often daily and with passion. These discussions ultimately resulted in the FDA providing the following statement in their FAQs for testing:

> Although the current available literature suggests that symptomatic individuals with COVID-19 and asymptomatic individuals without known exposure may have similar levels of viral genetic material, there is limited data on the distribution of viral loads in individuals with and without symptoms across demographics, different settings,

and specimen types. Therefore, when screening asymptomatic individuals, health care providers should consider using a highly sensitive test, especially if rapid turnaround times are available. If highly sensitive tests are not feasible, or if turnaround times are prolonged, health care providers may consider use of less sensitive point-of-care tests, even if they are not specifically authorized for this indication (commonly referred to as "off-label"). *For congregate care settings, like nursing homes or similar settings, repeated use of rapid point-of-care testing may be superior for overall infection control compared to less frequent, highly sensitive tests with prolonged turnaround times.*[5]

Next, we needed to address the CMS and their CLIA regulations. Seema Verma was highly motivated to protect nursing home residents and thus suggested a work-around to the CLIA standards of only using tests in the way they were approved or authorized. And that work-around was "enforcement discretion." I had never really heard that term before I became the assistant secretary, but it was used regularly in the context of the FDA and now by the CMS. Although the agency could not unilaterally change the law or the official regulations, the CMS would not *enforce* those regulations for a period of time. And that is what Seema Verma stated explicitly: "CMS will temporarily exercise enforcement discretion for the duration of the COVID-19 public health emergency under CLIA for the use of SARS-CoV-2 POC antigen tests on asymptomatic individuals. Specifically, CMS will not cite facilities with a CLIA Certificate of Waiver when SARS-CoV-2 POC antigen tests are performed on asymptomatic individuals, as described in the FDA FAQ."[6]

Next was the issue of conflicting state laws, rules, and regulations. I had the ability to fix those problems myself. With new authority based on the secretary's PREP (Public Readiness and Emergency Preparation) Act declaration on March 10, 2020, I extended coverage to licensed health-care practitioners prescribing or administering POC COVID-19 tests for screening in congregate facilities across the nation. The PREP Act guidance I issued included licensed health-care practitioners prescribing or administering FDA-authorized COVID-19 tests, *including for off-label (outside the authorization) use to screen asymptomatic individuals in congregate facilities.* More importantly, as I stated in the guidance, "This PREP Act coverage preempts any State or local provision of law or legal requirement that prohibits or effectively prohibits such licensed health-care practitioners from administering or prescribing FDA-authorized COVID-19 tests to symptomatic or asymptomatic individuals at congregate facilities."[7]

Now that we eliminated all the government and bureaucratic barriers to doing what was obvious from a public health point of view, we next had to deal with obtaining sufficient supplies and developing a national implementation plan. There were approximately 15,500 nursing homes in the United States according to the CMS, and about 12,000 of them had a CLIA waiver (meaning that they could perform the simple POC tests themselves on-site). Seema indicated that as long as the ~3,000 SNFs without the certification actually submitted the short paperwork to become CLIA waived, they could proceed with testing *even before* the CMS formally approved their applications. This was still another example of Seema Verma figuring out a way for the bureaucracy to work for Americans. So it was going to be likely, we thought, that nearly every one of the 15,500 SNFs would be eligible for the POC testing initiative.

There were many considerations going through my mind, and I discussed my thoughts with the team and especially with Seema. The OMB always had me in a budget squeeze despite the availability of billions of dollars in testing funds sitting in an account. In addition to the OMB's artificial constraints, there were real restrictions on the supply of tests. And I did not know whether testing was important for all SNFs or just the ones in "red areas" (those with high transmission and test positivity) as classified by Deb Birx. Initially, given the constraints, my decision was to supply instruments and tests only to the SNFs in the red areas or perhaps the red and yellow (moderate transmission) areas. That would have been the easy decision and was likely achievable without hiccups that could later be exploited by the media and the Democrats. Irrespective of Trump, who definitely wanted no more embarrassments related to testing, I did not relish the potential flogging in the media when we hit a speed bump because we were being as fast and aggressive as we could—which brought execution risk.

The public health data made the choice very hard. A green area could be yellow or even red the next day, and part of the goal was to keep the green areas green, and testing would be critical to make that happen. It was one of our only weapons at the time—no vaccines or widely available treatments.

Public health data notwithstanding, providing testing capability to some SNFs and not others did not sit right with my conscience—maybe it was some inner voice of my deceased grandmother. I had made enough choices already that needed to be made, like with ventilators, and those turned out right. I felt I needed to be bolder, even though supplying SNFs only in the hardest-hit areas of the country would have been a big win in itself at that time in the pandemic.

I talked to Seema. I told her that I wanted to supply *every single SNF* with a testing instrument and testing supplies. Seema was fully supportive and wildly enthusiastic. I also briefed Secretary Azar about this because he had always been careful about making "unforced errors," which this program could become. But as expected, he was fully supportive because the need was so great and likely because his personal code of ethics prioritized protecting the vulnerable (ages, races, socioeconomic groups). I presented the plan to the vice president, who was surprised and a bit incredulous that we could actually do this, but he was extremely enthusiastic about the program once I recommended it. He implicitly understood the risks involved in "overpromising" but had faith that we would get it done. I wish I had the confidence in myself that he did at the time . . .

We announced the program on July 14, 2020, just twelve days after the authorization of the BD test. The program would begin the week of August 3. We initially supplied 2,500 nursing homes, but then at the end of July, we announced that *all* nursing homes would receive instruments and tests. I requested invoking the DPA, which was approved by the White House and the president, so that nursing homes would get all the available tests they could use (and be at the front of the line). There was no argument at all from the companies—they were "all in"—but using the DPA made sure there would be no possibility of pushback from their traditional customers, who of course wanted these tests and instruments as well (and for good reasons).

Actually, implementing this initiative turned out to be extremely challenging, both because of its importance to save our seniors and because of the spotlight we were in. I needed someone to live and breathe this program night and day who I could trust both professionally and politically. Rachel Kellogg was the person I wanted as point guard on this project, under my daily direct supervision. Rachel was very young—in her midtwenties young. I met her when she was in the Immediate Office of the Secretary working as a briefing coordinator. This was a thankless job, making sure people far above her pay grade were submitting what the secretary needed to see when he needed to see it and with every relevant stakeholder included at decision meetings. She did well with this, but Rachel was more importantly a nurse—a clinician—and she wanted more clinical challenges. We got along well together, and I needed more clinically trained staff members in my immediate office. She and I both independently talked to her boss—Ann Agnew—who agreed this was an important and appropriate move for my office and for Rachel. I had already taken one of Ann's top people a year earlier and felt it appropriate to discuss personnel changes with her as a colleague. Rachel joined my office in October 2019 as a policy coordinator working on the major issues in my portfolio—most importantly, sickle cell disease.

But when COVID hit, I needed her to jump into the response. She recalled the specific circumstances to me later. The day I became testing czar, I called her late that night during a White House meeting and said, "OK,

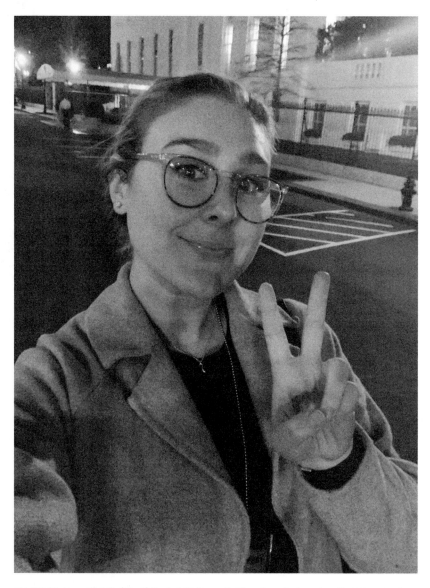

OASH Deputy Chief of Staff Rachel Kellogg. Selfie taken during the all-nighter in the West Wing on March 13 (sent to her family at midnight; "Peace from the West Wing," personal photo).

Rachel, are you ready to do some scut work for me?" The next morning at 6 a.m., Rachel was in the West Wing of the White House helping build out the testing strategy and pulled an all-nighter there.

When we began the nursing home project, Rachel's perspective as a nurse was vital—oftentimes, physicians are not as in touch with the needs of staff and training as nurses are. It is hard for some doctors to accept that, but it is a fact. That sensitivity was especially important when starting up the nursing home initiative, because staff were nearly always overworked and undertrained, even in normal times. I also appreciated Rachel because she would never take no for an answer. In July 2020, I appointed her as my deputy chief of staff. She never let me down and deserves a lot of credit for the success of the SNF program.

In total, we delivered POC testing instruments to 15,300 nursing homes along with 5.3 million tests. After the first distribution of tests, we made sure that nursing homes would receive first priority from the test manufacturers as well as discounted pricing. The nursing homes could use their recent allocation of billions of dollars to purchase additional POC tests as they needed them. Even if they did not purchase a single additional test and found other ways to meet CMS standards, we knew that even a two-month testing surge would identify thousands of positive staff and temporarily remove them from the workforce while they were infectious. And this would deal a blow—perhaps not a mortal wound but a significant one—to the virus's attack on our seniors. We also knew there would be new technology just around the corner, what we had been working toward since day one of the pandemic: simple card-based antigen tests that were as cheap as a Starbucks latte and did not require any instruments or particular training to perform.

BINAXNOW

On September 27, 2020, I stood on the podium in the Rose Garden of the White House next to the president of the United States, stuck a swab up my nose (both nostrils, actually), and performed a rapid antigen BinaxNOW test on myself—in front of the media and the world.

There was a lot of discussion in the Oval Office about whether I should do that or not. Several of the White House communications staff told me I absolutely could not do that. What if I messed up the test? What if I blew a snot ball onto the podium with the president? It would be a total embarrassment to the administration. What if I were positive and had just been on stage with the president and everyone saw that?

I understood their concerns. But BinaxNOW was a major advance in the United States' fight against COVID-19 and an important win for the Trump administration. On that day, we were averaging over nine hundred thousand tests per day reported to the CDC and had cracked the one-million-tests-per-day mark on thirteen separate days. These were essentially all PCR tests except for the BD and Quidel tests we had provided to the SNFs. Our national testing capacity far exceeded demand by close to three times. But we wanted to increase testing even more and could best do that by making testing easy, convenient, and quick, with immediate results. This would finally enable the screening of high-risk asymptomatic people across the country and be the foundation for eventual home testing.

BinaxNOW was the first lateral flow antigen test that could be made in bulk—meaning it was just a simple card, a dropper of solution, and a swab. This was the same test that would later be available over the counter in pharmacies and sent to millions of homes. So it was a big deal. We had been working with Abbott and several other companies to get this type of test available as soon as possible, but Abbott was the first to achieve FDA authorization. They received their authorization one day before my Rose Garden appearance. Results were available in fifteen minutes or less with no instrumentation and with a demonstrated sensitivity of over 97 percent and a specificity of 98.5 percent. The cost was $5, and Robert Ford (CEO of Abbott) had assured me that they could have twenty million per month to start but could scale to fifty million per month within a few months. For our testing program, this was truly *the* game changer that we had talked about for months and Birx had talked about since her first day as the coordinator. This type of rapid test was very difficult to develop and validate, but we had just cut years off from the normal process.[8] This was "warp speed" before the term became popularized as the official name for the vaccine initiative!

This was our biggest game changer, and it was built on months of effort, investment, and collaboration. Knowing that the EUA was imminent, we set up a contract with Abbott to purchase the first 150 million BinaxNOW tests for a cost of $750 million plus an extra $10 million for shipping. This was still not a "home test." It needed to be done (or supervised) by a "laboratory" with the result interpreted by a trained technician or clinician. This was OK because all nursing homes were laboratories (meaning that they had a CLIA waiver because of Seema's flexibility); almost all pharmacies were "laboratories" by federal standards as well. School clinics either could function as laboratories because they were one already (i.e., they had their own CLIA waiver and a school nurse) or could function under the umbrella of a pharmacy or the local public health department. In March 2021, the BinaxNOW test was authorized by the FDA for home use. So while President Biden's claim that there were no home tests available when he took office is technically correct, the Trump administration actually did all the work and made all the investments needed for home tests to be available in Biden's second month in office.

On that September day in the Rose Garden, I announced our purchase of the 150 million BinaxNOW tests by the federal government. We had thought long and hard about what we would do with them. This was a precious and unique resource, and we were buying the entire global supply for the next several months. That was a burdensome responsibility, but it was the absolute right policy to implement.

We decided to allocate fifty million for the highly vulnerable because that was where the most lives could be saved, and it was the best way to relieve hospital overcrowding. This meant we would deliver eighteen million to nursing homes to supplement the instrument-based antigen testing already provided; fifteen million to assisted living centers that also had highly vulnerable residents but no POC tests; ten million to home health-care and hospice agencies, for obvious reasons; and one million to historically Black colleges and universities (HBCUs) and tribal universities. We made the decision to include HBCUs and tribal universities because African Americans and American Indians were at high risk of hospitalization and death, and even though the college students would probably have no complications of COVID-19, they might bring the virus home with them to their parents and grandparents. BinaxNOW gave the universities the ability to test students before they spread the virus to their own at-risk family members. The remainder of the fifty million would be flexible; we could allocate more to any of these groups while saving tranches for disaster relief operations, like hurricane emergency shelters. Hurricane season was just beginning, and we did not want our emergency shelters to become superspreader events.

For the remaining 100 million tests in this initial 150-million-test purchase, after consultation with the vice president, secretary, and task force, we decided to send them to the governors of all states and territories, based on their populations, in order to support efforts to reopen their economies and schools as fast and as safely as they could. We gave the governors and their health staffs an enormous amount of technical assistance, written recommendations, and a one-stop number to call for questions. Governors also knew that I was personally available 24-7, and several called me frequently about testing and every other issue.

The 150-million number was not an empty promise. I had always been very careful not to overpromise; I wanted to overdeliver. By the time I made the announcement in the Rose Garden, my team had already shipped 65,000 tests to disaster operations in California, Oregon, Texas, and Louisiana (wildfire rescue and hurricane shelters), 2.1 million tests to 7,600 nursing homes, 900,000 tests to assisted living facilities, 300,000 tests to the Indian Health Service, and 339,000 tests to HBCUs.

BACK TO THE ROSE GARDEN

On September 27, as I stood next to the president in the Rose Garden preparing to demonstrate this new rapid test, I knew that I was going to test negative for COVID-19. I had already undergone an Abbott ID NOW test at the WHMU just two hours before. I had already practiced the BinaxNOW test on myself at least three times that day, so I felt comfortable that I knew what I was doing. I felt it was critical to demonstrate to the American people how easy and painless this test was in order to motivate them to get tested when

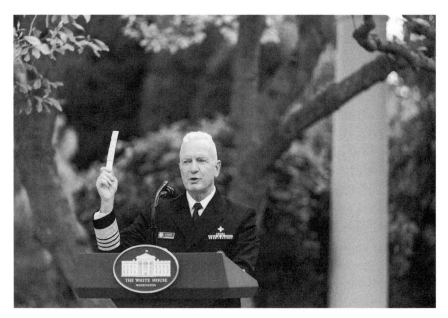

Admiral Giroir performs "self-swab" and BinaxNOW test on himself in the White House Rose Garden with President Trump (White House photo).

they were sick or exposed or undergo screening testing when asked to do so. I wanted to create more demand. The national testing issue was no longer supply; it had already transitioned to the *demand* for that supply.

I opened up the BinaxNOW card, put six drops of liquid in the first hole, unwrapped a Puritan swab (I had just invested another $120 million into Puritan to increase swab production), stuck the tip in one nostril and rotated five times, stuck it into the other nostril and rotated five times, put the swab into the second hole in the card, rotated it three times, closed the card, and that was it. There was a sigh of relief from the communications staff at the White House; I did not lose the election for Trump by botching the self-swab or flipping a booger onto the presidential podium. The vice president was elated. Of course, the reporters asked me later what the result was, and I told them *negative*. It was a good day for the testing program and for the administration.

On January 12, 2021, Abbott completed our order for 150 million tests—close to schedule, despite ongoing challenges in the supply chain, especially for swabs. I did not want to leave the Biden administration with a cliff, so before I left, I ordered another thirty million BinaxNOW tests and had the budget allocated for an additional sixty million BinaxNOW or equivalent tests—there were a few that were close to FDA authorization, and the Biden team might want to diversify their suppliers. I left them with that flexibility.

We also did something that was novel but has been completely forgotten: we placed BinaxNOW on the government (GSA) purchasing schedule and made all states and territories eligible to purchase BinaxNOW off that schedule at the same low price ($5) without having to negotiate and execute separate contracts with Abbott. The states had literally tens of billions of federal dollars for testing that was unspent, so money was not an object for them. All the states had to do was place an order over the internet. It could not have been any easier. Unfortunately, few states took advantage of this program, and that failure combined with the Biden administration's failure to continue federal purchasing of rapid tests led to the profound shortages of tests in the summer and fall of 2021.

FINAL THOUGHTS ABOUT TESTING

Could Testing Have Prevented the Pandemic in the United States?

Testing during COVID-19 was uniquely important because unlike influenza, Ebola, or even SARS or MERS, where disease spread was from symptomatic people, the spread of COVID-19 also occurred in people who were entirely asymptomatic or who had not yet developed symptoms (presymptomatic). Still today, most people who contract COVID-19 have no idea from whom they got it. Thus, before vaccines, the only way to stop the spread was mitigation for everyone, like masking and lockdowns (with all their inherent problems and horrible consequences), or to test as many people as possible—especially those likely to spread the infection in their communities (like college students). Our nation had never faced a challenge like this where testing was so important, and we were not prepared for the challenge. There would never have needed to be a testing czar if this had been an influenza pandemic.

When I say that we can't test our way out of this pandemic, I mean that. But that does not mean we can't test our way out of *any pandemic*. If in the future there is, say, a COVID-23, and we had five hundred million to one billion tests per week available, and if nearly every person tested themselves once or twice a week and voluntarily stayed at home if positive, then we *could indeed* test our way out of the next pandemic. And such a system would work even with a test that is only 70 percent sensitive, which is much less than the 90 percent sensitive tests we have today for COVID-19. Professor Mike Mina is a big proponent of this type of testing, and he has been mostly correct since the early days of the pandemic.

The remaining questions are whether people would voluntarily self-test on a mass scale, repeatedly, and if they did, would they self-isolate for seven to ten days if they were positive. During COVID-19, we repeatedly saw an unwillingness to undergo testing among high school students during our pilot programs and a similar unwillingness during our pilot strategic surveillance programs in many states. Indeed, most governors did not even use all the Abbott BinaxNOW tests that we had distributed. And when the Biden administration took over, testing plummeted (down by >50 percent by summer 2021) because there was decreased demand from the American people, which was exacerbated by a deprioritization of testing by the Biden administration. Testing picked up again when the Delta variant hit, but so many manufacturing lines were already disassembled that it took months to catch up;

the CDC even issued a notice on September 2, 2021, that there was a shortage of rapid tests. This time, the shortage was artificial and avoidable—the Biden administration did not keep the production lines open with federal orders, and the United States paid the price. It was even worse when the Omicron variant hit and there were no tests available for the holidays of 2021.

The lesson here is that we need to build flexible capability for testing at a large scale and be prepared to use it when needed at the earliest stages of the "next pandemic." I talk about the types of public-private partnerships that are necessary to achieve this in chapter 12. We certainly used serial screening testing for those going into the White House, for critical infrastructure like power and meat packing plants, for military units, for UPS and FedEx pilots, and for many other situations. Many universities that required testing (or highly incentivized it) dramatically drove down infections in their communities—not just within their universities.

Even if we can't supply a billion tests per week to the American public, we can absolutely dampen a future outbreak—even if there are asymptomatic spreaders—if the nation is better prepared. There was no way to have that type of testing available during the first six months of COVID-19 given where we (and the Obama administration before us) were in regard to preparedness. We did not have the technologies, the infrastructure, the supplies, or the supply chains.

I absolutely wanted the CDC tests to be more available in February 2020 and for the FDA to allow academic laboratories to begin testing without burdensome regulatory approvals. That could have helped in several local outbreaks and saved lives. But with dozens of US cities already seeded with COVID-19 and the overall frequency of asymptomatic transmission, it would have required tens or hundreds of millions of tests ready to go to dent the rise in cases in our country during those first months—and still, having those numbers of tests may not have made a difference at all. I say this because even though we had as many tests "as we needed" in the summer of 2021, including home tests, the Biden administration could not dampen the Delta outbreak with testing. Delta was controlled by immunity—vaccinations for many and natural immunity for the rest. Americans were getting the Delta variant of COVID-19 at a rate of a half million per day. Delta burnt itself out primarily because of population immunity. The same was true for Omicron. Even with home testing widely available, the impact on the overall outbreak was limited. The impact on high-risk individuals, however, whose testing led to treatment with oral antiviral medications, was likely profound—reducing hospitalization and death by as much as 80 percent.

Did Trump Tell Me to Slow Down Testing?

Trump knew that more tests would mean more reported cases, and he stated so many times. Especially early on, he was watching the scorecard. *His* scorecard. He even specifically stated that he was concerned about repatriating Americans from cruise ships because their cases would "count" against *his* numbers, but he supported repatriation anyway.

In the beginning, we had enough testing to perhaps detect one out of every seven cases of COVID-19, and even in October 2021, the nation was detecting less than half of the cases. So it is true that if you test more, you will detect more cases, and the numbers will go up. But testing was not the reason we were seeing more cases during the early summer and winter surges during the Trump administration. Those of us actually implementing public health policy and making recommendations to governors and the American public followed three parameters to make the conclusion that actual cases were indeed going up: the estimate of the actual cases (not just the reported cases to the CDC that were dependent on testing), the number of daily COVID-19 hospitalizations, and the number of daily COVID-19 deaths. I informed the president directly—and I certainly told the media many times during the summer and fall—that numbers were going up because we had a real spike in cases; it was not the fault of more testing. Hospital numbers (at least the way HHS collected them) were fairly accurate and could be used to see trends. The same is true for COVID-19 deaths.

Trump never told me to slow down testing—ever. But he did ask me if the number of cases was actually going up or if the increase was due to testing. I provided my honest assessment and conclusion. He understood.

As far as the opinion of the vice president and every task force member (except perhaps for Scott Atlas), more testing with rapid turnaround times was always the goal. Jared Kushner specifically told me to only consider slowing down when we had one billion tests per month—and that was a serious statement. So we never slowed down. When we hit one hundred million tests reported to the CDC on September 20, Pence wrote me a little "Well done, Admiral Giroir" note and passed it to me across the Situation Room table. Even Chief Mark Meadows and Secretary Steven Mnuchin met with me separately on several occasions later in the fall of 2020 and provided me with resources and top cover so that I could place orders for more new testing technologies, like Cue and Ellume—both of which were breakthrough technologies (highly sensitive, web linked, done at home) in their own right.

Did I "Almost Quit" My Job as the Testing Czar?

On June 1, 2020, I gave an opening address to the President's Advisory Council on HIV/AIDS (PACHA). Even though I was committed full time to the COVID-19 response, I made the time to address PACHA, since my staff and I resuscitated the council after it imploded (due partially to internal resignations and partially because Trump fired the rest of the members who were intransigent in their opposition to the Trump administration). I was responsible for leading the Ending the HIV Epidemic in the US initiative and hoped to make good on my commitment to this national effort after COVID was contained. As was my custom, I wrote all my own speeches, and during this opening address, I specifically wrote and delivered the following phrase: "I expect to be demobilized from FEMA in mid-June and return full time to my former position and responsibilities—including HIV."

So the answer to whether I almost left the role as testing czar is yes. The most frustrating part of leading testing was that neither I nor Secretary Azar had control of the funds that had been allocated to HHS by Congress to implement a national testing program. The money was entirely controlled by the OMB, and every dollar I desperately needed had to be justified for weeks to thirty-something-year-old staffers with spreadsheets and no scientific knowledge or national urgency. Where their direction came from was unclear, but I assumed it came from higher in the White House and that the underlying concern was preserving money in case it was needed for OWS. I understood the primary importance of vaccines but always thought that Congress would have allocated more money if asked to for this effort. Honestly, it was not until the publication of Paul Mango's book on OWS in the summer of 2022 that I learned that Speaker Pelosi was indeed playing political games with COVID-19 funding and that sufficient funding to OWS was a real risk.[9]

But to me and my team in the summer of 2020, all we knew was that the OMB always had redundant, onerous, and incessant volumes of questions, most of them reflecting not only a true ignorance of the science but a complete dissociation from the urgency of the situation. The staff in the Office of the Assistant Secretary for Financial Resources, including (perhaps especially) the HHS chief financial officer, were at least as frustrated as I was but caught in a completely dependent (abusive?) relationship with the OMB. Tammy Beckham said multiple times, "What is wrong with those people?" There were billions of dollars in the bank, but the OMB would not let us spend them. More correctly, they would not let us spend money until I personally threw a fit and exclaimed that people would die and that American blood would be on the OMB's hands—and I would make those facts known publicly. Numerous initiatives were turned down outright or delayed until the initiative was no longer as impactful.

In mid-May, there was over $6 billion left of the $8 billion that Congress allocated to HHS for testing and diagnostics, and I assessed that we needed most of those funds to implement programs such as regional university testing hubs, community-based wastewater sampling, and infrastructure programs like those that invest in plastics and nitrocellulose (the paper strip that one does lateral flow antigen testing on). Weeks went by, and we could not even get approval for the funds to continue the operation of our Laboratory Diagnostics and Community-Based Testing Task Forces. Without money, these task forces would abruptly disappear—and that meant the national testing programs would disappear, all of them.

I gave the OMB a serious deadline after weeks of back and forth. But the OMB "wheel of pain" kept turning. The deadline passed with no OMB action, so in my mind, I was done. I was not going to be held accountable for a national testing system when I was not given the resources to build one— or even to keep my task forces operational. Since we were transitioning from FEMA back to HHS and roles and responsibilities could be distributed among HHS offices, this was a good opportunity for me to go back to my normal assistant secretary responsibilities. Remember, my official position was as a member of the DLG, but I had no responsibility regarding emergency response except for the leadership role of the Commissioned Corps. Bob Kadlec's office (Office of the ASPR) should have owned testing, but as we know, Azar put me in charge because of the well-publicized testing crisis caused by the CDC and the FDA. In any case, HHS and the OMB would just have to figure it out. As a point of reference, cases were relatively low at that time—we had no idea that there would be a winter 2020 resurgence of COVID-19.

My statement at PACHA had some effect—people noticed. The media noticed. An HHS spokesperson also confirmed that the responsibilities for testing (and other responsibilities) would be distributed among the relevant HHS operating divisions—and for sure, that was not going to be in my home office. Even Senator Murray noticed and sent a letter to Vice President Pence on June 4 stating that eliminating my role was "wrong" and then went into the typical partisan attacks on the failures of the Trump administration. She said there had been some improvement and then defended the need for my role to continue. Go figure, after all she had done to delay my nomination and delegitimize my position prior to COVID-19.

I had not talked to the VP about any of this, but I should have, even though my authorities for testing came from HHS. Pence never questioned me about my statement or the press, and perhaps he did not notice the perturbation at all because of his more important responsibilities. In any case, there was a sufficient "fog of war" in the transition from FEMA and changing roles back to HHS, and this was clearly my opportunity to punch out of a job that I did not have budgetary authority to fully accomplish. I did indeed want to get back to the public health initiatives that were core to my office. And all of these would become more urgent because of the pandemic: addiction and overdoses, HIV, childhood immunizations, weight management, and other critical health needs.

It was also unclear to me if Deb Birx wanted me to stay in the testing czar role. In retrospect, her opinion was probably as important to me as the OMB funding in deciding whether to stay or leave. I respected Deb, but we had some different thoughts on the way forward for testing in general and how testing could be used to reopen the country. I was not shy about disagreeing with her (in private) and debating the options. She tended to give orders and not explanations. And after all, I really did not work for her. Indeed, many times I had to work around her, and everyone understood that this was necessary because of some of her management issues. But she was extremely smart, I respected her, and almost always, we came to an agreement. If we couldn't come to an agreement, which was rare, I would always defer to her because she was the coordinator, and I recognized that with so much uncertainty surrounding the virus, success depended much more on disciplined implementation than any given high-level plan.

One day during the summer of 2020, prior to going on stage in the White House press room with the president, I told Deb in no uncertain terms that I thought of the six billion people on the planet, she was the only one who could possibly do the job she was given and maintain the trust of the American people while doing it. But we had some ongoing professional disagreements (never personal), and I assumed she probably wanted to run testing herself. This would be her opportunity, and anyway, she might have been able to get more out of the OMB than I was getting.

I took a couple of days to think about it and regroup. If I left as testing czar, there was really no one else who could take the lead, even in the Office of the ASPR. And the two task forces related to testing were being run by Dr. Tammy Beckham and Rear Admiral Schwartz—both from my office.

And certainly, by that time, I had about as much clout as any medical person in the White House and certainly with the vice president. The VP trusted me and knew that I would get things done; he could rely on me, and I thought (and still think) he liked me personally.

I spoke to Azar, who was always a great mentor, and discussed the general situation. He could not help me with the OMB because, for testing and diagnostics, the OMB was dealing with me directly because of my role on the White House Coronavirus Task Force. This was quite different from the typical HHS budgets that all go through the secretary and are mainly under his control. I also asked Azar to speak to Birx candidly about whether she wanted me to stay on in my role. She would be honest with him, for sure. She would have been honest with me too; perhaps I just did not want to hear a lack of confidence from her directly. Azar did speak with Deb, and to my surprise, she stated that she really wanted me to stay and actually was surprised I would even consider leaving the job. That made an enormous difference to me. Why? I am not sure. But it did—everyone needs a little affirmation, particularly when you are often the piñata at the party. After that, Deb and I got along extremely well—with her support, my team created a testing "machine" that was increasingly effective.

I stayed on as testing czar and continued to fight the daily battles against the OMB. It was the right decision. I needed to remain "in the fight," especially in retrospect, because there was another dramatic increase in cases in the fall and winter. There was much more to do for testing, and moreover, I was able to appear frequently on the national media to deliver critical public health messages.

Dr. Beckham took a lot of the OMB burden off my shoulders, answering the endless questions on a day-to-day basis and pushing aggressively to minimize any further delays. Once Russ Vought was officially confirmed to lead the OMB, things became somewhat better. Russ was an outstanding guy who understood that the OMB was there to provide the whiskey and fresh horses to those of us in the field. I pressured Russ on occasion when the lower-level bureaucrats stalled efforts. I felt bad about that because Russ was one of the good guys and a great collaborator. I wish he would have been the OMB director two years earlier. Nonetheless, even with Russ in the lead role, budgets remained very tight. Chief Meadows and Secretary Mnuchin helped me with testing projects that they were particularly interested in, but the majority of the efforts remained piecemeal because we did not have the agility and flexibility to fully build out the testing program the way I wanted to do it. Make no mistake, we spent a lot of money and I believe made a huge impact, but I felt I could have done more, particularly in the July–December time period.

It was not until December 2020 that much of what I requested was approved, albeit often at lower funding levels than I needed. I assume the money shook loose so that we would not leave money unspent. Money that was easy to spend we spent, like sending $50 million to the CDC for a national wastewater surveillance program. But by that time, it was too late to put out competitive solicitations and organize major national programs like regional testing centers at universities and more infrastructure for the supply chain. I briefed all of these to the Biden administration transition team, and they—to their credit—picked them up and increased the funding to the levels that I had originally asked for. But after their initial efforts, it appeared that testing was no longer the Biden team's focus, and thus it was essentially neglected for a critical nine months, which led to the testing shortages in the winter of 2021–22. It seemed they already forgot the lessons that all of us learned just one year earlier.

11

Inside the White House Coronavirus Task Force

Wikipedia indicates I became a member of the task force on March 13, 2020. There actually was never an official announcement; it just happened. March 13 was the day when I appeared on stage in the Rose Garden with the president and vice president, a few members of the task force, and CEOs from major US corporations. But for me, I felt I became a task force member during the Sunday, March 15, national briefing from the White House press room, during which I announced the implementation of the national drive-through testing program with Trump and Pence.

During the national press briefing, I stated, "This is not make-believe. This is not fantasy. We will have the capability of testing tens of thousands of people through the sites every week." That comment was not scripted by the White House communication staff (none of my comments ever were); it just spontaneously came out of my mouth. The public had received so much conflicting information up to that point that their patience was already growing thin; they needed assurances. And after forty-eight hours with my newly formed testing team, I felt certain that the community-based testing program would kick off within days and then rapidly grow in the following weeks. And it did.

When we left the stage, the vice president literally patted my shoulder and said he really loved that line—"This is not fantasy"—it made the point that we were going to get this done. To me, that was the moment I knew I was going to be on the task force and assume a more prominent role at the White House level. I would have many more transparent, blunt moments from the White House podium and on national media. I always tried to give the American people the best information we had at the time, along with all the uncertainties and complexities. To this day, people still stop me on the streets and thank me for my honesty and candor.

From March through the midsummer of 2020, task force meetings occurred multiple times per week and even daily. Whether by design or de facto, there were "core members" who were always present and participated in the entire range of discussions and decisions, and I was fortunate to be one of those core members. The vice president always led the task force meetings. The agenda was finalized by Marc Short, chief of staff to Pence, which was generally fine but was sometimes a problem as the doctors occasionally struggled to get items on the agenda that we felt were critical. But in general, Marc was solid—no unnecessary drama and no unforced errors under his watch.

Olivia Troye, before she went rogue against the administration, often gathered materials for the meetings. I had no idea that she had an official title on the Pence team because she functioned only administratively with regard to the task force. She never said a word about policies or issues. While speaking of "whistleblowers," I should at least mention Dr. Rick Bright, who was the BARDA director and then moved to the NIH to run a component of the Rapid Acceleration of Diagnostics (RADx) testing program. His allegations against HHS claimed, falsely, that we prioritized the political agenda over the health agenda. Let me first say that no one in the White House or on the task force ever knew who Rick Bright was (aside from Azar, Kadlec, and me) or needed to seek his opinion. He was a PhD with reasonable scientific experience in vaccine development, and I had often worked productively with him on a limited range of issues. But Rick was not a public health professional, did not have a medical degree, and completely lacked a national strategic perspective. He had never cared for a patient, nor would he ever. After his complaint against HHS, President Trump said he did not know Rick Bright and actually never heard of him; I am certain that was true. And Rick's decision in early 2020 not to fund a promising oral antiviral drug, molnupiravir (which was later proven to be highly effective and lifesaving in treating COVID-19), attests to his lack of perspective and practical clinical expertise. From my point of view, his decision probably cost tens of thousands of lives. What he perceived as "pressure" to fund the development of molnupiravir was absolutely appropriate, evidence based, and completely nonpolitical.

Birx was the task force coordinator and officed in the West Wing. Her small support team was an eclectic mix of perhaps six to eight individuals. Tyler Ann McGuffee, a public health professional originally from Louisiana, had worked for many years with Pence in Indiana and then moved on to HHS focusing on reducing the price of drugs. Tyler Ann was Deb's right-hand person and implemented Deb's external and internal priorities. She was indispensable. The remainder of Deb's team were all detailed from other departments, including the Department of Defense—Deb felt very comfortable with military personnel (in uniform or not), since most of her career was spent in the US Army, and they would do everything she would tell them to do, without discussion or comment.

Although preparations started at the crack of dawn, the actual task force meetings generally occurred in the afternoon. This was appropriate because we could complete our morning operational meetings at FEMA and then be in position at the White House for the afternoon task force meeting. The task force meeting would conclude about an hour before the evening press conference, which gave us some time to gather our thoughts and jot down a few notes before addressing the nation.

Birx, Fauci, Redfield, and myself were always seated at the main conference table in the Situation Room. As the coordinator, Birx always sat next to Pence, Fauci next to Birx, and myself next to Fauci. Redfield generally sat on my right at the end of the main table near the video screens. Commissioner Hahn rarely physically attended because of the distance between the FDA and the White House, but he was almost always on the phone. In general, cabinet members sat on the other side of the main conference table from the doctors. Secretary Azar was the most frequent cabinet attendee, physically present at most meetings. Depending on the agenda, Secretaries Carson (Department of Housing and Urban Development), Scalia (Department of Labor), Mnuchin (Department of Treasury), and Perdue (Department of Agriculture) and Acting Secretary Wolf (DHS) would also attend. FEMA Administrator Gaynor participated by videoconference. Rear Admiral Polowczyk was almost always on the agenda, although not officially a member of the task force. As the supply chain lead, Rear Admiral P's updates were critical to everything we were trying to accomplish. Finally, Seema Verma was nearly always present, for good reason. Her agency, the CMS, regulated and provided reimbursement for nursing homes, hospitals, and essentially the entire US health-care system. She had all the carrots and sticks, and Seema was not afraid to use them to achieve national objectives.

Around the wall of the Situation Room in the White House were also important individuals who variably attended depending on the agenda. Marc Short (VP chief of staff) was always present. Other senior staff included the surgeon general (Jerome Adams), Larry Kudlow (director of the National Economic Council), Matt Pottinger (deputy national security advisor), Lt. Gen. (ret.) Keith Kellogg (national security advisor to the VP), Brad Smith, and Russ Vought (OMB acting director and then director). Jerome was one of the first docs on the task force, tapped before I was. He had a long history in Indiana with the vice president and was making enormous contributions as the "nation's doctor" in media and through personal travels around the United States. I was particularly fond of Larry Kudlow—he was very practical and logical with a dry sense of humor. The year before the pandemic, I explained to him in public health terms what he already inferred from his training: that the health outcomes of Americans actually depended more on jobs and the economy than any individual medical care issue and that Trump might be remembered as "the public health president" because life expectancy was increasing across all races and ethnic groups—primarily because of Trump's economic policies.

At least one communications professional from the White House team also attended the task force meetings—often that was Katie Miller from Pence's office. Katie was often abrupt in the way she interacted with task force members but a serious communications professional; we appreciated her skill set. Communication to the American people was among our biggest challenges, and Pence frequently would highlight points that needed emphasis in the media or directly to the public.

Most people think of the Situation Room as a large futuristic room with 3D electronics and digital screens all over—more like the NASA control room. It is not. It is a simple, small conference room with two screens at the

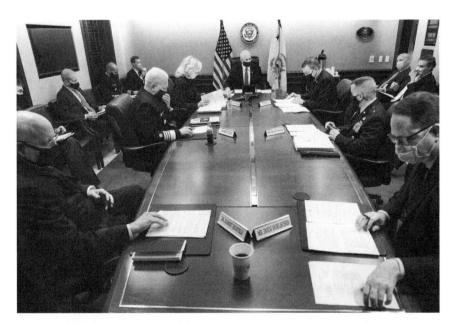

Task force meeting in the Situation Room. Vice President Pence at the head of the table. Admiral Giroir is seated next to Dr. Birx on Pence's right. CDC Director Redfield at bottom left of photo (White House photo).

end of the table (opposite the head) and digital clocks indicating the time of day at strategic locations, including wherever the president is located. We were always concerned about the cramped quarters and risk of COVID infection, despite the daily testing required to enter the White House if you were in close contact with Pence or Trump.

For the task force meetings, Pence always made opening remarks—sometimes an update about an issue, a comment about a potential press briefing, or just a congratulatory note. He often requested one of the task force members lead a prayer—typically that was Ben Carson or Bob Redfield—but he called on me once to lead prayer, and I did.

Immediately after the opening remarks, the floor was given to Deb Birx to provide a data-intensive update on the pandemic. By the time of her remarks, there had already been substantial discussion and evaluation of the day's data by the doctors on the task force. Specifically, every morning at about 6 a.m., Deb provided the task force doctors with an email briefing containing about one hundred PowerPoint slides detailing the most recent data on cases, fatalities, hospitalizations, and mitigation. The data provided information on every level, from the national to the state and even down to the metropolitan. I faithfully consumed this briefing every morning over two cups of coffee in my apartment. Immediately after, I put together a daily report on testing, including overall numbers, turnaround times, supplies, and state allocations of resources, and then walked the mile or so to HHS or FEMA.

For the task force, Deb prepared a shortened version of the entire data set consisting of about fifteen to twenty key slides. At the end of her presentation, everyone on the task force had a snapshot of the status of the pandemic and where we anticipated the next regional outbreaks or other problems (like hospital bed shortages) would occur.

Even early on in the pandemic, we saw an important pattern that proved true almost in every geographical location. An early rise in the percentage of tests that were positive foreshadowed an increase in reported cases, followed by increased hospitalizations in three to four weeks and then increases in deaths. When there was an increase in test positivity, we knew there was going to be an outbreak that would follow. We acted on that intelligence whenever we saw it and urged state and local officials to do so as well; often they did, but sometimes they did not.

Right after Pence's opening remarks at each task force meeting, Deb went through her data and conclusions, which usually took about ten minutes. Fauci then generally provided some color commentary on the data. Typically, the vice president tried to look for positive signs in the data, but Deb was brutally honest with her assessments. Pence was never in denial—he wanted the unfiltered facts—but there were occasional silver linings, and he wanted to understand those as well. Deb always seemed hesitant to provide any positive news. Next, the VP would generally turn to Pete Gaynor and Rear Admiral P, who would highlight any important regional issues from the daily FEMA UCG meeting and also provide a detailed report on the supply chain—how much we needed, how much we had, and where everything was going. There was always an emphasis on nursing homes and the vulnerable.

Early on, testing was always prominent on the agenda. I reported factually about the numbers of tests, the weekly shipments of supplies to states, turnaround times (from the large commercial labs that were doing 50 percent of the national testing), the status of shipments to nursing homes, and a look forward to when the next inflection point might be—like when we were preparing to have the Abbott BinaxNOW tests available for distribution.

Bob Redfield typically talked about infection control strategies and pending CDC guidance, like mask wearing or the approach to crowded indoor spaces and school openings. We all had input into those recommendations, but Bob "owned them" from the CDC point of view and always had the last pen on the paper.

The remainder of the meeting really depended on the priorities of the day and week. Early on, Secretary Perdue had a critical role, successfully endeavoring to keep the food supply intact. Secretary Azar was generally the lead to overview the development of vaccines and therapeutics within OWS. Steve Hahn provided regulatory updates for EUAs, including plasma, hydroxychloroquine, remdesivir, and vaccines. Bob Kadlec (ASPR at HHS) worked across many domains but was the lead in the distribution plans for remdesivir and monoclonal antibodies. Secretary Scalia discussed the protection of the workforce but also the importance and strategies to maintain employment—this was frequently an important topic and persisted across the entire duration of the pandemic. Secretary Mnuchin rarely attended, but when he did, he typically updated the task force on the congressional funding packages and took input over what we needed the packages to contain.

Frequently, the task force docs (Birx, Fauci, Adams, Hahn, Redfield, and myself) met prior to the task force meetings, and when the task force meetings became less frequent in the late summer and fall, we would meet on our own to assess progress and develop new plans. These meetings were absolutely essential when Scott Atlas joined the task force and was apparently advising the president independent of the other doctors. Scott had made it very clear that he was not going to budge from his positions, and he and Birx did not exactly have a collegial relationship, so we proceeded with our "docs cau-cus" meetings without him. We would always have the benefit of his views at the actual task force meetings.

Aside from the times when Atlas attended the task force meetings, there was very little high drama in the Situation Room. But there were exceptions, like the occasional appearance of Peter Navarro. Peter Navarro is a really smart guy, a PhD economist who served as an assistant to the president, the director of Trade and Manufacturing Policy, and the national DPA policy coordinator. Although this was not my area of expertise, I thought he was appropriately aggressive in these areas—we needed US supply chains, and he was obsessed with developing them and getting critical supplies necessary for implementing an effective public health response. Peter was also a ferocious defender of the president always and everywhere. He had a lot of history with members of the task force, especially Fauci, before I joined the group. There had already been a lot of water under the bridge, much of it turbulent. For example, it is widely reported that Navarro was the main advocate for shutting down travel from China, which was opposed by Fauci and perhaps others. Peter had been right, and he had also been right on the need to push the DPA and the domestic production of supplies. My impression was that he was doing an outstanding job in his domain despite his eccentricities.

But Peter did not understand the limits of his expertise, or perhaps he truly believed that his qualifications as an economist made him an expert in all things medical as well. He wasn't. One day in April, we were having a typical task force meeting, reviewing the data and dealing with policy alter-natives. I was not sitting in my normal spot but was at the opposite end of the conference table from the vice president. All of a sudden, from the door to the immediate left of where the vice president sat at the head of the table, Navarro burst in with a stack of papers about two feet thick. He passed behind the vice president and started yelling something like, "You doctors say there is no evidence to support hydroxychloroquine, but here it is." He then threw the papers down on the Situation Room table and continued to carry on.

My first thought was that Navarro could be a character in a new sequel to the classic movie *Dr. Strangelove*. I fully expected Pence to utter the famous line from the movie, "Gentleman, you can't fight in here. This is the war room!" Peter was really worked up. His rant was initially directed at Fauci, who actually made a polite but accurate comment stating that the evidence had not proven any benefit of the drug. Peter quickly retorted, and then I jumped into the argument. I thought there was enough bad blood between Navarro and Fauci, and some of the fire needed to be diverted—so

I diverted it to me. I stated similarly that early in March and April, we were all hopeful about hydroxychloroquine, especially me, but the appropriately controlled clinical data was increasingly disappointing. A few more verbal jabs were delivered by Navarro, and then he left the room as quickly as he had entered it.

Navarro's overt attacks on Fauci and less public attacks on the rest of the doctors continued. His well-publicized op-ed against Fauci in *USA Today* was entirely inappropriate—whatever you think of a person, if that person is in your boss's administration (and Fauci was in Trump's administration), you don't write an editorial like that.[1] Bottom line, in his fervor to protect and defend the president, he likely did more damage by going public about his personal rift with Fauci. It implied—incorrectly, from my point of view—that Trump could not keep his senior team in order and that there was "chaos" in the White House, exactly the message that the Democrats were trying to sell to the public.

On August 2, 2020, I had a good interview on the Sunday morning show *Meet the Press* on NBC. It was a typically tough interview, but near the end, the host asked me about the president and hydroxychloroquine. I tried to never overtly contradict the president, but I had a responsibility to provide the best information to the American public. I said, "Most physicians and prescribers are evidence based, and they're not influenced by whatever is on Twitter or anything else. And the evidence just does not show hydroxychloroquine is effective right now. We need to move on from that and talk about what is effective."[2]

Of course, my "breaking with the president" was the only headline in the national press after that interview, and Peter Navarro attacked me publicly the next day. He said I had not read the data and that medical doctors' opinions were a dime a dozen. Of course, I had read the data, and he knew that. So again, his fervor to defend the president combined with his shotgun dismissal of anyone who was even partially aligned with Fauci got in the way of the scientific truth. I was not as mad at him as I should have been because I knew (hoped?) that no one would take his medical opinions seriously. I stated later during one of my media calls that if there comes a time when patients with appendicitis call an economist for help, then they should take medical advice from Peter Navarro. Ultimately, the decision about treatment with hydroxychloroquine or any other FDA-approved medication is a decision between a doctor and a patient; the job of the task force doctors (and the CDC and the FDA) was to generate data and help interpret the evidence. The media-fueled hydroxychloroquine debate highlighting those with extreme views (on both sides) wound up diverting public focus from the other promising therapies that were rapidly coming online.

Fauci was neither as bad as Navarro said he was nor as good as "the national treasure" or "Saint Fauci" narrative that the media portrayed him to be. Tony has had a stellar scientific career, and his contribution, especially to HIV research and treatment, is well known. But Tony is also a political animal and survivor and was not going to jeopardize his national standing or scientific reputation for any president or specific issue. I know that Tony was personally harassed by many scientists for even being seen in the same room as Trump; this bothered Tony a lot, as it would bother most people to be ostracized from their professional peers—even if completely unjustified.

During the Trump administration, Tony only rarely got over his head about topics for which he was not an expert, but that became much worse during the Biden administration. From my perspective, during the time we served together, Tony was generally a good colleague who tried to work within the system. He never disrespected President Trump in public or in private and had a solid working relationship with Pence. He and I interpreted the pandemic data similarly, although we differed frequently on federal actions in response to the data, and all the docs shared the same concerns about the potential for viral resurgence in the winter of 2020–21 and beyond.

Despite those few notable moments of drama, the task force meetings were very evidence based and mostly wonkish. I was profoundly affected by the number of deaths and the ongoing tragedy, but being an ICU doctor, I could compartmentalize those feelings (at least temporarily) to focus on the work at hand. I am sure the other doctors also compartmentalized their feelings to stay on task. We would deal with our emotions at a later time, and that time—at least for me—came soon after I left Washington, DC.

THE CDC DOES NOT MAKE NATIONAL POLICY

In February 2020, it appeared to the world that the CDC was in control of the overall decision-making process in our country in addition to their core responsibilities for quarantining and testing. Certainly, they were in the spotlight and fairly autonomous in their communications. The one caveat is that Secretary Azar was fully engaged daily and had significant oversight on most of the actions and decisions the CDC communicated.

But after the declaration of a national emergency and the implementation of the White House Coronavirus Task Force, the specific role of the CDC was demonstrably clarified in the Situation Room. In one of the few times that Jared Kushner attended the task force meetings, he stated something that absolutely needed to be stated, and that is (paraphrased), "The CDC does not make policy. The CDC provides facts and recommendations to the policy makers—and they make the policy." This was important on so many levels, and I agree with that position completely and for many reasons.

First, the CDC "experts" had a narrow worldview that primarily encompassed infection control. To make the point in its most extreme form, the best way to "control" COVID-19 was to lock each family unit in its own home, turn off the economy, and wait it out for a perfect vaccine or a divine intervention. This is not so far-fetched, since many nations around the world tried to institute this type of zero-COVID policy. That type of infection control comes with the unintended public health consequences of increased depression, suicides, and substance-use disorders and overdoses; missed cancer and early heart condition screenings; profound weight gain and its consequences; and numerous other public health consequences that we are facing in the United States despite our relatively moderate national approach to lockdowns. The infection control experts at the CDC did not take any of these other public health issues into account.

Second, the CDC had no idea about the effects of infection control on our economy and jobs. Over the long term, the most important influencers of public health are jobs and economic prosperity and all the social determinants of health that spring from these, including education, food security, and a safe physical environment. The CDC did not know what was needed to maintain the power grid or to keep the shelves stocked in grocery stores. It was bad enough to not have enough toilet paper, but if the store shelves had no bacon and chicken, Americans might have truly panicked.

Third, the CDC was not concerned about strategic weaknesses, including vulnerability to terrorist attacks. Many of our adversaries would have relished hitting us while we were down. Such an attack could have had psychological consequences far beyond the actual physical destruction involved. And who in the CDC was an expert in our armed forces and military readiness? Or nuclear deterrence? Or operational readiness among the Special Forces?

Finally, infection control decisions could potentially infringe on our cherished freedoms and liberties—neither of which is the domain of the CDC. Americans are by nature independent and bristle at federal restrictions and overreach. All of us should be careful about the slippery slope of the federal infringement of rights (like freedom of movement, speech, and worship) that seemed to be forgotten by many in the media and Congress and rarely, if ever, was considered by infection-control career experts at the CDC.

The bottom line is that the CDC should never make policy because the pandemic response is not merely about infection control. The pandemic response is also not as simple as "following the science." Science doesn't inform about trade-offs that are always present—for example, balancing some risk of infections in order to maintain the food supply and the mental health of children. The phrase "following the science" makes no sense anyway. Science is a *process* that generates hypotheses that are proven by data to be mostly true or mostly false. We have seen many times that the science was wrong—such as when Fauci advised against masks in the early pandemic and when Walensky told us to take our masks off after being vaccinated (and then changed her position abruptly soon after). Every infection-control recommendation must be looked at holistically for its effects—and that is why whenever a policy was on the table, the relevant cabinet members were around the table, and their staffs had outlined every detail and all implications before a decision was made.

For all these reasons, the CDC (or any other unelected agency with a narrow focus) should never make policy. And if anyone now says they are just "following the science," they are either misinformed, have tunnel vision, or are trying to misdirect you.

There is a risk to this approach, however, and that risk is that the pursuit of votes could tip the scales in decision-making—so there must be transparency and objective evaluation. Closing the southern border may mitigate COVID-19 spread, but it also stops illegal immigration. That would be appealing to many voters, independent of its consequences on the pandemic. Opening the cruise industry would economically help Florida, an important swing state, and so on and so on.

By my assessment, Vice President Pence played it straight. His direction of the task force was never politically motivated, meaning he did not make decisions in order to get votes. In terms of President Trump, while he was fully engaged with the task force up until the early summer, he almost universally heeded the advice of the medical experts. The last thing he wanted to do was "shut down" that big, beautiful economy that he had built. But he did shut it down for fifteen days on the advice of the task force. And he certainly did not want to continue that for another thirty days, but he accepted that recommendation as well. He didn't like testing so many people because we would indeed uncover more cases, and that made *his* new case numbers look bad. But he supported all the advances in testing that we were able to accomplish. He never told me to slow down testing and indeed celebrated our progress in the Rose Garden.

Yes, Trump was certainly too optimistic about the pandemic just going away, but if you look at many of the graphs he was shown, the "science" actually predicted that COVID-19 would go to very low levels by Easter 2020. Biden was also optimistic, declaring independence from the virus in July 2021. That declaration was followed by the Delta and Omicron variants, which far surpassed the case numbers and carnage ever experienced during the Trump administration.

Early on, the "science" indicated that Americans were in no immediate danger—and that was said by every public health professional, including Fauci and Redfield. That was true; it wasn't imminent, but it was an inevitability down the road. Early on, we all had every reason to believe that hydroxychloroquine could help the pandemic. The in vitro data, published in top medical journals, showed that it was as effective as remdesivir to combat viral replication. There were clinical studies, albeit poorly controlled ones, that suggested a benefit. And physicians had been using the drug for decades. Also, I am certain that Trump got earfuls of anecdotal experiences from his friends and well-meaning clinicians across the country and continued ardent support of the drug from people like Peter Navarro. I don't blame Trump so much for his initial embrace of hydroxychloroquine because I cautiously embraced it too; he just couldn't give up on it despite the data suggesting otherwise.

It was Trump's "campaign persona" that got sideways with task force recommendations and caused all the doctors on the task force great stress and distress. Trump's campaign persona began to dominate the scene in early summer when he was on the campaign trail; during that time, he did not attend task force meetings and only rarely was directly briefed by the core task force doctors. It was clearly not a good example to hold rallies with tens of thousands of yelling supporters in the middle of a pandemic hot zone, especially since masking was optional and few if any chose to wear one. It was also counterproductive for core members of Trump's team, especially Peter Navarro and Scott Atlas, to publicly attack Birx and Fauci and occasionally me.

What happened on the campaign trail never influenced our recommendations to the American people. It also never seemed to affect Trump's support for the task force's ongoing recommendations to governors and the public. Trump's actions and policies for the nation were often contradictory to his practices on the campaign trail.

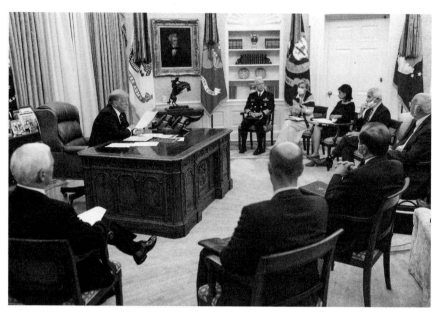

Briefing of President Trump by task force members, late summer 2020. In order, Admiral Giroir, Dr. Birx, Seema Verma, Dr. Fauci, Secretary Perdue (on sofa), Dr. Redfield, Secretary Azar, possibly Secretary Scalia, and Vice President Pence (White House photo).

I continued to promote masks and enhanced testing and the avoidance of unproven therapies. I did take some personal psychological solace in the Hatch Act, which forbids active political participation (like in political rallies or fundraising) by all government officials with rare exceptions (like cabinet members). This was even more relevant for me in uniform, where political neutrality was an expectation and obligation. I had no connection to—or control over—what happened at the rallies or anywhere else on the campaign trail. It was a legal prohibition and certainly an ethical one.

The president did not have such restrictions, however. He was always the president, and what he did as a candidate for reelection he also did as president of the United States. And that was the essence of the problem.

TASK FORCE SUPPORT TO STATES

I honestly became incensed at anyone who repeated the political talking point that "the states were left on their own." The absolute logistics miracle of expanding the supplies of PPE and distributing them according to need to every single hospital and nursing home in the nation deserves to be the topic of another book—not mine. As of September 2, the last day that FEMA was in charge as the lead agency, we had distributed 249 million respirators, 1.1 billion surgical masks, 46.7 million eye and face shields, 432 million surgical gowns, and more than 28.6 billion gloves to the states. I am certain that some states interrogated the overseas markets to obtain more, but Rear Admiral Polowczyk pretty much had it covered. He brought all the distributors into one room, assured allocation according to need, and accelerated the supply chains by using air bridges instead of sea transport. The distribution of supplies continued to increase in the fall and winter—but those final statistics are not publicly available.

In terms of testing, I already described how my team expanded, controlled, and distributed every aspect of COVID testing supplies, including swabs and media, and all POC tests. We also assisted in the allocation of PCR tests and worked individually with each state—on a concierge basis—to assure that they could source any remaining deficits through suppliers with excess capacity. All of this was done with full transparency and frequent collaborative calls with state public health and political leaders. We never competed with states for limited supplies; on the contrary, we used our federal authority to enhance and amass those supplies and then distribute them to states according to their needs and state plans. However, we were not able to create matter out of nothing, so the states could only get what actually was available in the real world, not the make-believe world of the Harvard School of Public Health or the Democratic National Committee.

In relation to the task force, due to the efforts of Deb Birx and her White House team, a several-hundred-page guide was sent from the task force to governors every week detailing the status of the pandemic down to the county level, with specific recommendations for testing, mitigation, the opening of schools, and all other details. Every chart a state needed to have and every recommendation the state needed to implement were sent to each governor every week like clockwork. That typically occurred on a Monday or Tuesday, and then the vice president hosted a videoconference with all governors in the afternoon on that day or the day after.

Pence had several of us do technical briefings on the governors' calls on various matters—for example, the distribution of POC tests or the allocation of remdesivir. The governors shared best practices. The governors' calls were very beneficial up until some governors covertly and inappropriately invited media to listen in (probably a national security violation, actually). Inevitably, those governors would have a two-minute rehearsed "rant" against the president during the governors' call, and that two-minute soundbite would show up later that day on national media. I hated that because our valuable working calls were becoming political theater, and that was going to cost more lives.

But most governors participated honestly and with no ulterior motives, and I liked and respected them on both sides of the political aisle. But Gov. Larry Hogan made me nauseated. He would typically give a flowery, grateful, and obsequious statement about the administration on the vice president's calls and then within an hour of the call skewer the president and every member of our team. If he had issues, we were all available to problem-solve on the call or at any other time. But he decided generally to go it alone, which led to multiple debacles—not the least of which was purchasing millions of junk Korean tests when there were millions of quality USA-made tests available instantaneously—many actually stored in Maryland warehouses.

In addition to these formal interactions, all the task force doctors frequently took calls from governors or their staffs. My most frequent calls were from Gov. Phil Murphy of New Jersey (always polite, professional, and gracious) and Gov. John Bel Edwards of Louisiana (equally professional and always trying to get as much help as he could for his state). I also spoke frequently to Gov. Inslee (Washington) and occasionally to Gov. Pritzker (Illinois)—honestly, all my interactions were professional and productive. We also went on the road. Deb Birx covered the most ground during the "Atlas time," which was the period when she mostly stopped doing national media appearances. I don't know how many states she visited, but it was at least thirty. She would fly somewhere, then drive for days and meet with governors and health officials and honestly anyone who would sit down and talk with her.

I also frequently flew on Air Force Two with Pence to meet with governors in their states, including Arizona, New Hampshire, Louisiana, and Massachusetts. Gov. Charlie Baker (Massachusetts) and Gov. Chris Sununu (New Hampshire) were both wicked smart and were thinking very strategically about minimizing infections while keeping their economies and employment as robust as possible. They asked tough questions, and I liked that. I did not have all the answers, but they appreciated my candor and perspective. For some of the larger states, like Florida and Texas, I spoke mostly to the state health officer or emergency management chief, like Chief Nim Kidd in Texas—and that was fine with me. They had the technical knowledge and were empowered to make decisions by their bosses.

What we could not do—and did not ever want to do—was force the states to comply with our recommendations. In the first place, we did not have the authority to force compliance; that is not the way public health works. Public health is a state- and county-level activity with rare exceptions, such as the international quarantine authority, which lies within the CDC. But in general, the governors or mayors had the authority for public health decisions, depending on the individual state laws. This was *federally supported, state managed, and locally executed*, like all other emergency responses. The federal government made recommendations, but then we supported the decisions of the governors in any way we could. Even President Biden in December 2021 finally understood the role of the federal government and the critical importance of state action when he finally admitted, "Look, there is no federal solution. This gets solved at a state level . . . and it ultimately gets down to where the rubber meets the road, and that's where the patient is in need of help or preventing the need for help."[3] All Biden's campaign promises of how the federal government would "shut down" the virus were false promises—as I knew they were all along.

Although we all understood and respected the federal system, the task force docs were frequently frustrated by extremes in state policy, and we worked hard to normalize these to a reasonable compromise level. Some states put in place much less mitigation than we recommended, but other states or cities banned everything (like school attendance and outdoor dining), which was equally as dangerous as undermitigation. We were also very distraught at times because state leadership did not act on a rise in positivity rates for testing, despite our warnings and pleas. Both Democrat and Republican states, from time to time, did not follow the advice we provided.

To my knowledge, we never said, "Told you so." If states needed surge testing to help salvage a situation, we sent it. That happened often. If they needed supplies or personnel, we sent them. Personally, I felt at peace with the situation. No one elected me to anything. The system was there for a reason, and the governors were elected to be responsive to their state constituencies. They weighed factors that were not in my immediate expertise or experience.

We really won't know the actual long-term impact and successes/failures of many of these governors' decisions for some time in the future. And when we do, we need to be careful not to make it a partisan witch hunt either way. We need to learn from our policy choices so we will have better evidence for the next pandemic. A few more deaths in the short term could be balanced by fewer deaths in the long term, from either COVID or the consequences of shutdowns, like suicides and drug overdose deaths.

An obvious failure among many states and certainly by the Biden administration until the data were overwhelming was the refusal to acknowledge the importance of natural immunity. Natural immunity is real and powerful—and, at least for the Delta variant, much more protective than vaccine immunity.[4] However, getting naturally infected intentionally is not a good choice compared to taking a vaccine and lessening the risk of hospitalization or death during that initial infection.

The bottom line is that no state got everything right, and we really don't yet know with certainty what "everything right" actually means. Let's be humble and transparent and improve for the future.

I respect the federalist system—and certainly that was Pence's view as a former governor. Each state had a CEO, the governor, and while the federal government had many enabling roles like funding, supplies, vaccines, and recommendations, the CEO was ultimately in charge. People in states should trust their governors more than they trust the federal government. The governor is closer to the people he or she serves and could be replaced in the next election or even immediately in a recall. I believe that the federal system served us well, but in any case, it *is* our system, and I swore to defend it.

ATLAS SHRUGGED

I had never heard of Dr. Scott Atlas. To my knowledge, he had never been involved in any pandemic preparedness meetings over the two decades I had been in and out of government focusing on those issues. He did not have an infectious disease background or training in immunology or public health, aside from the rudimentary training everyone receives in medical school. And apparently, I was not watching the cable TV shows that he was featured on—because I had never seen him. He was a neuroradiologist with a distinguished career in that field, a former professor at Stanford, and at the time a senior fellow in health policy at the Hoover Institute at Stanford. But these impressive credentials did not necessarily translate to expertise in infectious disease epidemiology or leading a pandemic response. However, in late July 2020, he showed up at the White House.

I don't remember the exact date in early August, but I remember the meeting vividly. I was called to a small huddle in the vice president's office in the West Wing. There were perhaps five or six people there, but notably not Deb Birx. Fauci was not there either. Pence introduced Atlas as a new advisor to the president and member of the task force. OK. I thought we could always use another doctor, perhaps one with a different perspective who could bring new insights. But the meeting was strange and a little awkward. Perhaps it was just one of those premonitions you get when things are about to go awry.

At the end of the meeting, Atlas gave me a written copy of his approach to testing and to the pandemic. There were many points aligned with our overall strategy at that time, including prioritization of the vulnerable and the need for more POC testing. Unlike what he later claimed, these were not *new* ideas, nor were they *his* ideas. We had been progressively implementing this strategy to protect the vulnerable and dramatically enhance rapid POC testing since the end of March. But nonetheless, there was strong alignment here. Good start, I thought!

But there were several points that were contrary to our guidance and, indeed, indicative of his belief that we should let the virus broadly infect the healthy so the country could get back to normal. His document specifically stated, "Broad population testing of asymptomatic people is not a priority—tens of millions of people have been infected; the action item if positive (quarantining asymptomatic, low risk people) would be both hugely disruptive to society, and interfere with the critical population immunity need to eradicate the threat (not to mention contrary to American values of personal freedom)."[5] This is by definition a "herd immunity" approach but with some important caveats, including the explicit objective to shield the vulnerable.

There was, however, a very serious problem with his concept of shielding the elderly. Atlas was not fully accounting for the fact that the vulnerable are all around us, not just in nursing homes, and that we could not protect them without a larger, more comprehensive strategy that also decreased infections among the young and healthy, at least until there were safe and effective vaccines and antiviral medications. In addition, large swaths of our US population live in multigenerational homes, especially racial and ethnic minorities. One-third of Americans are obese, and millions have hypertension or lung disease; few of these reside in nursing homes.

The ubiquitous presence of vulnerable people was obvious to me the few times I went to the neighborhood Harris Teeter grocery store during the pandemic—there were people of all ages shopping, including the elderly. Some of the stockers and cashiers were in their sixties, many obese and likely with underlying health conditions. There were homeless outside the front door, maskless and interacting with everyone. And who knows how many people had cancer or HIV. My favorite apartment concierge was a slightly overweight African American man probably in his early fifties—high risk—and he lived with a sister who was on immunosuppressive therapy. Bottom line, letting the infection spread among the young and healthy would create a killing field for all the elderly, obese, chronically ill, and immunocompromised who live throughout our communities. So to protect the vulnerable—before vaccines and antiviral medications—it was absolutely imperative to minimize community spread through testing and quarantine.

Atlas displayed a troubling combination of science and political ideology, evidenced by his views on individual liberties and how testing and quarantine violated these freedoms. These were very appropriate concerns: we all had them and debated them regularly in the task force. But the primary job of the task force doctors was to outline the best course of action *to limit the impact of the virus* (infection control and saving lives), and then the entire multi-disciplinary task force would debate the implications of potential actions to control the virus on the economy, education, mental health, national security, individual liberties, and so on. But Atlas was weighing all those considerations in his head and coming up with a conclusion about actions. If you don't like Fauci getting out of his lane when he dismissed the importance of individual liberties, Atlas did the same at the opposite extreme. Neither Atlas nor Fauci is a constitutional scholar, and neither should have positioned his views on liberty behind the veil of medical science.

Atlas could read and interpret scientific data with extraordinary rigor. And in truth, he often made relevant arguments and challenged conventional dogma when the task force docs became complacent and stale in our assessments. We always needed new ideas and approaches, especially prior to vaccines and oral antiviral therapies. More importantly, Atlas was apparently the only medical professional regularly briefing President Trump at that time. If he had Trump's ear, we needed to engage with him. I felt strongly that I needed to interact with him as productively and collegially as I could. Only one thing mattered—saving American lives and ending the pandemic. At least during that time, I perceived the road to doing so went through Atlas and not around him.

Atlas characterized Birx and Fauci as advocating for "lockdowns" and subsequently railed against these policies as well as Birx and Fauci personally, both during and after his time in the White House. To me, this was a strawman argument because none of us individually or as a group *ever* advocated Draconian lockdowns. As stated earlier, the fifteen days and then thirty days to slow the spread were stopgap measures at the beginning of the pandemic when there were no vaccines, no medications, and no good data on masking or physical distancing. They were intended to, and succeeded in, keeping the hospital systems from being overrun and preventing tens of thousands of Americans from dying without an available ventilator. Furthermore, over fifty million essential US workers were advised to go to work with a mask even if they had close exposure to a person with COVID-19—that is *not* a significant lockdown.

In addition, well before the end of the thirty days to slow the spread period, the task force developed and presented the *Guidelines, Opening Up America Again*[6] because we recognized the extreme collateral damage of stringent lockdowns. President Trump was out front in this effort to get Americans back to work and back to school. The document recommended certain very reasonable conditions that should be met in order for states to open up safely and progressively. But in our federal system, it was ultimately up to the states to craft their own policies. And the reality was that there was little the federal government could do or should have done to coerce state-level actions.

Recognizing the potential harm to children, the CDC *never* recommended closing schools. Despite that, many school districts closed their doors, perhaps indelibly harming the underserved. When in the summer of 2020, certain large school districts around the country indicated they had no intention of reopening, Trump threatened to cut their federal funding. To my knowledge, no funds were ever withheld. I was pleased with both the intent to keep schools open and the fact that the federal government wound up never "heavy handing" local school district decisions. Moreover, the task force doctors (myself included) spent substantial time on governors' calls and in the national media emphasizing the irrevocable harms of school closures, especially to the underserved.

We advocated mask wearing—Atlas disagreed. He argued with the evidence and vociferously stated what he perceived as the consequences. But to me (and to the other docs), the preponderance of the data showed that mask wearing in indoor crowded spaces was a reasonable step to provide some level of protection against transmitting the virus or becoming infected yourself. Masks are not perfect and became less so during the Omicron variant, but we assessed that they were overall of benefit in specific situations—especially prior to vaccines being available.

At his first task force meeting, Atlas initially listened attentively to the proceedings. But then when prompted for his opinion by the vice president, he unloaded on Birx, essentially arguing every point she made and challenging the data and her interpretation of it. There were many heated arguments, even in front of the vice president. Birx resented being challenged, especially in such an overt way.

Personally, I did not have any public or even private heated arguments with Scott, and we spoke many times away from the other docs, reviewing the evidence and discussing alternatives. The reality was that Atlas was in the White House and speaking with Trump and had made some important arguments that we needed to consider. So I tried hard to be a moderating force between him and Birx/Fauci. Unfortunately, the fact that I worked with Atlas and did not avoid him or his sometimes helpful input fueled Birx's paranoia that I was working against her. This was obviously false. I was never against Birx in any way, although I did sometimes disagree with her conclusions and proposed actions. We generally worked those issue-oriented debates out privately and amicably.

I don't know how much Atlas actually influenced the president. He apparently briefed Trump regularly, which the other doctors had only rarely done after the early summer of 2020. Atlas was on national TV shows and talked to many governors. Soon after he arrived, Deb decided she would never be in a meeting or roundtable discussion with him because she felt it lent him credibility that he did not deserve. I thought that was a terrible decision because only one side of the scientific issues was heard. And as coordinator, Birx should not have ducked controversy like that. Not lending credibility seemed like an excuse to avoid engaging in debate about complex issues. Whatever the reason, Deb started spending more and more time on the road working directly with governors and state and local officials. I continued to work with Atlas and every other member of the task force because we all had to be part of the solution and would soon have the tools—including vaccines and medications—to begin truly defeating the virus.

Atlas resigned at the end of November 2020. He left as quickly as he had shown up.

WHO "NEEDS A TEST"? THE TRUE STORY OF THE CDC'S AUGUST 2020 TESTING GUIDANCE

The media relished stories of conflict within the task force. And Scott Atlas's time in the White House fueled more than a few. But vigorous scientific debate in the context of policy making shouldn't be perceived as dysfunction. Rather, it is an important part of the process. One such difficult and intensely discussed decision in August 2020 needlessly mushroomed into a media-fed, misrepresented controversy. To this day, the House Select Committee on Coronavirus and even Dr. Birx in her book have mischaracterized this CDC testing guidance—both the reasons why it was developed and how it was actually approved.

In the summer of 2020, testing numbers had been growing dramatically; that was great and consistent with the national testing strategy. But we had a problem, and I first saw it through my daily monitoring of turnaround times (TATs) from large commercial labs like LabCorp and Quest. These labs were performing about half the testing in the United States, and TATs were increasing. Really increasing! And that was because of the huge growth in demand from not just people who "needed" a test but also those who "wanted" a test. Those who "wanted" a test included those traveling abroad or even to other states for nonessential purposes as well as those who were told they were required to have a negative test before returning to work or school (which was contrary to the science and inconsistent with CDC guidelines). In addition, we could see that many people were being tested perhaps a dozen times over a few weeks, which did not make any sense at all. Finally, a growing number of Americans just wanted to be tested, and while that was good in some sense, the national supply could not handle that amount of demand in the summer of 2020. And for context, the nation still could not handle such demand in the fall of 2021 when the Biden administration presided over shortages of their own doing.

In July 2020, TATs had increased to five or six days in many areas of the country, and there were anecdotal reports of eight- to twelve-day turnarounds. If this continued or worsened—and communications from the companies suggested that it could worsen in the near term—such delays in receiving results could threaten nursing home testing as well as the diagnosis of the sick within hospitals. Nursing homes and many hospitals were still highly dependent on the large commercial labs—and would remain so until we could get millions of POC tests distributed. We knew some relief was on the way. We had finalized the purchase of point-of-care tests that would be shipped with instruments to nursing homes in early August. We anxiously anticipated card-based point-of-care antigen tests (like BinaxNOW). We estimated that they would be available sometime in the fall, but we did not know when. So at that point in August, we had to take action, and quickly, to prioritize testing.

Prioritization of testing to those in greatest need was the sole aim of the August guidance—it was never to decrease testing. Indeed, the opposite was the case: we intended to both increase testing and prioritize it.

The first thing I did was communicate expectations to the commercial labs. I indicated that all hospitalized patients, health-care workers, and residents and staff of nursing homes (which we classified as "high priority") needed a turnaround of two days or fewer. Clinical specimens ordered by health-care providers, including those in our community-based sites and for public health tracking and tracing (classified as "priority"), needed to be four days or less. All other testing (classified as "routine")—including for travel and returning to work, and asymptomatic surveillance testing—needed to have results in fewer than seven days. And importantly, routine tests were not to be completed *at all* unless high-priority and priority TATs met the objectives I set out. The labs not only complied but appreciated the guidance. They were caught in the middle and needed a federally mandated way out. In fact, LabCorp and Quest were already in the process of dramatically expanding their capabilities and scale, so they would have the capacity within weeks. But in the short term, they were in trouble, and that meant the nation was in trouble.

At the same time that I prioritized testing to the commercial labs, the CDC needed to update its testing guidance both because of the evolving science and to account for the priorities of the nation at that moment—including the squeeze on testing—until BinaxNOW or other similar tests could be authorized sometime in the future.

When Redfield discussed an initial draft of the guidance at the task force level, there was significant debate and discussion. And yes, Atlas had a point of view that differed from the other docs—so Pence told us to go offline to gain consensus on the guidelines before they came back to the task force and ultimately to the CDC to pass their internal clearance and approval processes. As the testing czar, I assumed the responsibility of gaining consensus—not all that easy because of the strained relationship between Birx and Atlas. "Strained" is an understatement.

Redfield and I had an initial two-hour meeting with Atlas where we discussed many issues and came to an agreement on a number of them. We also identified many considerations that had not been part of the original document. Very few items were actually controversial or even debatable—for example, the fact that people did not need to be retested to return to work after completing the recommended period of isolation.

In terms of testing those who had been exposed to the virus (close contact with an infected person within six feet or less for fifteen minutes or more without appropriate masking) but who were not symptomatic, we wanted to make a few critical points with the new guidance. We had strong indications that people who were exposed and tested negative once (at any time after exposure) were returning back to the community and interacting with the vulnerable without further precautions. That was a terrible situation because one negative test could become positive any time within ten to fourteen days after exposure. A negative test only meant it was negative at that moment in time. Whether negative or positive, that individual needed to quarantine according to CDC guidance (fourteen days at that time).

The second point was that if exposed but asymptomatic people were around vulnerable individuals (or vulnerable themselves), it was important to be tested. For these individuals, testing positive could lead to specific treatment for the individual or their vulnerable contacts. However, for healthy individuals who were *not* vulnerable and *not* advised to take a test by their doctors, we stated that such individuals did "not necessarily need a test." And that was absolutely a correct statement, even in retrospect, for August 2020. The rationale was straightforward: once a person was exposed, that person needed to quarantine for fourteen days. A positive test or several negative ones did not change the recommendation for a fourteen-day quarantine. If the person became symptomatic or was in a high-risk group, testing became a high priority because of the potential need for specific anti-COVID treatment.

The new guidance was released by the CDC on August 24. Within days, the media bombardment began. The revision to the guidance was characterized by blaring headlines: "This Change in Policy Will Kill"[7] and "CDC Was Pressured 'from the Top Down.'"[8] And unfortunately, Fauci, instead of explaining the reasoning for the new guidance and admitting he had been fully involved for three weeks during the revisions, told CNN's Jake Tapper that he was under anesthesia for vocal cord surgery when the guidance was approved and suggested that he wasn't part of the discussion.[9]

Despite what the press said at the time or how some try to revise history today, there was very little controversy about the issue of not necessarily testing healthy asymptomatic people who were not specifically recommended to be tested by public health practitioners or physicians. Official emails—which I saved copies of—clearly indicate that although there was debate and discussion over several other items, there were *no edits* to the "you do not necessarily need a test" recommendation by either Dr. Fauci, Dr. Walke (CDC career staff and incident commander in Atlanta), Dr. Redfield, or Dr. Birx—although there was ample opportunity for edits to be made. In fact, Birx wrote back to me after reviewing the draft guidance on August 5, "Just a couple of comments. Thank you for your support and encouragement."[10] She made absolutely no comments about the "you do not necessarily need a test" language.

Indeed, the final document was affirmatively cleared by all the doctors except for Dr. Birx, who made no written comment either way during the final clearance process despite being sent the document multiple times. Once the document was affirmatively cleared and without any objections, the document was sent back to the CDC for their final review and clearance, at which time the CDC could have approved or disapproved it.

The misstatements about the guidance in the media and by political operatives (some wearing white coats) did more to fuel misinformation about testing than the guidance ever did itself. But why be constrained by truth if it fit the anti-Trump political narrative?

The CDC ultimately changed the guidance—I think probably just to stop the irrational critiques and the consequences of media misinformation. The CDC went back to recommending tests for anyone in contact with a person with COVID, even though it did *nothing* to change outcomes or courses of action. That goes against a century of medical wisdom, which states that you don't perform a test if it makes no difference to the patient, especially if there is sufficient overall surveillance going on to detect regional outbreaks (which there was). The guidance was also blind to the reality of test availability, which meant that the guidance *could not* actually be followed. Again, why offer guidance that is impossible to implement?

But then, as if by design (which it wasn't), the CDC's rerevised guidance was issued right after I announced the FDA authorization of BinaxNOW and the distribution of 150 million free rapid tests, exactly what we needed to assure testing of the vulnerable with appropriate turnaround time. Lab-Corp and Quest were also gaining control of their turnaround times because of rapid expansion and internal prioritization, as we directed.

The guidance was never meant to decrease testing, although it was spun that way by administration opponents and by a complicit media. Remember, testing never really experienced a substantial and sustained decrease until after Biden was inaugurated. My team battled every day to increase testing volumes and effectiveness, and that continued throughout the remainder of the term right up until January 20. The August guidance was needed to prioritize testing for those in highest need while preserving and advocating for asymptomatic testing within the context of public health surveillance or medical advice. We preserved and guaranteed the availability of truly life-or-death testing in hospitals and nursing homes at a time when the testing ecosystem was still expanding and diversifying to meet demand. By the end of September, rapid POC tests were being distributed in the tens of millions each week—and the problems of August were gone forever.

OPERATION WARP SPEED

OWS was a major success for the Trump administration but certainly not the only one. I give credit to the Biden administration for taking the baton and at least initially continuing with the Trump administration playbook, up until the point Biden attempted to implement vaccine mandates and demonize the unvaccinated. That was exactly the opposite of what the United States needed at the time because it entrenched the vaccine hesitant in their opposition and also stifled scientific debate among objective physicians and scientists.

By the end of our administration in January 2021, we had already contracted to buy nine hundred million doses of vaccines with an option to purchase up to two billion more; we had procured over one billion needles and associated products, like alcohol swabs; we had signed up over forty thousand pharmacy sites and an additional thirty thousand other sites to administer the vaccine. I personally provided regulatory guidance that overrode state laws so that pharmacists, pharmacy interns, pharmacy technicians, and emergency medical technicians (especially those in the National Guard) could vaccinate Americans against COVID. There was no shortage of vaccinators as the Biden administration claimed, nor had we neglected actually getting vaccines in arms. Nonsense! And the data show that the Trump administration rollout had already achieved a rate of vaccination on the day of inauguration (1.59 million shots in arms) that exceeded the rate required to achieve the Biden goal of one hundred million shots in one hundred days.

The details of OWS have been fully described by Paul Mango, who worked daily with Azar to develop and implement OWS.[11] But from my point of view, the successes of OWS stem primarily from two factors. First, the United States had intensively invested in vaccine technology and infrastructure for almost two decades, so both the technologies (like mRNA vaccines) and the infrastructure (bulk manufacturing and filling the individual vaccines into vials) had been reasonably well thought out prior to COVID-19. Second and most important, Azar engaged the private sector in a true partnership with multiple HHS components for rapid development, clinical trials, scale-up, and distribution. This lesson and model need to be built upon and expanded in order for us to adequately prepare for the next pandemic.

COULD 130,000 MORE LIVES HAVE BEEN SAVED IN THE TRUMP ADMINISTRATION?

On October 12–13, 2021, the House Select Subcommittee on the Coronavirus Crisis conducted a closed-door interview with Deb Birx. In May 2022, they conducted a similar interview with me that lasted six hours. Why these were "closed door" is a mystery and an injustice to every American who wants to hear our opinions for themselves instead of just being supplied with months of partisan spin by the Democrat and Republican members.

Deb made several very important, substantive statements that were carried widely in the media. These deserve detailed analysis, and I hope that Deb is able to explain her meaning in a nonpartisan forum so that we can improve upon the future national response. But her most provocative statement, highlighted by the subcommittee to the public, is the following: "I believe if we had fully implemented the mask mandates, the reduction in indoor dining, the getting friends and family to understand the risk of gathering in private homes, and we had increased testing, that we probably could have decreased fatalities into the 30-percent-less to 40-percent-less range."[12] When you do the math, that reduction turns into 130,000 additional lives that could have been saved.

In other parts of her interview, Deb stated that with regard to the White House, the election "just took people's time away from and distracted them away from the pandemic in my personal opinion." Furthermore, when asked if she thought that President Trump did everything he could to try to mitigate the spread of the virus and save lives, she responded, "No. And I've said that to the White House in general, and I believe I was very clear to the president in specifics of what I needed him to do."[13]

The conclusion of the liberal press, whether stated explicitly or implicitly in all their coverage, was that *Trump was responsible for 130,000 avoidable deaths*. It doesn't get much more explicit than a headline in the *Hill* on October 27, which read, "Top Pandemic Official Claims Trump Could Have Saved 130K People from Preventable Deaths."[14]

In addition to my final chapter that details reforms at the global, national, and local levels, the proposition that Trump could have saved 130,000 more lives just by listening to the scientists deserves a full and transparent analysis—and I will do it here, at least from my point of view.

First, let me make two comments that need to be stated for the record. When Deb Birx talks about "White House failures," it should be obvious that she was, in fact, "the White House." OK, she was not the president or vice president, but she was the task force coordinator. Her office was in the West Wing, her team was there and controlled most of the incoming data, and she led every White House Coronavirus Task Force meeting and nearly every governors' call. Nonetheless, it is also true that if she was failing at her coordinator role, Trump should have replaced her—so it is back on the president, at least in that context.

Second, I don't think her comment that she told the president what she needed him to do should be taken literally. Telling a president what she "needed him to do" is a declaration that is never made to any president, much less Trump. Her role (and my role) was to make recommendations and advise the president and vice president and communicate evidence-based recommendations to federal and state officials and to the public; we don't tell the president or vice president what we need him to do.

Let's analyze this specific statement: "I believe if we had fully implemented the mask mandates, the reduction in indoor dining, the getting friends and family to understand the risk of gathering in private homes, and we had increased testing." Here, she means the royal *we*. Implementing these measures was not in the purview of the federal government. Mask mandates and reductions in indoor dining are state and local measures. The task force made specific recommendations, every week at the county level, to governors regarding these mitigation measures. The "we" is not the task force or the federal government or Trump; it was the state and local leaders who made these decisions. That was not a "Trump thing" to implement.

If Birx and the press are going to have that standard, then the Biden administration is at least as culpable or more so than the Trump administration. During the Delta surge in August 2021, mask wearing was down from 70 percent during early January under Trump to ~30 percent nationally under Biden.[15] And there were *no* states that mandated bar or restaurant closures in August 2021. Only a handful had indoor gathering limits. So are we to say, "If only Biden had fully implemented masking and indoor dining restrictions, he could have saved 250,000 more lives in 2021?" Or how about, "If only Biden had fully implemented the vaccine recommendations from the scientists, he could have saved 400,000 more lives during Delta and Omicron outbreaks?" That is exactly what is being projected onto Trump, and I don't believe that is fair in Trump's case or Biden's.

Getting families and friends "to understand the risk of gathering in private homes" was her next point. I would argue that we communicated that point frequently and clearly. My assessment is that the American people *understood exactly* what we were saying but often made a different decision because they weighed the risks and acted appropriately for their families. Perhaps the families that gathered did indeed follow the recommendations to distance and protect the vulnerable, or maybe they weighed the emotional harm (and the impending wave of suicides and drug overdoses) and decided to have a Thanksgiving meal together instead of virtually. In any regard, there was no surge in cases following Thanksgiving or Christmas 2020 according to CDC-reported cases. Cases had been on the rise, and there was no increase in the slope following holiday travel. On the contrary, the week after the New Year holiday 2020–21, cases started to plummet.[16] So the risk of family gatherings was probably grossly overstated.

Finally, the reports that Birx took a trip to her Delaware home accompanied by three generations of her family to celebrate Thanksgiving do not support her premise that family gatherings were inherently unsafe. As for Jill and me, we stayed by ourselves for Thanksgiving and Christmas in Washington, DC, if for no other reason than I needed to work on the pandemic. There was no time for a break. But equally important, it did not seem right for me to be on national media every evening asking Americans to make sacrifices that we were not willing to make ourselves. We had already seen the damage done by political leaders who, after issuing restrictions on individuals and businesses, were spotted flaunting noncompliance with those same guidelines. Americans are quick to spot hypocrites and tune out their messages.

For Birx's next point—"if we had increased testing"—she should know that the administration (and I) did everything in our power to increase the supply of tests, and the rate-limiting factor from early summer onward was *not* the availability of tests but how many people wanted to be tested. From the task force, we strongly supported surveillance testing in at-risk populations or for specific segments, like college students, who could spread disease within their neighboring community. We doubled down on testing the vulnerable in nursing homes, assisted living facilities, tribal nations, and HBCUs, sending the new POC tests to these locations. When there were outbreaks or potential outbreaks in the summer and fall of 2020, we established 644 federal surge sites in twenty-three states to supplement the approximately nine thousand retail sites and community health centers already under the federal program. This was in addition to the tens of thousands of routine health-care clinics that offered testing. And we sent one hundred million BinaxNOW tests to governors with the specific intent that they use them to increase testing. And finally, Birx absolutely misstated the truth when she said that testing decreased after the CDC's August 2020 guidance concerning testing asymptomatic contacts—testing went up dramatically over the next months, not down. By the way, the CDC guidance delivered under Biden on December 28, 2021, stated explicitly that someone exposed should test *only if possible*![17] That was not so different than the CDC guidance that Birx has questioned.

Although I imagine it is theoretically possible that we could have increased testing even more, I don't know what we could have done. And let's again make the analogy with the Biden administration: testing plummeting after his inauguration—down by over 50 percent by the early summer of 2021.[18] More importantly, he let the industry involute because of his failure to reorder tests and keep the manufacturing lines working seven days per week. BinaxNOW factories went offline, and only in September 2020 (after Delta blew through the country) did the Biden administration again invest in testing. As a result, testing was in much worse shape in December 2021 than it was in December 2020. So if there is blame on the Trump administration, it is double on the Biden administration.

As to the concept of 130,000 preventable deaths, it is unclear to me how much of an impact mask mandates or restrictions on indoor dining would have mattered. Mask wearing actually went down dramatically in 2021 under the new administration. It is also unclear (still) whether mask *mandates* (as opposed to public health messaging about masking) actually increase proper mask use and limit the spread of the disease. And if there had been more bans on dining, even outdoor dining like what occurred in several states and localities like California and Washington, DC, more people would likely have had crowded indoor parties at home with takeout food. I saw that daily from my apartment window in DC, where thirty people crammed into a small apartment across the street because they couldn't go out together. That was much more dangerous than outdoor dining or indoor dining with reduced capacity. So I don't know, nor does Deb, how much these mandates would have changed the trajectory of the pandemic and the ultimate death toll if they had been adopted by the states and localities.

Now in terms of Trump, the argument can be made that if he had been more forceful about supporting the task force recommendations (and indeed practiced what we preached on the campaign trail), there would have been more uptake of the measures we were publicly recommending in writing every week to every governor. That is a completely fair hypothesis and one that should be debated. The task force doctors all wanted the Trump campaign machine to follow our public health recommendations. But again, if we applied the standard for Trump to Biden, perhaps we should also state,

"If only Biden had worn a mask when he went to a DC restaurant and prac-ticed what his administration preached . . ." "If only the Biden team didn't get ahead of the FDA and state there would be boosters for everyone by a specific date when there was no data to support it or ignore the science and insist on vaccine mandates even for those naturally immune (who did far better during Delta than those with two vaccine doses) . . ." "If only Biden had not been distracted by climate change summits in Europe or weekends in Delaware or campaigning for his social spending bill . . ."

And if we are going to assign blame for excess deaths, we should also be fair in assigning responsibility for lives saved. Without the leadership of Trump and Azar's involvement in OWS, vaccines would have been delayed by months or years, and there could have been tens of thousands of more deaths, maybe even hundreds of thousands. In terms of testing, I am quite certain that with-out the audacity of Trump and his White House to fully engage the private sector, testing would have continued to flounder at the CDC. And finally, without the Trump team's emphasis on reopening the United States, the num-ber of suicides, drug overdoses, child abuse victims, and missed cancer and heart attack screenings might be double or triple what it is now. If people want to do a scorecard, they should count the runs in addition to the errors. We need a complete, honest, nonpartisan analysis—and we haven't yet gotten it.

We all must realize that political scapegoating, which continues today during the closed-door subcommittee interviews—like the one I was sub-jected to—does not actually lead to solutions: ending this pandemic is not as easy as merely replacing a president or "following the science." The public health professionals in the Trump administration followed the science to the best of our abilities, given the uncertainties in the data. And no matter who is in the White House or wearing US Public Health Service uniforms, our nation's response will always be dictated by the adequacy of our public health and societal preparation before the pandemic begins, the capabilities and rela-tionships of our leaders, and the inevitable politics of the day. The solutions are not easy. But there are solutions—feasible ones that will not disrupt our society or infringe on our liberties.

If we don't want a repeat of COVID-19 in the next decade, we need to abandon the politics and get serious about the solutions. I am committed to doing that with any administration at any time. Every day that passes is precious time wasted. My hope is that this book can potentially bring people together, across party and socioeconomic and ethnic divides, to learn from our successes and failures and begin the process of making our world biosafe for the next century.

12

Keeping the United States Biosafe in the Twenty-First Century

To me, the most concerning issue that will stifle future progress is the incessant blame game, even while the pandemic is still ongoing in the United States and throughout the world. There continue to be statements like "If only Trump had not been president, this would not have happened." "If only more people followed the science, no one needed to die." "If only the American people sacrificed more, this could have been prevented." Scapegoating only leads to a false sense of security and the belief that simplistic solutions will keep us safe in the future. They won't. In fact, this type of thinking puts all of us at even higher risk.

We also cannot turn back the clock. Travel and global connectivity will continue to increase and should. Techniques for the genetic manipulation of natural organisms and synthetic biology (creating entirely human-made genes and organisms) will continue to advance at a startling pace and will become simple enough (as many already are) that a graduate student is fully capable of dangerously tinkering with Mother Nature. Rogue nations like China and Russia and perhaps radical extremist groups will seek a strategic advantage by weaponizing biology—even exploring the possibility of creating pathogens that selectively target particular racial or ethnic groups.

To state the obvious, we need to cut the political bullshit and focus on real solutions to prepare for the next pandemic threat. "Those who cannot remember the past are condemned to repeat it."[1] So in this, the last chapter of my book, I want to offer practical suggestions and feasible solutions so that we don't repeat the past. There are no easy answers, no silver bullets, and no guarantees. But we can dramatically lower the potential for a new pandemic emerging in the first place and certainly can improve our national and global responses to contain any emerging threat. It is the least we can do in honor of the millions worldwide who lost their lives to COVID and to future generations who will need to survive in this exhilarating but dangerous world we leave them.

PREVENTING EMERGENCE: MINIMIZING THE SPARKS

The best way to control a pandemic is to prevent it in the first place. While complete prevention is impossible, several initiatives can reduce the risks—perhaps substantially. And we can achieve them in a multilateral way, respecting the autonomy of nations and the importance of their cultures and social fabrics.

Wet Markets

The term *wet market* has many different meanings, and we must be careful to define our policies in such a way that they are evidence based and implementable in diverse cultures. A wet market may be nothing more than an open-air market (or another nontraditional market) that sells perishable produce. Millions of people (and perhaps billions) rely on wet markets for their food, and without this access, feeding their families would be threatened. Wet markets, especially in China, are also an important aspect of the community, where people meet and socialize. These types of wet markets are no more of a threat than the French Market in New Orleans; the Eastern Market in Washington, DC; or the thousands of farmers markets that make fresh foods available across the United States every day.

There are *live animal markets*, which sell live traditional food sources, especially chickens, ducks, and other fowl. Crowded conditions and exposure to animal waste increases the chances of transmission of viruses from bird to bird within and across bird species and to humans who are in close contact with them. Live animal markets are particularly concerning because of their incubation and spread of avian influenza viruses, which have regularly decimated the poultry industries of many countries, as is happening at the time of this writing in 2022 in the United States and around the world, and risk human pandemics caused by the bird flu. The 1997 H5N1 influenza outbreak in Hong Kong was thought to arise from such a live bird market.

Finally, there are *wild animal live markets*, where diverse wild species are sold live for food or traditional medicines. The animals may be captured or bred in captivity by small producers. The types of animals in these markets that have a high risk of spreading new diseases include bats, civets, foxes, wolves, badgers, squirrels, hedgehogs, cats, dogs, pheasants, crows, snakes, and many other species—some of which I have not even heard of. The Huanan Seafood Wholesale Market in Wuhan, China, was such an establishment, with diverse wild animals for sale. Although the Huanan Market was likely not the origin of SARS-CoV-2, live animal wet markets are extraordinarily risky because of the close contact of wild species to humans and to other wild species, risking genetic recombination of diverse viruses and perhaps direct infection of humans by animals.

Our policy objective should be *not* to eliminate wet markets but to minimize or eliminate wild animal markets and, to the degree possible, live bird markets. I have no concern about live fish in a tank, since fish are evolutionarily distant and very unlikely to have their pathogens infect humans or other mammals.

Here, there is common ground between China and the United States. In early 2020, China prohibited the sale of wild animals for food and, in July 2020, announced a plan to phase out the sale of live poultry in wet markets as well. China has not banned wild animal sales for traditional medicine. While that would be ideal, there are still targeted steps that could be accomplished to reduce risk, including limiting the number of animals sold, separating different species, utilizing sanitary wildlife farming practices (as opposed to wild capture), and enhancing hygiene and sanitation in a controlled environment. The Chinese may not be ready to give up their three-thousand-year-old medicine traditions, but we should also not let the perfect be the enemy of the good. The world needs to get done what it can now and then continue to work in the future to further minimize risks.

The United States should vocally support China if they consistently and transparently implement these reforms, and both countries should work through the WHO to establish these as model practices. The United States and China should then encourage at-risk countries to adopt best practices through technical assistance and grants and as a condition of direct financial support.

Most importantly, the Global Health Security Agenda (the master plan and playbook) adopted by the WHO should formally include risk mitigation in wildlife and live animal markets as a component of its Joint External Evaluation (JEE) process. The JEE is specifically designed to help nations evaluate how well they are implementing the Global Health Security Agenda. The JEE process begins with a national self-assessment followed thereafter by an objective, external evaluation conducted by representatives from multiple nations who are members of the WHO. The evaluation assesses many aspects of human and animal health, food safety, agriculture, defense, and public safety.

Although voluntary, the JEE process has been tremendously beneficial for promoting global health security, with approximately one hundred countries having completed their evaluations, including the United States, and another twenty already scheduled. Of note, China has not undergone a JEE and should be encouraged to perform one in light of the COVID-19 pandemic. But even a successful JEE does not ensure transparent notification of the global community about an emerging killer infection like COVID-19. But it would make the emergence of such a disease less likely in the first place. And that is at least a start.

BSL-4 Maximum Containment Laboratories

Biosafety level 4 (BSL-4) laboratories are designed and constructed to "safely" work with the most dangerous microbes on earth. These pathogens cause serious diseases for which, in general, there are no treatments or vaccines. Examples of pathogens that require BSL-4 safety measures include the Ebola virus, the Nipah virus,[2] and the Variola virus (smallpox). But in addition to these highly dangerous organisms, certain types of experiments on less dangerous organisms must also be conducted at BSL-4 safety levels. A relevant example is the controversial gain-of-function research (performing experiments to actually make an organism *more dangerous*) on novel bat coronaviruses. Constructing and operating a BSL-4 laboratory indicates the operator's desire to work on such extraordinary pathogens but in an environment that protects scientists and researchers (and thus humankind).

The Wuhan Institute of Virology is now perhaps the most widely publicized BSL-4 laboratory in the world. But it represents only the tip of the iceberg. According to a new nonprofit organization that tracks BSL-4 laboratories, there are sixty-seven such labs in operation, under construction, or planned around the world, including twenty-six in Europe, fifteen in North America, nineteen in Asia, four in Australia, and three in Africa.[3] The great majority of these are in large urban areas, like Wuhan, where an accidental leak could potentially expose millions of local residents essentially overnight.

Of the twenty-two countries that host BSL-4 laboratories, only about one-quarter of the countries score high on biosafety and biosecurity preparedness; the remaining countries have medium or low-level preparedness. But independent of these overall national scores is the actual operation of the laboratories. To err is human, and facilities and processes are only as good as the staff working within them. For example, even within a BSL-4 laboratory, experiments can be conducted at lower levels of biocontainment than recommended. There is some evidence to suggest that this was the case in Wuhan. But even at appropriate levels of care, mistakes happen. These are some of the most infectious agents on the planet, and it only takes a few organisms to infect a lab worker through the respiratory system or a tiny break in the skin.

Unfortunately, lab leaks are not rare. In 2004, a SARS outbreak in Beijing was traced to a lab leak. SARS has also infected lab workers in Taiwan and Singapore. In 1978, smallpox infected a worker in England but was not further spread because of aggressive quarantine and public health interventions. In 1979, at least one hundred died near Sverdlovsk in the Soviet Union as the result of an accidental release of anthrax spores by a military bioweapons facility. There have also been troubling incidents and near misses in the United States with agents including pandemic flu strains, anthrax, and smallpox, even occurring within laboratories at our premier national agencies like the CDC and the FDA.

Several lines of evidence implicate the Wuhan Institute of Virology as the origin of the COVID-19 pandemic. First, an extensive investigation conducted by the WHO seeking a natural animal origin—taking samples from over eighty thousand animals from throughout China—produced no virus within decades of evolution related to SARS-CoV-2. Second, unlike a "normal" transmission from animals to humans that smolders for months or years before human-to-human transmission occurs, this virus was nearly perfectly adapted for human-to-human transmission from the outset; that suggests laboratory manipulation or evolution and not a natural event. There are multiple other concerning indicators, including documented lab safety lapses, gain-of-function research resulting in the creation of novel highly infectious viruses, reports of lab workers becoming ill in September and October of 2019, and the undisputed massive cover-up of information and prohibition of CDC access by the Chinese government. And bottom line, isn't it just a little too coincidental that a pandemic caused by a novel bat coronavirus not found in nature started just a few miles away from a secretive Chinese laboratory studying (and performing gain-of-function research) on highly infectious novel bat coronaviruses?

Complicating everything is the very nature of the research being conducted at BSL-4 laboratories, which can almost always be interpreted as "dual use," meaning that while generally intended for appropriate humanitarian reasons, it can also be used to inflict harm. Having spent decades associated with the US government and with the highest level of national security clearances, I can assure everyone that the United States does not have an offensive

bioweapons program. We are transparent and honest with all treaty obliga-
tions. The same is unfortunately not the case with many other countries for
which offensive military applications are a by-product—if not the primary
objective—of their research. In such circumstances, as may be the case in
Wuhan, there is every reason for the country *not* to be transparent about
its research program and to intimidate and subjugate all scientists and staff
involved in the program to ensure state secrecy.

Because of the many countries and cultures involved and the intentionally covert nature of research within some countries, there are no easy
answers. And, of course, we only know about the labs *that we know about.*
There are undoubtedly hidden laboratories doing secretive experiments that
are not known to the public and therefore are beyond external scrutiny. These
potentially include makeshift laboratories within rogue states or extremist
organizations for which there is no "dual" to the research—it is only meant
to inflict harm. So what can we do?

1. *Develop and formally adopt international standards for safety at biocontainment laboratories.*

   Standards establish best practices. Even covert national programs
   would find it in their self-interest to follow these standards because it
   does no good to have an accidental release of an experimental agent,
   risking deaths within the homeland and exposing the covert program to the world. If COVID-19 began in the Wuhan Institute of
   Virology, it almost certainly was released accidentally. If this were an
   intentional Chinese attack, they could have started the outbreak in
   the United States and not in China and blamed the United States for
   it—but that is not what happened.

   Today there are multiple organizations that provide technical assistance related to biosafety practices. Also, the International
   Organization for Standards (ISO) has recently published an international standard for any organization that tests, stores, transports,
   works with, or disposes of hazardous biological materials. ISO has
   165 national members, including China, Russia, the United States,
   and most European countries. Formal adoption of these standards
   should be accomplished multilaterally through WHO and added as a
   component of the JEE process.

2. *Export controls.*

   The United States and aligned countries should implement comprehensive export controls on devices and biological materials, at least

at some level and in certain circumstances. While this is very difficult in practice because of the very nature of dual-use research and the presence of multiple suppliers, there is no reason for the United States to assist in building a BSL-4 laboratory for a country that may have covert intentions, engages in dangerous practices, lacks all transparency, and covers up emerging outbreaks. Indeed, France established a partnership with China, and the French led the design, construction, and commissioning of the Wuhan lab, but the Chinese ended French participation as soon as the laboratory became functional, possibly to hide covert Chinese research from the external world.

The same can be said for *genetic information*. China does not allow the export of genetic information about its people, but China aggressively seeks and gathers genetic information on citizens of other countries. This information could be used for any number of nefarious purposes, including blackmail using personal health information or potentially the development of bioweapons that specifically target one or more ethnic or racial groups.

It is remarkable to me that the great institutions of US science, including the NIH and the CDC, seem oblivious to threats caused by the disclosure of our genetic information. Such disclosures occur daily, sometimes even by direct federal sponsorship but more frequently through Chinese acquisitions of US companies doing genetic analysis or offering below-cost gene-sequencing services to ancestry companies. And even easier, it is likely that our DNA databases (perhaps even the NIH's All of Us program) are being cyberattacked by China and other nations. That is one reason why Secretary Rick Perry, when leading the Department of Energy, offered to store all US genetic information gathered by the NIH and the Veterans Health Administration in the most secure computers on the planet—those in Department of Energy labs like Los Alamos and Oak Ridge National Laboratory. I do not know if that is being done, but Congress should mandate that this happens—immediately—or the president should issue an executive order.

3. *Limit funding to suspect programs and nations.*

The NIH and other agencies like USAID should not fund potentially dangerous research in countries that are neither transparent nor accountable to the United States. Transparency includes open access to the facilities conducting research; access to information systems detailing the research, including all-natural and synthetic gene

sequences; and unfettered external access to scientists and staff conducting the research. *Potentially dangerous* must be defined broadly
and include the collection of dangerous microbes (like bat coronaviruses from distant caves), whether they are further genetically
manipulated or not. Congress, in conjunction with the intelligence
community, should categorize which countries should and should
not be eligible for funding, and US agencies should comply with
those designations.

4. *Strengthen the United States' internal review process on gain-of-
   function and other potentially dangerous research.*

   The review of the safety and appropriateness of gain-of-function
   research cannot be left to the scientists alone. Scientists will always
   err on the side of scientific discovery and underestimate global risks.
   Furthermore, scientists and academics are mostly naive to the ill
   intentions of rogue nations that truly seek world domination and
   have no hesitancy to use biological weapons or assassinate "dissi-
   dents" with chemical weapons if it is to their advantage.

   Although I am less concerned about the nefarious intentions
   of US researchers, unintentional lab leaks are possible even at the best
   US institutions. So before we accidentally (or intentionally through
   gain-of-function research) create the next pandemic coronavirus
   or 1918 flu strain, Congress needs to establish a detailed, transparent, accountable process to determine whether the true benefits of
   such research clearly outweigh the potential harms. The criteria for
   which research gets reviewed and how decisions are made should
   be explicit, including the characteristics of the research, the safety
   record of the institution, and the experience and loyalties of the laboratory staff. Moreover, any decision panel should include diverse
   stakeholders, including policy makers, nuclear and other scientists,
   citizen representatives, counterproliferation experts, and ethicists.

   It is entirely possible that US tax dollars, through the NIH
   and the private nonprofit EcoHealth Alliance, directly or indirectly
   funded research at the Wuhan Institute of Virology that ultimately
   caused the pandemic. Whether it did or didn't, we should have those
   answers by now—definitively. We don't, and that is a problem.

The United States needs to take these steps seriously, meaning being
willing to implement economic and other sanctions against noncompliant
nations. The United States should also offer generous incentives and technical

assistance for nations who cooperate and fully subscribe to the Global Health Security Agenda under the World Health Organization.

DETECTING A RISK: WHERE THERE IS SMOKE . . .

Once a new pathogen like SARS-CoV-2 reaches our shores, it is absolutely imperative for us to identify as many cases as possible as soon as possible. There are two scenarios for which we must prepare:

1. *The identification of infected people in the United States from a disease that has already been identified in another country.* This was the scenario for COVID-19; the first US case was diagnosed on January 20, 2020, in a man with a cough and fever who had recently returned from Wuhan (a fairly easy diagnosis).
2. *The identification of a new pathogen first arising and circulating in the United States.* This could be from an infection emerging here (like the 1918 Spanish flu), a traveler arriving from a foreign country, or perhaps a deliberate attack on our homeland.

For COVID-19, as discussed extensively in this book, testing in the United States was woefully insufficient because we were unprepared for the diagnostics challenge presented by this type of virus. The CDC and the FDA created the perfect storm for an early testing failure. But because we started out so wrongly with testing for COVID, it is fairly easy to fix (or at least substantially improve) for the next pandemic.

What I am most concerned about is detecting a pandemic pathogen that is new on the world scene (emerging disease or attack) that manifests itself first in the United States. I am not worried about diseases like Ebola. Ebola is contagious through blood and bodily fluids but not through the respiratory route. You are not going to get Ebola by walking in the grocery store or riding on public transportation. As viral loads go up in Ebola patients, they become seriously and visibly ill—universally. And although the clinical syndrome of Ebola can masquerade as other common diseases, honing in on an Ebola diagnosis would be done rapidly by clinicians. And we have vaccines and treatments for Ebola in the stockpile.

Similarly, anthrax is a reasonably straightforward diagnosis for astute clinicians, even if there is no history of a "white powder." Anthrax is also not contagious from person to person, and we are now well prepared with vaccines and medical countermeasures. If smallpox emerged, the first patient who displayed the clinical syndrome (with pox covering their skin) would be immediately identified, and the decades of US preparation and stockpiles of vaccines and countermeasures would be unleashed.

What if the next coronavirus pandemic starts here in the United States without warning, particularly during the winter flu season? How would we know that the virus was here before it ignited the next global pandemic? The answer is, right now, we would need to be extraordinarily lucky.

The CDC relies on what is called "syndromic surveillance" through the National Syndromic Surveillance System. This system now includes over six thousand health-care facilities and over 70 percent of emergency rooms, which send information on patient symptoms—like fever, respiratory distress, or vomiting—back to the CDC. The idea is that if many more patients start showing up in Texas (or anywhere else) with fever and vomiting than usually show up during that time period, this observation gives a heads-up that something is going on and needs to be investigated. Dozens of disease detectives from the CDC would rush to the scene and eventually have their names emblazoned on an upcoming issue of the *MMWR* reporting their findings.

The National Syndromic Surveillance System is critically important but terribly insufficient. First, it assumes that people will be sick enough to go to the hospital or emergency room early in their illness, before they have spread the disease widely. Second, it is horribly insensitive to a new respiratory pathogen like COVID-19. In other words, if someone comes in with a cough and fever in the winter, the likely diagnosis is influenza; most centers don't even perform an influenza test, and if the flu test is negative, health-care providers treat you for the flu anyway. So to detect a signal from a new respiratory infection, especially in the winter, is very difficult and won't occur until it is "too late."

The system (even in retrospect) did not detect a significant spike in respiratory illness caused by COVID-19 until the end of February, at least six weeks after the virus had begun circulating in the United States. If we were not actually looking for COVID, it might have been attributed to a spike in influenza or another typical winter virus. I asked the CDC in February 2020 to calculate how many cases of COVID in the United States would be required to trigger an unusual spike in the system. The answer was tens of thousands or perhaps even a hundred thousand—far too many to provide sufficient early warning to control a new pandemic. So our warning systems performed poorly even on a pathogen that we knew would be heading our way from China and Europe.

Therefore, in addition to these syndromic systems, we need a much more sensitive and comprehensive system that utilizes modern technology (most of which is now commercial off-the-shelf and supplemented by other technologies and informatics systems that need to be developed and optimized).

Vision

There should be a new national system that analyzes clinical samples from patients presenting with respiratory symptoms (and perhaps other symptoms) throughout the country. The analysis would include a molecular screening test to determine whether the sample harbors no pathogens, a typical pathogen, or a totally novel one. This would not be done as a clinical test but as part of a national surveillance system framework implemented at the state or regional levels.

Given appropriate sampling and pooling, a novel virus (or bacteria or fungus or anything else) would be identified among the first patients, not after the first hundred thousand. Even if no *pandemic* microbes were ever detected, such a system would revolutionize our understanding of annual diseases and help us better treat patients by knowing the prevailing organisms in our communities at that time. This is even more important now because we are in a golden age of developing medicines that can combat viruses in the way that common antibiotics combat bacteria. We would save lives starting on day one and would gain insights into human health never before imagined. It would also give us weeks or months of a head start on developing POC diagnostics.

This Is Not Science Fiction

The system can be based on existing technologies, including next-generation nucleic acid sequencing coupled with artificial intelligence and machine learning. It would cost only a small fraction of what we have already spent to support clinical COVID-19 testing. The system would be anonymized so that patient confidentiality is respected. Eventually, when more therapies are available against viruses, the results could be accessed by patients and their physicians to inform potential treatments.

Fifteen years ago, under the vision and leadership of Special Projects Office director Dr. Amy Alving, DARPA invested and succeeded in developing and commercializing a "universal biosensor" through the TIGER Program (Triangulation Identification for the Genetic Evaluation of Risks). Initially marketed as the Ibis T5000, this complex device had multiple components that resulted in the identification of any organism, known or unknown.[4]

As an initial proof of this concept, one of the first two cases of 2009 H1N1 was actually detected and identified using the Ibis T5000 at the Naval Health Research Center in San Diego, California. In this groundbreaking scientific paper, the authors state, "The ability of this high-throughput tool to correctly identify both well-characterized and novel influenza strains offers the possibility to integrate surveillance for emerging strains with on-site rapid diagnosis used for patient management, shortening the times between the emergence of new strains, their detection and identification, and appropriate public health response activities."[5] The T5000 technology is already outdated but could undergo another round of innovation to reduce cost and size and enhance its capability. Alternatively, more modern technologies—namely, next-generation sequencing (NGS)—have the potential to upgrade the initial DARPA vision and fully integrate molecular surveillance into routine clinical laboratory systems.

In this regard, Illumina (a global leader in NGS) has already developed an assay that, in a single sample in a single tube, detects the presence of 280 respiratory pathogens. It is entirely feasible for Illumina to develop a panel in a single tube that would cover all known human pathogens and their variants, enabling the detection of new influenza strains and novel coronaviruses and anything else lurking in the infectious sphere.

Further development of a modern surveillance platform and the national system to deploy it is the exact type of project that the newly approved ARPA-H (Advanced Research Projects Agency for Health), a health-focused clone of DARPA, should lead. ARPA-H recently received $1 billion in funding from Congress and will be a component agency within the Department of Health and Human Services.

The Proof Is in the Pooing

During the pandemic, I championed another technology that could be profoundly important if further developed and implemented nationally—sewage screening. The concept of screening sewage is not new. Back in my DARPA time from 2004 to 2008, we flirted with options to perform covert surveillance on potential Iraqi biological weapons sites by sampling and analyzing wastewater. The vision was good, but the detection technologies and implementation strategies were not yet mature.

In 2018, I was reacquainted with sewage sampling by a highly innovative company out of Cambridge, Massachusetts, named Biobot, led by two young superstar women, Newsha Ghaeli and Mariana Matus. They combined their expertise in urban design and chemistry to create a very flexible platform for sampling sewage wastewater, from square blocks or square miles to whole communities. With their system, they could provide a remarkably specific view of what was happening in a community without divulging any personally identifiable medical information.

One potential application was to determine whether there were spikes of dangerous drugs being used, most notably fentanyl or its one thousand times more potent analog, carfentanil. This could be done because the metabolic products of these drugs are eliminated in urine, and that urine gets flushed. If we knew these dangerous drugs had entered a community or were at an increased level compared to normal, we could surge resources, such as naloxone and syringe and needle exchanges to prevent HIV and hepatitis, and convince teams of practitioners to encourage addiction treatment with medication-assisted therapy (like Suboxone).

In addition, Biobot had already perfected their technology to perform nucleic acid amplification on microbes to determine if new patterns of antibiotic resistance were present in a community—something every clinician needed to know to better treat pneumonia or meningitis or even ear infections in children. Newsha suggested that they could also detect new outbreaks of hepatitis (a viral infection of the liver affecting millions in the United States)—just by sampling sewage.

Early in the pandemic, sewage sampling surfaced as a potential way to detect outbreaks in a community. The virus causing COVID-19, like many other respiratory viruses including influenza, is shed in the gastrointestinal tract. Early data from several communities indicated that a spike in COVID-19 nucleic acids could be detected in sewage up to four days before emergency room visits would begin to increase. This could be a powerful tool to warn communities about new potential outbreaks so they could surge resources (docs, nurses, antibodies, other treatments) and provide warning to vulnerable residents.

In March 2020, the CDC had begun to do pilot work on wastewater surveillance but was only investing $2.5 million to begin coordination efforts at eight sites in the United States. I became a vocal cheerleader for this effort and, through my authority as the assistant secretary, convened an interagency leadership group beginning in July 2020. With the assistance of Russ Vought (newly confirmed director of OMB), my request for $50 million to fund a national wastewater surveillance system was approved in late 2020. The CDC announced this program on a national scale in late November 2021.

Creating an Integrated Alert System

No single alert system, including wastewater surveillance, can be allowed to regress into another stale, insensitive, bureaucratic, and siloed CDC warning system. The system has to be "real time" in its readouts, fused with syndromic information from hospitals and health systems, and informed by universal biosensor data on clinical samples.

The fusion and integration of intelligence sources is the way our defense and intelligence communities develop high-confidence conclusions amid uncertainty. In fact, this is exactly what we needed early in the response at FEMA, but instead, we had nothing but sparse data and poor analytics. In general, I had to develop the packages I needed by crunching numbers myself and getting modeling input from volunteers like Dr. Blythe Adamson and the IHME at the University of Washington. The armed forces personnel assigned to FEMA task forces (including junior officers) were incredulous that our disease "intelligence" was as primitive as it was. They immediately saw the need for an analytics group built on top of comprehensive and fused data sources.

Specifically, US disease data must be combined with all sources of intelligence from other countries, especially those in Asia and other high-risk regions. When our intelligence community saw a surge in the number of cars parked at Wuhan hospitals in October via satellite reconnaissance, that information did not get transmitted to me or anyone in the USPHS Commissioned Corps to inform our preparations, even though we had a clear need to know. Two months more of preparation could have made a world of difference.

Let's not repeat the intelligence silos that blinded us to 9/11 for yet another threat to our country—pandemics. Data from all sources need to be collected, assessed, fused, and communicated by an experienced interdisciplinary disease intelligence team to leadership at the White House, the HHS, and the Department of Defense. The United States needs a new, modern approach to early warning; the CDC will participate but cannot own the process.

TRANSFORMING THE FEDERAL BUREAUCRACY

The opportunities to improve our national response to future pandemics begin with organizational reform at the federal level. Our major agencies need a reboot, and many need a complete overhaul. Some of the successes during the pandemic, like the turnaround in testing that began on March 12, 2020, were due to a recognition of the ineffectiveness of traditional bureaucracies and the building of a new model using a combination of federal officials who "get shit done," volunteers from the private sector, and logistics and contracting expertise from the Department of Defense. There was no playbook to inform this essential pivot in approach. In the future, the country should not count on the presence of a Jared Kushner and a Brad Smith or the presence of a testing czar who had worked on pandemic preparedness and response for two decades.

The decades of preparation to develop and manufacture vaccines against pandemic viruses paid off in 2020. Yet still in April of that year, there was a high risk of failure because the traditional processes of sequential vaccine scale-up, clinical trials, FDA authorization, and allocation were going too slowly to meet our national needs. The likelihood of "failing" was evident to all of us in a meeting conducted in the Roosevelt Room attended by HHS principals, including Secretary Azar, Paul Mango (deputy chief of staff), Deb Birx, Peter Marks (FDA), myself, and several members of the White House staff.

As a result, Secretary Azar conceived the concept of OWS and, based on his experience in government and in the pharmaceutical industry, appointed leaders outside the typical public health community who were the absolute best in their fields: Moncef Slaoui for commercial vaccine development and Gen. Gustave Perna for logistics and distribution. OWS immediately and massively leveraged US industry by assuming all financial risks, which enabled OWS to do simultaneously within months what the industry would have done sequentially over years. The CDC immediately began working on state plans for vaccination, far in advance of any vaccine being available. And the NIH and Surgeon Gen. Adams led efforts to conduct clinical trials rapidly and with unprecedented racial and ethnic diversity, upon which the FDA could assess the safety and effectiveness of the vaccines for all Americans.

For distribution, OWS (and specifically General Perna) utilized preexisting US companies for packaging and distribution of supplies, including giants like McKesson, UPS, and FedEx. And through the use of the PREP Act in my role as the assistant secretary, I provided guidance that superseded any state regulations to allow pharmacists, pharmacy technicians, pharmacy interns, and emergency medical technicians to administer COVID-19 vaccines. That enabled OWS to utilize retail pharmacy chains to provide shots in arms at forty thousand pharmacy locations around the country. This pivot in organizational approach was essential for our nation's vaccine success but happened instinctively without any direction or organizational guidance from the Obama playbook or any other planning document.

The CDC

There is no single organization involved in the pandemic response that needs reform and reorganization more than the CDC. Not just during the COVID-19 pandemic but for many years before, issues with the CDC were readily apparent and a source of frustration to many of us, including CDC director Bob Redfield, who began to reform the organization immediately after taking charge. If Trump would have won reelection, my "ask" to Secretary Azar would have been to help turn around this storied organization and help fight the battles within the CDC and externally that need to be won in order to restore the luster of this great institution.

There are many outstanding professionals within the organization, including highly capable career staff like the acting chief of staff (and former chief operating officer) Sherri Berger and public health experts like Dr. Debra Houry (now principal deputy director), Rear Admiral Michael Iademarco, Dr. Mitchell Wolfe (rear admiral, USPHS, retired), and hundreds of others. But even with such incredible people within the organization, the performance of the CDC with regard to COVID was, and continues to be, woefully lacking.

During the evacuations from Japan and China, CDC staff had little operational capability. The CDC could not provide health-care utilization models when we on the leadership group at FEMA most needed them to allocate scarce resources like ventilators. The CDC could not (and still can't) provide the data the nation needs to make policy and often does not have the national strategic perspective to even understand why we need that type of data. Despite constant pleas from Dr. Birx, CDC genomic and serologic surveillance was almost nonexistent and lagged far behind the rest of the developed world. In 2022, more than two years after we first learned of COVID-19, we still lack critical information that we need to finally defeat COVID-19, much less prevent the next pandemic. In its current iteration, the CDC is totally averse to any risk-taking or "pushing the envelope" and, as a result, is glacially slow in its responses and guidance.

So I offer a few recommendations to change the organization and its culture:

1. *The CDC must focus on its core mission—namely, the prevention and control of infectious diseases, both domestically and globally.*

   The CDC has become bloated and ineffective because of mission creep, partially by its own doing and partially because of Congress's legislative mandates to dedicate resources to members' pet diseases and causes. During the peak of the pandemic, I was told that as many as 80–90 percent of the CDC staff was on telework, and the majority were still on telework in late 2022. How can it be that during a pandemic, CDC staff were mostly working from home? In fact, despite having eleven thousand employees and additional thousands of contractors, the CDC leaned heavily on deployed USPHS officers (in addition to the nine hundred officers permanently assigned to the CDC) to support CDC missions like airport screening and border checkpoints. In fact, the CDC could not find enough doctors and nurses even to staff their own employee clinic at their headquarters in Atlanta and thus requested additional USPHS officers to do that (officers who had generally been on the front lines for months battling the disease across the nation—not teleworking). Why? Because so many CDC employees and staff are not focused on their essential mission to control infectious diseases and respond to pandemics.

   Here is one simple premise: until the CDC can effectively prevent and/or manage infectious disease outbreaks, including pandemics, it really should not be doing much else. Chronic diseases are a problem—no doubt. But we don't need over one thousand CDC employees working on preventing heart disease and diabetes when the CDC can't handle COVID, especially when there are professional societies and nonprofits, like the American Heart Association, that have more scientific expertise and public reach than the CDC.

   Another example is maternal health and mortality. This area should be owned by the HRSA in their maternal and child health bureau, coordinated through their system of HRSA-funded health centers that take care of one in three people in poverty and one in five uninsured in the United States. The HRSA can not only generate the knowledge and recommendations but also put those into direct action for patient care and through sponsorship of clinical training for doctors, nurses, and varied health professionals. The current funding at the CDC for these programs should be reallocated to the HRSA.

2. *The CDC must become more operational and less academic.*

The lack of operational know-how, whether for Ebola in Texas or COVID-19, was astounding. The CDC was not always that way. Part of this is mindset, part is leadership, part is training, and part is the expectations of the nation. The CDC needs to start up a cell in the director's office whose sole responsibility is to assure operational readiness. The CDC has a Board of Scientific Counselors that helps with strategy and scientific rigor. The CDC needs a board of operational readiness counselors, composed of individuals like Michael Callahan and James Lawler, operators from the Department of Defense, and first responders on the front lines in communities. This board should set expectations, require training and drills, evaluate staff, and hold leaders accountable. The US Marines pride themselves on a saying from my former Department of Defense mentor, Gen. Al Gray, who stated, "Every Marine is, first and foremost, a rifleman. All other conditions are secondary."[6] An equivalent philosophy should be developed for the CDC, perhaps something like "Every CDC staff, first and foremost, is able to don and doff PPE, investigate and medically assist sick people, perform basic infection control, and provide clear health communications. All other conditions are secondary."

3. *The CDC must hold states and localities accountable.*

A primary function of the CDC is to fund state and local public health infrastructure, and this is vital to overall national biosecurity. In general, the CDC funds are distributed in the form of "grants," whether or not they are officially termed that. What I mean is that money is distributed to states with no formal strings attached, no metrics for success for additional future funding, and rarely any objective deliverables. As a result, billions of dollars are distributed, but there is a poor return on our national investments.

I think everyone means well here, in that restricting funds to a poorly functioning region might further adversely affect public health, so a strange codependent relationship has developed between the CDC and the states it serves. Nonetheless, specific deliverables, outcomes, metrics, and timelines need to be established and enforced across the board. This is the only way that the United States will know what we are getting for our national investments and whether we will be ready for the next pandemic.

The CDC cannot hold states accountable on their own because much of the problem begins with Congress. For example, with regard to federal funding for testing provided by Congress during the Trump administration, the language was clear—send the money to the states within a certain time (for the last tranche during my tenure, it was three weeks). By law, the states were entitled to the money, and the HHS / the CDC was essentially just a pass-through. Even though that was the case, in May of 2020, with $11 billion from the Paycheck Protection Program and Health Care Enhancement Act pending allocation, my team insisted that states and territories submit a testing plan and provide overall goals prior to receipt of funds. Dr. Beckham and I, with consultation from CDC experts, created a template that included numerous critical parameters that needed to be covered by state plans, including testing in nursing homes and for the underserved. All states and territories submitted their plans to be assessed and scored. Most were outstanding, but a few were dismal and received feedback and technical assistance from my team. But everyone received their money, no matter what, because that was the law.

Congress needs to provide CDC with the flexibility to actively manage the precious public health funding they receive, and the CDC needs to be obsessive about demanding performance and improving their expertise in project management. This is a very different mindset but one that is no longer an option if we are to keep the United States biosafe in the twenty-first century.

4. *The CDC needs more funding and more flexible funding for infectious disease and pandemic preparedness.*

More money to a dysfunctional organization will not yield results. Throwing money at a problem rarely does anything productive unless it is spent wisely. I am assuming here that the general reforms I propose and others will be implemented and the CDC will be held accountable for tangible progress.

While the overall CDC budget grew substantially in the late 1990s and early 2000s, it has been essentially flat when adjusted for inflation for the past ten years. But even that "flat" spending belies cuts in the tip-of-the-spear programs, such as the CDC's Public Health Emergency Preparedness program that supports states and local areas in their preparations for pandemics and other emergencies. The funding for this program had decreased dramatically from $940 million in 2002 to $675 million in 2020.[7] Even back in 2014 when I testified to Congress after the Texas Ebola crisis, I identified CDC hospital preparedness funding cuts as a major issue that needed to be remedied.

Our nation has a short memory of pandemics: smallpox, polio, HIV, H1N1, Ebola. I am not certain whether it is memory lapse or subconscious wishful thinking that something "like this" will never occur again. We tend to increase public health funding only after a crisis has occurred, but then we cut it again before the next crisis can be averted. This cycle of dysfunction needs to stop.

I had the opportunity to have an insider view of the process as the only senior public health expert who was a member of Secretary Azar's internal budget review committee. This committee evaluated and prioritized agency requests and also attempted to align, as best as possible, budget requirements from the OMB—for example, reducing the HHS budget by 5 percent or a CDC division by 10 percent. No matter what the CDC or HHS proposes for a budget, it must ultimately meet the OMB guidelines—hopefully after some give and take on specific high-priority programs. Budget decisions are made at the White House level through the OMB and detailed in the president's budget submitted to Congress. Ultimately, Congress has the power of the purse and approves its own budget, which may or may not include the salient features of the president's proposal.

The budget guidance we received from the Trump-administration OMB was ruthless in its cuts to the public health budget at the CDC. On the good side, they identified the CDC as bloated and less capable than what the nation needed. But the OMB's solution was just to cut the budget, which would fix nothing and actually make all matters worse.

Even more troubling to me, the CDC and NIH budgets became more of a game for the OMB and the people who controlled the OMB like Mick Mulvaney. By cutting the president's budget for the CDC and the NIH, the OMB would fulfill its ideological "deal" by pretending to balance the budget, but we all knew (and so did the OMB) that such cuts would never be sustained by Congress. The money was always preserved or even increased. But because the executive branch did not set priorities, congressional leadership frequently allocated the restored funding for their own constituents' projects—often less strategic or critical than what we would have proposed. Perhaps this was done by individual members of Congress for political self-interest, but I believe it was mostly because members did not have the perspective of the executive branch's public health and pandemic preparedness leadership, so they did the best they could given the information they had.

In addition to budgetary consistency, the CDC needs *flexible* money. I was shocked at the hundreds of funding lines and sublines that require the CDC to spend funds only in certain restricted ways. I get it. Congress has the power of the purse. But pandemics and other health crises, like acute paralysis in children or Zika or e-cigarette lung injury, are emergencies and do not fit into the two-year process required to establish an agency budget line. The CDC director needs a pool of multiyear funds (meaning money can be spent any time over five years, as an example) that can be allocated for whatever public health emergency (or imminent emergency) may arise. I don't know the right number, but it should be at least $100 million per year as a start.

But how much money does the CDC need? This calculation has to start with a mission and requirements—core requirements for infectious disease control and pandemic preparedness—and then work backward for budgetary implications. This is how the Department of Defense operates in its budget cycles, and I believe it is appropriate here. Let me give a few examples of potential requirements:

- The United States must have a nationwide system of reporting test results and vaccinations for specific infectious diseases within twenty-four hours electronically, and it must include pertinent information like age, sex, race, ethnicity, zip code, and other essential information.

- The United States must have a system so that the ages and underlying conditions of all hospitalized patients during a pandemic are reported within twenty-four hours. (Even in mid-2022, only twenty-four states reported the ages of those hospitalized, so we were trying to make policy on schools and child immunization without the most critical information.)

- The CDC must develop and implement a structure for public-private partnerships around diagnostic testing so that for any new outbreak, the United States can scale to one hundred million tests per week within four weeks of the identification of an outbreak.

- The CDC must maintain a global presence in regions of risk to provide technical assistance and frontline intelligence for ongoing public health emergencies before they reach the United States. (Prior to COVID, Dr. Redfield was being forced to reduce the global CDC presence because of budgetary pressures, exactly the opposite of what is needed in an interconnected world.)

While requirements for *every* disease are unreasonable, core requirements for pandemic preparedness and response are not only reasonable and feasible but essential for assuring biosafety in this century. Less money should go to named buildings in Atlanta and more money to frontline public health preparedness and response.

5. *The CDC needs to expand its primary stakeholder communities.*

Probably because of the way money is allocated by Congress as well as the alignment of culture and the revolving doors of government, there are several siloed constituencies served by siloed agencies within HHS—and this was a critical issue in the COVID-19 pandemic response.

In "normal times," the primary recipients of CDC funds are state and local health departments and their affiliated public health laboratories and, to a much lesser degree, select federal and international laboratories. Let's think about this in terms of the COVID-19 response.

State public health laboratories are government or government-affiliated laboratories that perform disease surveillance and monitoring, workforce development and training, reference testing for unusual pathogens, and some clinical and diagnostic testing. The CDC interacts with and supports public health laboratories as a priority. This makes total sense. When there is a foodborne outbreak or a potential Ebola victim, the public health laboratories are there to provide the needed diagnostics and related services. Many also perform newborn screening for genetic disorders, which is of vital public health interest. Related to COVID, the CDC provided testing kits first to public health laboratories, and they would in turn perform testing on potential COVID patients on a limited basis. But independent of the fact that the CDC failed to provide public health laboratories with the supplies they needed, public health laboratories were never meant for this type of massive scale.

The CDC—as far as I could tell—had zero interaction with large commercial laboratories (like Quest and LabCorp) that would need to bear the brunt of the US testing burden. They also had no interaction with test manufacturers, like Abbott, Cepheid, or Thermo Fisher, or reagent suppliers, like Promega and Qiagen, who were responsible for actually providing the critical reagents and materials. Although there was some coordination with major academic health center laboratories, this was also quite limited in scope.

The problem was that an overall large-scale national testing plan required the CDC to engage all segments of the ecosystem, not just the public health laboratories. And that did not happen. In fact, an internal memo from the CDC in February 2020 suggested that the major commercial labs might be needed by August or September 2020, which was incorrect if not entirely delusional.

So the CDC needs to broaden its primary stakeholder interactions and do that formally. The structure should include representatives from large commercial labs, suppliers, academic labs, and public health laboratories, together with clinicians who will actually employ testing capacity. I tried to lay the foundation for this type of entity by implementing the National COVID-19 Testing Forum.[8] The forum's first meeting was in July 2020; it included representatives from across industries, academia, and government; and it had the goal of getting the right tests to the right people at the right time.

This forum was a good start, but it did not have the authority, structure, or luxury of time in the middle of a pandemic to do the appropriate coordination and planning. This forum was a place for disparate opinions to be heard in a relatively public setting. What I envision for the future is more of a select group, with the ability to discuss confidential information in a setting with antitrust protection using Title VII of the DPA, as was done for PPE and other critical supplies.

It is possible that the CDC will be incapable of breaking its old habits, but they are the logical choice for this function. There will need to be seamless coordination with the ASPR, which owns the federal responsibility for the stockpiling of tests. BARDA, the NIH, and the new ARPA-H will remain responsible for funding the research-and-development program to provide novel testing technologies to fill the stockpile.

The linchpin, however, is the coordination of the entire ecosystem, not just limited components, and the establishment of objective requirements that drive an integrated plan to keep the United States biosafe.

HHS

The US Department of Health and Human Services has approximately ninety thousand employees and a budget proposed for the fiscal year 2022 of $1.63 *trillion*, which is more than double the requested budget for the Department of Defense. In the HHS organizational structure, there are eleven operating divisions—including the NIH, the FDA, the CDC, and the CMS—and sixteen staff divisions, such as the OASH (my previous office) and the ASPR (primarily responsible for public health emergency responses and the SNS). So by my count, the secretary of HHS has twenty-seven direct reports. The average and optimum number of direct reports for a Fortune 500 company CEO is somewhere between seven and nine. So the leader of the largest department in our government—and certainly one of the most important—has a span of control that is impossible to manage effectively for any human being. Moreover, the secretary needs to respond to the constant barrage of inquiries and needs from the White House—especially the Domestic Policy Council and often the president or vice president. This was especially the case during the Trump administration.

Secretary Azar was one of the most intelligent, capable, experienced (within both HHS and the pharmaceutical industry), and insightful leaders I have ever worked with. He focused on specific goals and tangible objectives and lived by *The 4 Disciplines of Execution* to assure tangible outcomes and not just rhetoric.[9] He had an excellent staff. But in my view, my boss (who is also a friend and colleague) was forced to spend much of his effort making this massive bureaucratic structure work during normal times. When the pandemic began, organizational effectiveness became even more challenging. Early in the pandemic, the CDC and the FDA made recommendations and significant policy changes with ripple effects across the department (and the country) without the secretary weighing in or even knowing about them until after the fact. For example, the FDA reasserted enforcement against LDTs for COVID-19, which tanked innovation and delayed testing at universities and academic medical centers for at least six weeks. I imagine managing the department became even more challenging when Azar started leading the White House Coronavirus Task Force and later was the driving force behind OWS. There is only so much time every day, and each of these tasks was a full-time job.

To get the organization right for pandemics and other public health emergencies and to improve function during "routine times," HHS should be restructured in a way that resembles (but does not exactly duplicate) the early HHS organization in the 1980s. Such a change would provide the secretary with a more appropriate span of control and thus the ability to remain externally facing while still driving the internal strategic direction.

Title 42, section 202 of the US Code states, "The Public Health Service in the Department of Health and Human Services shall be administered by the Assistant Secretary for Health under the supervision and direction of the Secretary."[10] The "Public Health Service" includes much more than the USPHS Commissioned Corps. It actually includes all the major HHS operating divisions (like the CDC, the NIH, and the FDA) and three staff divisions (the OASH, the ASPR, and the Office of Global Affairs). In fact, the only major HHS divisions not part of the Public Health Service are the human services agencies, specifically the Administration for Children and Families (ACF), the Administration for Community Living, and the CMS. Until 1995, the assistant secretary for health (ASH) had full authority over all the Public Health Service agencies that were in existence at that time, including setting priorities and adjudicating budgets. The ASH, in turn, directly reported to the secretary. This allowed the secretary to have a reasonable number of direct reports but also clearly enabled the coordination of public health initiatives across HHS divisions. That coordination was led by the ASH, typically a medical doctor who was confirmed by the Senate following presidential nomination.

In 1995, the ASH and the OASH were subsumed into the Office of the Secretary, and the leaders of the Public Health Service agencies (like the CDC, the FDA, and the NIH) became direct reports to the secretary. The OASH remained responsible for formulating many of the critical national plans, including the Vaccines National Strategic Plan, the National HIV/AIDS Strategy, the Physical Activity Guidelines for Americans, the Dietary Guidelines for Americans (in conjunction with the Department of Agriculture), and the national health objectives outlined in Healthy People 2030, but the

ASH had no direct authority to implement these plans through the operating divisions.

In the Trump administration, as the ASH, I was still tasked with organizing and leading many of the major health initiatives—such as the Opioids and Substance Use Disorder Policy, Ending the HIV Epidemic in the US, and the National Youth Sports Strategy—and related to COVID, I served as the testing czar, which included having the authority to issue EUAs for diagnostics independent of the FDA. So de facto, I had assumed much of the former ASH role, but without the direct authorities within the organization.

What I think makes sense for the future is for several of the public health divisions to be aligned again under the ASH, including the CDC, the HRSA, and the Indian Health Service. However, the FDA and the NIH should remain direct reports to the secretary because of their size and influence and also the nature of their missions. With this structure, the secretary would be better able to lead HHS and be free to provide more strategic direction during a pandemic. In routine times, the structure would also allow more technical coordination and disciplined execution to deliver on public health policies that might improve our miserable health status as a nation.

Under no circumstances should the responsibilities and operational leadership of the ASPR be moved to the CDC—or even worse, the NIH, which is being discussed in some circles. The NIH is perfectly adapted for its current mission, and the CDC can be reformed to achieve its traditional mission. But these missions are both very different from actual *emergency response*. To make a very loose analogy, when there is a Category 5 hurricane and flooding, and you are sitting on your rooftop with water coming into your attic, you want a swift-water rescue squad, not a professor who can mathematically model the effects of climate change on severe weather. Both are critically important, but you can't substitute one for the other.

US National Leadership Structure during a Pandemic

Starting with my initial involvement in biosecurity issues in the 1990s and continuing to today, no question has been more important than "Who is in charge?" A second question, which I believe has been answered by the COVID-19 response, is "Who should be in charge, and when?" We wound up in mostly the right place but did so without a playbook and by a circuitous route that cost time and effective decision-making.

As a first principle for organizing a disaster response, there needs to be a clear chain of command. Without this, the situation becomes a nightmare of frustration for those trying to carry out operations and follow strategic directions. From my perspective, at no time in our COVID response was there truly a clear chain of command from top to bottom, although at certain times and levels (like FEMA with the UCG), the organization was highly structured and functional. Overall, we made it work because of the talent and flexibility of those involved, but the nation cannot count on that being the case in the future.

As a second principle, the organization should resemble, to the degree possible, the typical ICS in the National Incident Management System (as discussed in chapter 8). This is indeed the all-hazards (wildfires, hurricanes, mass casualty events, etc.) playbook for a response structure that has functioned extraordinarily well from the local to the national level. Everyone in emergency response at all levels knows their roles and responsibilities, the organization, and the fact that the structure can scale from a small local response to a national or even global one.

Essential to the ICS is the incident commander—the *someone* who is in charge of the response. That person has overall leadership responsibility, including managing the implementation of the incident action plan, communications, safety, and the delegation of duties to others. The incident commander, however, takes policy direction from executives and senior officials, often termed a *policy-coordinating committee*. A good example of this functionality was at FEMA, when Josh Dozer was the incident commander for the response—he was in charge of the response, without a doubt. But major strategic decisions and direction on the allocation of scarce resources like ventilators were approved by the UCG, composed of Pete Gaynor, Bob Kadlec, Dan Jernigan (CDC), and myself.

Early in the pandemic, until Secretary Azar declared on March 2, 2020, that Dr. Bob Kadlec (ASPR) was officially the incident manager (also referred to as the incident commander) and I was the deputy incident manager, the CDC was in charge—at least it seemed. Perhaps the best way to describe it prior to March 2 was that there were two parallel structures, brought together by the daily leadership of the secretary. On January 20, the CDC activated its EOC in Atlanta, an impressive facility fully equipped with state-of-the-art communications and visualization tools, and put literally hundreds of people on the response. The CDC had a designated incident commander and assumed the leadership role for pandemic epidemiology, public health recommendations, and external communications. In parallel, the ASPR organization had activated the SOC, was preparing hospitals, was endeavoring to increase supplies of PPE and develop countermeasures, and was organizing the evacuations of Americans from Wuhan and cruise ships. From the beginning, the secretary was briefed multiple times per day and provided overall direction to the department. He was fully engaged.

On March 2, the secretary affirmed that the ASPR was formally in charge of the response. And then on March 19, Trump declared FEMA to be the LFA, and the UCG was formed, incorporating both FEMA and HHS leadership into a single structure.

In addition, layered on top of these response structures was the White House Coronavirus Task Force, which was officially created on January 29 with Secretary Azar as chair. On February 26, the vice president was put in charge of the task force and Dr. Deborah Birx was named coordinator. Those roles were never defined, but at least it was clear that the vice president was in charge of the task force meetings, even if his chief of staff controlled the task force agendas and policy options we could actually discuss.

As we plan for the future, let's first discuss the CDC. What I first realized during Ebola in Texas six years earlier was that the CDC is not in charge of anything. During any regional outbreak, the CDC must be invited to participate by the state and local health departments (no, the CDC cannot just come to New York or Texas when they want to). Their primary role is to provide technical assistance to state and local public health authorities. The CDC does not provide command and control or engage in decision-making. The CDC also assists in outbreak investigations with its disease detectives and then of course writes the findings up in the *MMWR*.

The CDC is ideally suited for these supportive roles because they are indeed the subject matter experts with an unequaled knowledge base. Their incident manager is not the actual leader of the national, regional, or local responses—only the CDC response operations. The CDC has a vital role—and their role needs to be increased and further supported—but the CDC is not in charge of the response.

As stipulated in the PAHPA, passed by Congress in 2006 in response to Hurricane Katrina, the ASPR is charged with leading the United States to prepare for, respond to, and recover from public health emergencies and natural disasters from the medical and public health point of view. The ASPR is by no means perfect. It needs to be less insular and identify and remedy the factors that made it less effective and influential during COVID.

The president and the Senate also need to be sure that the nominee for the ASPR is truly operational and highly qualified, as I believe Dr. Kadlec was, given his stellar military career and lifelong dedication to biosecurity at all levels. The ASPR cannot be an academic plucked from a university, nor can the role be assigned to a donor as a reward for political support.

When a local issue transforms from one that needs CDC consultation to one that needs national coordination and response, the ASPR needs to be in charge. This applies to the public health and medical aspects of essentially every natural disaster and public health emergency related to infectious diseases.[11] This is detailed in operating procedures within the ASPR and the National Response Framework and is understood and accepted by most interagency partners.[12] Early in the pandemic, there should have been no confusion that the ASPR was in charge, not the CDC, under the policy guidance of the secretary and other key HHS leaders.

Depending on the nature and scale of the public health emergency, the ASPR should implement a formal policy coordination committee chaired by the secretary of HHS and include, as relevant, the ASH or surgeon general and perhaps a lead from a human services agency, such as the assistant secretary for the Administration of Children and Families, which was (at least initially) the lead agency caring for Americans once they arrived on US soil from Wuhan and the cruise ships.

In the case of an emerging infectious disease with pandemic potential, ASPR coordination with FEMA is essential, and indeed that is exactly what Bob Kadlec did. FEMA was at the table and represented fully in the initial ASPR response, which made the eventual transition to FEMA as the lead agency more seamless.

In addition, the nation should formally codify that in the event of a presidential declaration of a national emergency, FEMA becomes the lead agency and operations move from the Secretary's Operations Center at HHS to the NRCC at FEMA. The FEMA team should be infused with expertise from HHS, as was done during COVID, with the UCG consisting of the ASPR, the ASH (or surgeon general), and the CDC in addition to the FEMA administrator. FEMA task forces should be populated by experts from throughout FEMA, HHS, Defense, DHS, and other departments within the US government, as they were during COVID.

A major issue that remains unresolved is when and how to demobilize from FEMA back to HHS. On June 15, 2020, as FEMA prepared for another hurricane and wildfire season and COVID-19 cases waned, the center of operations moved back to HHS under the leadership of a Joint Coordination Cell (JCC), which consisted of Secretary Azar, Dr. Birx, and FEMA Administrator Gaynor. Having Birx involved assured some level of coordination with her personal White House team, which tracked and presented overall data but generally acted autonomously with minimal input from HHS. The JCC was obviously focused on the development of vaccines through OWS, which was a tremendous success, as we all know. But at least as far as testing and diagnostics, deployment of USPHS officers, budgets, and similar issues, the JCC was irrelevant and provided no value whatsoever. I actually don't recall ever attending a JCC meeting or being invited to one, as opposed to being in the daily decision-making meetings at FEMA with everyone around the table.

In addition to the JCC meetings, the secretary held a daily morning briefing with the HHS principals (including myself, the CDC director, the FDA commissioner, the CMS administrator, the surgeon general, the NIH director, the assistant secretary for public affairs, and other principals). This served as the primary means of information sharing and planning for the near term. At a much higher level, I was also on the White House Coronavirus Task Force, which continued to provide the overall policy direction for the response. In addition, the task force docs (Birx, Hahn, Redfield, Fauci, Adams, and myself) frequently met separately on medical and public health issues not only for internal deliberations of the science but also to strategize on how to vector the overall task force so that it remained true to the best science and public health recommendations. When I had an issue, my primary lifeline was the task force doctor group and then ultimately the White House Coronavirus Task Force itself. Secretary Azar was also always engaged, available, and supportive; he remained my immediate boss, not the JCC.

The demobilization from FEMA was as unprecedented as the initial mobilization to FEMA but was much rockier because of the amorphous leadership structure and chain of command—and this needs to be fixed before the next pandemic. What is the trigger for demobilization from FEMA, and what does the organization look like? How does it keep the continuity and operational tempo without inhibiting the operational work that would be highly evolved and efficient by that point? Demobilization from FEMA is a solvable issue, but it is just not solved yet.

White House Coronavirus Task Force

The White House Coronavirus Task Force was unprecedented in its successes but also suffered notable failures.

The establishment of the task force in and of itself was a critical step and a milestone. Because the pandemic impacted nearly every aspect of US life, multiple departments needed to be at the table, including the Department of Labor, the Department of Treasury, the Department of Agriculture, the Department of Housing and Urban Development, the Department of Transportation, the Department of Veterans Affairs, and the Department of Defense. Discussions also required White House coordination and leadership, which is why the task force also included members from the Domestic Policy Council, the national security advisor, and the OMB to provide funds for initiatives. The only entity with the gravitas to convene cabinet members whenever needed and make decisions above the department level was the White House.

That is probably why Secretary Azar's term as chair was short lived; he was a peer to other cabinet members and, to some degree, subordinate (if not in the official line of succession, then in terms of the Trump administration's power structure) to the White House senior staff, who were also on the committee. The vice president was the precisely correct official to lead the task force. He was clearly of higher rank than anyone in the room (except when Trump attended) and could make decisions that were binding on cabinet members. In the future, the VP should assume this leadership role even before a national emergency is declared.

The vice president's leadership cannot just be in name. For Pence, COVID was his primary responsibility—morning to night—and he personally chaired every task force meeting and interacted with members before and after meetings. He held weekly governors' calls and personally fielded incoming questions and criticisms from every level of leadership in communities, states, and other federal agencies. As I previously noted, he called me frequently during all hours of the day and night to discuss issues or point me to a governor who had specific needs. For a couple of months, my most frequent caller after 9 p.m. was the vice president of the United States!

Deb Birx was the White House Coronavirus Task Force coordinator, but that role was never precisely defined, and indeed the role changed substantially over time. Deb officed in the White House and, at least early on, met with the president frequently. Deb led every task force meeting with a review of the data, state by state and often city by city, along with her projections and view of the issues. Early on, she led off national press conferences but then was much less prominent in the summer and for the remainder of the response. She also held "doc meetings" to discuss medical and scientific issues prior to the meetings with the vice president.

Key public health items were sometimes triaged from the agenda and never discussed because the VP's chief of staff controlled the agenda. Sometimes, there were White House meetings about policy and the overall direction that occurred without Birx, and sometimes that happened specifically to work around her well-known weaknesses as a manager. As hardworking and scientifically astute as Birx was, she was not the best organizer or consensus builder, which further complicated the multiple chains of command and led to the work-arounds I reference.

What is the future structure? The VP needs to chair the task force, but there needs to be a true coordinator with medical and policy training who acts essentially as the chief operating officer at the right hand of the VP. This person should manage the agendas, prioritize policy discussions, assure follow-up, lead the generation of messaging, and have the complete confidence and backing of the VP and the president in order to hold cabinet members and their departments accountable. The individual needs to be medically and scientifically capable but does not need to be the "expert" in any specific virus or vaccine—those individuals rarely can see the big picture and are often primarily interested in infection control in contrast to overall public health, national security, and constitutional rights.

A true coordinator cannot be picked on the fly in the middle of the crisis, nor can that person engender the confidence and relationships within the White House without building them over time. So I recommend there be a position in the White House administration, at the assistant to the president level, for biosecurity. This is analogous to the position held by Dr. Bob Kadlec in the Bush administration and eliminated by the Obama administration. But it should be elevated in stature from a special assistant to the president to an assistant to the president. This distinction has important meaning both in and outside the White House. There is no need for a large staff or duplicated bureaucracy, but there is a need for an accountable individual.

The assistant to the president for biosecurity would be the single point of contact for all biological, chemical, radiological, and nuclear threats, including emerging diseases and pandemics. That person would assure that all US assets from varying departments—including the HHS, the Department of Defense, the DHS, and others—were coordinated, synergistic, and ready. That also means that research-and-development investments done by the NIH, DARPA, BARDA, and ARPA-H must take into account threat assessments and policy considerations, and major aspects of response (like testing and genomic surveillance) must be adequately resourced and effectively implemented. This person would help define the requirements for systems and agencies, including the CDC.

Moreover, the assistant to the president should be the primary contact of the Domestic Policy Council, the National Security Council (NSC), and the national security advisor in relation to US preparedness for and response to chemical, biological, radiological, and nuclear threats—with the emphasis on biological threats, both natural and man-made. This individual would assure that the NSC has sufficient expertise and intelligence related to pandemic threats to support presidential decision-making. Whether that requires an independent directorate in the NSC or not is less important than having a single person in charge at the White House level. Obviously, the assistant to the president would be perfectly situated to become the White House Coronavirus Task Force coordinator in the event of an emergent pandemic.

CREATING SUSTAINABLE
PUBLIC-PRIVATE PARTNERSHIPS

Perhaps the most important realization of the Trump administration, which likely happened sooner than it would have happened for any other administration, is that the typical agencies and mechanisms of the US government were insufficient to meet the demands of the pandemic. In the future, we must ensure that the private sector is front and center from day one, which actually means they need to be intimately involved in all prepandemic planning and exercises.

Testing was salvaged and eventually transformed by engaging large commercial laboratories like LabCorp and national retail chains like CVS and Walgreens; utilizing health-care delivery companies like eTrueNorth for surge testing; catalyzing and guaranteeing markets by large purchases of rapid tests from manufacturers like Abbott and BD; investing in domestic supply chains (like swab manufacturers) and utilizing the DPA to support commercial production lines while facilitating the importation of necessary supplies through air bridges; collaborating with Apple to develop in record time a user-friendly app to empower patients to know when they should be tested and what the results mean; coordinating with testing manufacturers and AdvaMed (the advanced medical technology trade association) to define the specific production and distribution of tests, reagents, and equipment; and investing in new technologies and platforms within the commercial sector through the NIH and BARDA.

In terms of medical equipment and consumables, Rear Admiral Polowczyk led the largest nonwartime mobilization of private industry in history, accelerating the manufacture and delivery of everything from ventilators to N95 respirators and gowns. He did this by expanding supplies through massive-scale air bridges until domestic manufacturing could be scaled up and most importantly by utilizing the robust health-care distribution chains already in existence through suppliers like McKesson and Henry Schein. By using the DPA Title VII, Rear Admiral P was able to have all of the national distributors around a single table to coordinate massive-scale delivery to every hospital and nursing home in the United States while enhancing the stock-piles of every state and the federal government.

And the most notable example of public-private partnerships is OWS and the overall vaccine enterprise. Scaling vaccines to hundreds of millions of doses, expediting clinical trials, and distributing vaccines nationally required the creation of OWS to spur typically conservative industry processes. McKesson was leveraged to package needed supplies—including a billion needles and alcohol swabs. UPS and FedEx were signed up to ensure rapid shipping to tens of thousands of locations under precise temperature control. And, of course, large federal vaccination sites were not needed (and they failed under the Biden administration) because OWS enabled forty thousand pharmacy sites, of which 95 percent of Americans lived within five miles. To put even more needles in arms, OWS also stepped up vaccination capabilities at an additional thirty thousand preexisting health-care sites, including federally qualified health centers (FQHCs).

While all of these accomplishments were historic in their significance, the system and relationships were built mostly on the fly by innovative leaders who were empowered to take (or just took them anyway) bold actions to right the ship. We need to prepare more holistically and broadly for the future. In general, the federal bureaucracies need to talk less among themselves in the echo chamber of DC and actively and formally engage the private sector, transparently and consistently, using authorities defined in the Defense Production Act. This engagement needs to be much more robust than just investing in a device or therapy that seems promising. We need something for the pandemic response that has multiple industry clusters, deals end to end with massive-scale problems, collaborates with private-industry leaders to solve the problems in a transparent way, and is sustained over time. The actual legal structure and organization need to be determined, but one could imagine building off examples like the partnerships between the government and power generation and transmission industries to manage the nation's energy grid and other key infrastructures that have been successful for decades.

When pandemic exercises and "war games" are played within federal agencies, the private sector needs to be present at the table informing federal thinkers and academics of the real-world limitations and possibilities. There also need to be serious discussions about approaches that would normally impinge on our free-market sensibilities. For example, does the federal government "let a thousand flowers bloom" for testing (there are still hundreds of EUAs waiting to be reviewed if not thousands), or should the federal government invest in and review only a handful of tests in the major categories (PCR, POC molecular, lateral flow, sequencing) developed by industry consortia that can be massively scaled in ultrashort time frames. This was the approach taken by South Korea early in the pandemic, which resulted in capabilities that initially far exceeded that of the United States. Of note, South Korea built their approach based on previous failures with SARS; it is up to us to learn the lessons of COVID and build for the future like they did.

GLOBAL COLLABORATION AND HEALTH SECURITY

The United States has no choice but to work directly with other countries individually and through multilateral organizations like the WHO. Future pandemics are unlikely to begin in the United States, and our experience over the past decade has definitively proven that an outbreak anywhere is a threat everywhere. The world needs every country to implement policies and preparations that will prevent a new disease from emerging in the first place or, when it does, be able to contain and control it while alerting the international community to any emerging threat.

Irrespective of the origin of the virus, the Chinese government's subsequent actions were exactly the opposite of what was needed to save millions of lives around the globe. They hid the massive health impact of the virus in the fall and winter of 2019. They covered up human-to-human transmission until it was no longer possible to sustain the misinformation; they hid knowledge of patterns of asymptomatic spread and, perhaps most critically, did not allow the CDC into China to support the response and gain knowledge that could be used to protect the United States and the rest of the world. China closed down its country but allowed thousands of potentially infected Chinese to travel to Europe and the United States, seeding the virus to such an extent that the pandemic was almost a fait accompli for the rest of the globe.

The United States and like-minded countries cannot deal with China and a handful of other repressive but technologically advanced nations only through the WHO or the United Nations. The United States and its allies need to work with China through all means necessary to prevent a repeat of COVID-19 and to make China understand that this is as much of a priority to the West as nuclear proliferation and deterrence.

China is not an easy problem to solve, but I do believe that there are ways to work with the Chinese collaboratively and productively in a framework of trust but with the constant need for verification and proof. We laid the groundwork for that trust with the 2015 George H. W. Bush Conference on US–China Relations, which I chaired during my time at Texas A&M University. This conference focused on the need for ongoing bilateral collaboration to prevent future pandemics and was attended by leading scientists and policy makers from both countries. At the very least, the United States should not enable nefarious and dangerous behavior by funding BSL-3 and BSL-4 research in China, and countries like France should not support China in building BSL-4 facilities to conduct such research—at least not until there is mutual transparency and collaboration and restored trust.

Our intelligence agencies should be tasked to collect as much information as possible on Chinese research, military plans, and individual scientists. We should also do everything we can from a policy standpoint to deter the development and use of biological weapons by any nation-state. Right now, US policy implies that an adversary nation can kill millions of our citizens through bioweapons, but we will only counter with conventional weapons. Absent a bioweapons program in the United States (and there is none), we should not exclude any of our military capabilities as deterrents to biowarfare—all options should be on the table.

There is also an important role for multilateral organizations like the WHO. I argued as strongly as I could that the United States should *not* withdraw from the WHO, and I still do not know whether Trump would have ultimately withdrawn or whether he was keeping his cards close to his chest in order to force desperately needed WHO reforms. As already stated, the WHO Joint External Evaluation process is working, and this process needs to be expanded to include pandemic prevention (like live animal markets) in addition to pandemic response and financial support to low-income countries. The United States should advocate the strengthening of the WHO according to the road map that I transmitted to the WHO Executive Board on behalf of the United States on September 2, 2020. This road map, which had overwhelming support from our allies, included numerous specific reforms to improve the "global capacity to prevent, respond to and defeat pandemics."[13] There are opportunities for progress in the near term under existing WHO mandates, including new warning designations short of an all-out public health emergency of international concern, further clarifying roles and responsibilities and specific time frames for action, improving transparency and oversight, and developing a framework that is much more effective than the current one for expediting the development of and access to medical products, including vaccines.

One easy reform is for the WHO to delink travel restrictions from trade restrictions under emergency conditions. Right now, the WHO process calls for the restriction of global trade if there are restrictions on individual global travel, making it much more consequential than if these were separate decisions. It makes much more sense to have a stepwise implementation of restrictions, as instituted by the United States early in the Trump administration, in which there were restrictions on individual travel while maintaining trade to support the global economy as well as international emergency responses. Finally, the WHO can improve its coordination with other international organizations within the United Nations, including UN developmental organizations like the World Bank and UNICEF (United Nations Children's Fund).

No set of WHO reforms will absolutely prevent the next pandemic, but they will strengthen the overall international response and yield tremendous benefits—as they recently have—for outbreaks like Ebola in Africa. These reforms need to be taken seriously by all signatories and member states, especially China. However, motivating the Chinese will take more than the typical resolutions and communications that are the product of multilateral organizations like the WHO. We will need US presidential-level leadership, which may include unilateral actions applied consistently across administrations, to assure global progress over time.

Aside from the need to strengthen the global health security agenda, there are many specific reasons why the United States needs to stay involved and provide leadership for the WHO. Without the United States in the WHO, we could expect a multitude of disastrous consequences, including international treaty concerns related to dangerous smallpox research, increased risks of poultry and human pandemic influenza, the resurgence of global polio, embargoes of US agricultural products, adverse classification and controls for narcotic drugs, and the further isolation and harassment of Taiwan and Israel.

CONCLUSION

Americans are inextricably part of an interconnected world, and microbes respect no boundaries. Keeping the United States biosafe must start on the front lines, whether that be in Liberia, India, or Wuhan. As COVID demonstrated, human beings are all in this together. The United States, as the world leader in innovation and a beacon of liberty and justice, has unequaled capabilities and resources and therefore exceptional responsibilities to keep our nation and our planet biosafe. The reforms outlined in this chapter are not a panacea, but they represent major steps forward based on our experience with COVID.

Pretending that COVID will be our last global pandemic or even the worst one is not a viable strategy for the future.

Notes

Chapter 1

1. Joe Biden (@JoeBiden), "I'm not going to shut down the country. I'm not going to shut down the economy. I'm going to shut down the virus," Twitter, October 30, 2020, https://twitter.com/JoeBiden/status/1322254443644026880?ref_src=twsrc%5Etfw %7Ctwcamp%5Etweetembed%7Ctwterm%5E1322254443644026880%7Ctwgr% 5Ea7aa9f8ce263f680cc82f020a175a7bb9ba72558%7Ctwcon%5Es1_&ref_url=https %3A%2F%2Fhannity.com%2Fmedia-room%2Fflashback-2020-joe-biden-vows-to-shut -down-the-virus%2F.

Chapter 3

1. *Hearing of the Committee on Health, Education, Labor, and Pensions, First Session on Nomination of Lance Robertson, Brett Giroir, MD, Robert Kadlec, MD, Elinore F. McCance-Katz, MD, and Jerome Adams, MD*, 115th Cong., S. Hrg. 115-390 (August 1, 2017) (opening statement of Senator Murray).

2. Including the American Society of Nephrology's President's Medal, the American Society of Hematology's Outstanding Public Service Award, the Sickle Cell Community Consortium's Healthcare Champion Award, the Society of Federal Healthcare Professionals' Tip of the Spear Federal Healthcare Leadership Award, the American Society of Health-System Pharmacists' Pharmacy Champion Award, Remote Area Medical's Distinguished Service Award, the Society of Critical Care Medicine's Founders' Special Recognition Award, and Secretary Becerra's Award for Distinguished Service for my team's work to improve maternal and child health.

Chapter 4

1. *Ebola in the Homeland: The Importance of Effective International, Federal, State, and Local Coordination: Hearings before the US House Committee on Homeland Security*, 113th Cong. (2014) (statement of Brett Giroir, director, Texas Task Force on Infectious Disease Preparedness and Response).

2. "First Global Estimates of 2009 H1N1 Pandemic Mortality Released by CDC-Led Collaboration," Centers for Disease Control and Prevention, June 25, 2012, https://www .cdc.gov/flu/spotlights/pandemic-global-estimates.htm.

3. David Metzgar, Darcie Baynes, Christopher A. Myers, Peter Kammerer, Michelle Unabia, Dennis J. Faix, and Patrick J. Blair, "Initial Identification and Characterization of an Emerging Zoonotic Influenza Virus Prior to Pandemic Spread," *Journal of Clinical Microbiology* 48, no. 11 (2010): 4228–34, https://www.ncbi.nlm.nih.gov/pmc/articles/PMC3020883/;

D. L. Ecker et al., "The Ibis T5000 Universal Biosensor: An Automated Platform for Pathogen Identification and Strain Typing," *JALA* 11 (2006): 341–51.

4. Brittany De Lea, "FLASHBACK: Biden's Chief of Staff Pick Admits Obama Admin Did Everything Wrong with H1N1," Fox News, November 11, 2020, https://www.foxnews.com/politics/flashback-bidens-chief-of-staff-obama-admin-h1n1.

5. There is also an asymptomatic spread of influenza, but it is much less pronounced than for COVID. Among asymptomatic individuals with the flu, household spread has been estimated at ~6 percent. For COVID-19, household spread from asymptomatic patients is >50 percent. Carlos G. Grijalva et al., "Transmission of SARS-CoV-2 Infections in Households—Tennessee and Wisconsin, April–September 2020," *Morbidity and Mortality Weekly Report* 69, no. 44 (2020), https://www.cdc.gov/mmwr/volumes/69/wr/mm6944e1.htm.

6. "The 2009 H1N1 Pandemic: Summary Highlights, April 2009–April 2010," Centers for Disease Control and Prevention, last modified June 16, 2010, https://www.cdc.gov/h1n1flu/cdcresponse.htm.

7. Of note, President Trump awarded the USPHS a second Presidential Unit Citation on January 19, 2021, "for extraordinary courage and the highest level of performance of duty in protecting, promoting, and advancing the health and safety of the Nation during the Coronavirus disease 2019 (COVID-19) pandemic." At that time, over 4,380 of our total of 6,100 had deployed 11,850 times.

8. A complete report of the Texas task force can be found here: *Texas Task Force on Infectious Disease Preparedness and Response: Report and Recommendations*, WTAW, December 1, 2014, http://wtaw.com/wp-content/uploads/2014/12/InfectiousDiseaseTaskForce120114.pdf.

9. "Ebola Virus Disease Cluster in the United States—Dallas County, Texas, 2014," Centers for Disease Control and Prevention, November 14, 2014, https://www.cdc.gov/mmwr/preview/mmwrhtml/mm63e1114a5.htm.

10. Steven Nelson, "Should Ebola Patient Nina Pham's Dog Be Tested?," US News, October 14, 2014, https://www.usnews.com/news/articles/2014/10/14/ebola-patient-nina-pham-dog-bentley.

Chapter 5

1. To the best of my recollection, this occurred on January 2, but the exact date may have been January 3 or January 4.

2. World Health Organization (@WHO), "#China has reported to WHO a cluster of #pneumonia cases—with no deaths—in Wuhan, Hubei Province. Investigations are underway to identify the cause of this illness," Twitter, January 4, 2020, https://twitter.com/WHO/status/1213523866703814656.

3. US Government Accountability Office, GAO-21-334 (Washington, DC, 2021), accessed October 3, 2022, https://www.gao.gov/assets/gao-21-334.pdf.

4. DISMA = disaster management; ICS = incident command system.

5. The team members included Cmdr. Julie Erb-Alvarez (executive officer) and five USPHS Service Access Team (SAT) officers: Capt. L. J. Belsito, SAT team lead; Lt. Cmdr. Nicole Carr (my former aide-de-camp); Lt. Cmdr. Bethanie Parrish-Salaam; Lt. Cmdr. Crystal McBride; and Lt. Adelaida Rosario.

6. "Coronavirus Quarantine Day 28—Release Date! Or Is It?," Coronavirus Quarantine, Torres Travels, March 2, 2020, https://www.thetorrestravels.com/category/coronavirus-quarantine/.

7. Mayor Ron Nirenberg (@Ron), "Today we learned that the CDC mistakenly released a patient from the Texas Center for Infectious Disease who later returned a positive COVID-19 reading. The fact that the CDC allowed the public to be exposed to a patient with a positive COVID-19 reading is unacceptable," Twitter, March 1, 2020, https://twitter.com/Ron_Nirenberg/status/1234287498181926912.

8. "Judge Denies San Antonio's Court Filing to Prevent Release of Coronavirus Evacuees: It's Unclear When Evacuees Will Be Released," KSAT News, March 2, 2020, https://www.ksat.com/news/local/2020/03/03/judge-denies-san-antonios-court-filing-to-prevent-release-of-coronavirus-evacuees/.

9. City of San Antonio et al. v. United States of America et al., SA-20-CV-0255-XR, order denying motion (2020), https://cases.justia.com/federal/district-courts/texas/txwdce/5:2020cv00255/1088068/2/0.pdf.

10. Robert Redfield, "CDC Response Letter to Texas 3-2-20," US Department of Health and Human Services, March 2, 2020, https://static.texastribune.org/media/files/9c8d9102fbe9c83ca67151ab1211b48a/CDC%20Response%20Letter%20to%20Texas%203-2-20.pdf?_ga=2.124041866.1214209272.1623797671-1161111328.1623797671:

> One individual met these criteria and was released only to learn that a pending test turned out to be positive; she was readmitted. For this individual, specimens were collected according to the CDC protocol. After her symptoms had resolved, specimen collections were started to determine that she had negative test results. The policy is that a person can have isolation precautions removed if there are two specimens that are negative, collected 24 hours apart. Her first specimen was negative. Her second specimen, which was collected 24 hours later, was inconclusive. Therefore, the protocol required a third specimen to be collected. Inconclusive results mean that the test is at the limit of detection, is neither positive nor negative, and needs to be repeated.
>
> While waiting on the results from the third specimen, the Infectious Disease Response Unit at TCID collected a subsequent fourth specimen without knowledge of the CDC team at Lackland. The prior confirmatory specimen (third specimen) was negative and, according to protocol, led to the release of the person. After the person was released, results of the fourth specimen were completed and showed a positive. Based on this last result, the patient was contacted and was returned to isolation at TCID.

11. "Coronavirus Quarantine Day 28."

Chapter 6

1. From a phone call I had with Speaker Gingrich (who was in Italy) on March 24, 2020.
2. Task force doctors included Birx, Fauci, Hahn, Redfield, Adams, and Giroir.

3. Whereas many budget professionals only care about spreadsheets, Jen had a true passion for public health; her skills with money were just a way to support public health—not vice versa.

4. "Transcript: Donald Trump Visits CDC, Calls Jay Inslee a 'Snake,'" Rev, March 6, 2020, https://www.rev.com/blog/transcripts/transcript-donald-trump-visits-cdc-calls-jay-inslee-a-snake.

5. Jake Sherman and Lauren Morello, "Trump Administration Rolls Out New Coronavirus Push, Names HHS Testing Czar," Politico, March 13, 2020, https://www.politico.com/news/2020/03/13/trump-coronavirus-testing-128048.

6. Each test kit included a positive control and a negative control. A positive control is a sample that should be positive if the test is run correctly; the negative control should be negative if the test is performing correctly. A positive result on a negative control could mean that the test was contaminated, either by the lab itself or back at the site of manufacture. Several laboratories simultaneously reported positive tests in the negative control, indicating conclusively that there had been contamination at the CDC level.

7. "March 13, 2020: Press Conference about the Coronavirus," University of Virginia Miller Center, March 13, 2020, https://millercenter.org/the-presidency/presidential-speeches/march-13-2020-press-conference-about-coronavirus.

8. "Laboratory Developed Tests," US Food and Drug Administration, last modified September 27, 2018, https://www.fda.gov/medical-devices/in-vitro-diagnostics/laboratory-developed-tests.

9. Extracted from HHS memo from Robert Charrow (general counsel, HHS) to Stephen Hahn, commissioner of food and drugs, June 22, 2020. Original document in possession of Admiral Giroir. A copy can be found at Politico, https://www.politico.com/f/?id=00000174-e9b2-d951-a77f-f9fe04fa0000.

10. Bill Whitaker, "Lack of Readiness, Questionable Federal Inspection Helped Fuel First U.S. COVID-19 Outbreak," *60 Minutes*, CBS News, November 1, 2020, https://www.cbsnews.com/news/covid-19-outbreak-nursing-facility-kirkland-washington-60-minutes-2020-11-01/.

11. Shawn Boburg et al., "Inside the Coronavirus Testing Failure: Alarm and Dismay among the Scientists Who Sought to Help," *Washington Post*, April 3, 2020, https://www.washingtonpost.com/investigations/2020/04/03/coronavirus-cdc-test-kits-public-health-labs/.

Chapter 7

1. Typically, attendees at the secretary's morning briefing would include the HHS chief of staff and deputy chief of staff; all the heads of relevant operating and staff divisions like the CDC, the FDA, and the ASPR; and the public affairs team.

2. Brooke Rollins was assistant to the president and a member of the Office of American Innovation. She later became the director of the US Domestic Policy Council in the White House.

3. "March 13, 2020: Press Conference about the Coronavirus."

4. The working groups included the *process* group, which developed and decided how to implement the actual processes for conducting testing at the community-based sites,

performed the tests, and provided results to patients and state public health officials; the *supplies* group, which secured PPE, swabs, media, and other supplies and distributed them to the sites; the *front-end* group, which developed and implemented a website, whether using Google as announced at the White House or another solution; the *communications* team, which communicated to the public, to patients seeking tests, to governors and state health officials, and to agencies in the government (my wife, Jill, volunteered and was an important contributor to the communications team); and the *scale* group, which worked with the retailers for initial sites and then scaled in subsequent phases to thousands of sites.

5. The tests consisted of tubes of PCR primers that matched sequences on the virus; these primers would result in the amplification of genetic material if the virus were present in the sample. Also included were positive control samples and negative control samples (which had been contaminated in the earlier CDC version) to assure that the test was performing correctly.

6. In addition to the primers and controls supplied in the CDC test kits, labs still needed additional reagents to "extract" the viral RNA from the sample—and these reagents were also in critically short supply. The CDC had none available and was not actively working on the problem. Many of these reagents came from small producers and foreign suppliers—many of which were in China.

7. The FDA granted authorization for tests stipulating a specific site of collection (nasopharynx) and a specific type of swab that could be utilized to collect it. Using a different site or swab type would violate the EUA and could result in faulty results (either false positives or, more likely, false negatives) or, more importantly, the wrath of the FDA regulators.

8. There are many more components needed for this "end-to-end solution," but they were not on my radar at that time, including laboratory robots to automate the process and pipette tips for those robots. Even the small test tubes eventually were in short supply, and we needed to call on the Department of Energy National Labs to fabricate them. And, of course, there were ubiquitous issues with finding trained laboratory personnel, especially in public health labs with tight budgets and high workloads.

9. David Lee and Jaehong Lee, "Testing on the Move: South Korea's Rapid Response to the COVID-19 Pandemic," *Transportation Research Interdisciplinary Perspectives* 5 (2020): 1–9, http://dx.doi.org/10.1016/j.trip.2020.100111.

10. Other USPHS officers included R. Adm. Estella Jones (veterinarian, FDA), Cmdr. Robert Horsch (environmental health officer, or EHO), Cmdr. William Pierce (pharmacist, FDA), Cmdr. Damon Smith (scientist and chief of the Readiness and Deployment Branch), Lt. Cmdr. Daveta Baily (EHO and Response and Deployment Team manager), and Lt. Alesya Van Meter (dietician and Response and Deployment Team coordinator).

11. Remember, tests were authorized by the FDA with a specific swab type and method of collection and, at that time, EUA-specified (and CDC-recommended) nasopharyngeal samples using a flocked NP swab, collected by a health-care provider. If an oropharyngeal sample was used, it would still need to be collected by a health-care worker and only done in combination with a nasopharyngeal sample.

12. "Coronavirus (COVID-19) Update: Daily Roundup," US Food and Drug Administration, March 23, 2020, https://www.fda.gov/news-events/press-announcements/coronavirus-covid-19-update-daily-roundup.

Chapter 8

1. Brian Naylor, "Known for Disaster Aid, FEMA Prepares for New Challenge with Coronavirus Relief," NPR, March 19, 2020, https://www.npr.org/2020/03/19/817903726/federal-emergency-management-agency-steps-up-incident-level-as-coronavirus-needs.

2. "Audio & Rush Transcript: Governor Cuomo Is a Guest on CNN's *Cuomo Prime Time*," New York State, April 15, 2020, https://www.governor.ny.gov/news/audio-rush -transcript-governor-cuomo-guest-cnns-cuomo-prime-time-4.

3. Brett Giroir and Jerome Adams, "Optimizing Ventilator Use during the COVID-19 Pandemic," US Public Health Service Commissioned Corps, March 30, 2020, https://www .hhs.gov/sites/default/files/optimizing-ventilator-use-during-covid19-pandemic.pdf.

4. Alex Eastman, unpublished situation report to Admiral Giroir, FEMA, March 26, 2020.

Chapter 9

1. "Transcript: Donald Trump Visits CDC."

2. "Playbook for Early Response to High Consequence Emerging Infectious Disease Threats and Biological Incidents," Executive Office of the President of the United States, accessed October 4, 2022, 50, https://s3.documentcloud.org/documents/6819268/Pandemic-Playbook.pdf.

3. "Total COVID-19 Tests per 1,000 People," Our World in Data, January 20, 2021, https://ourworldindata.org/grapher/full-list-cumulative-total-tests-per-thousand-map ?time=2021-01-20.

4. *Pooling* refers to combining samples from several patients into one laboratory test. Mathematically, this provides a significant multiplier effect when there is low or moderate community spread.

5. *Tracking US Coronavirus Testing Capacity* 3, no. 12 (October 6, 2021), https://www .covidresponseadvisors.org/_files/ugd/fd9688_2aed61b8c1a141b2aa19fbc1079f1d0e .pdf.

6. "Lab Advisory: Shortage of COVID-19 Rapid Tests May Increase Demand for Laboratory Testing," Centers for Disease Control and Prevention, September 2, 2021, https://www.cdc.gov/locs/2021/09-02-2021-lab-advisory-Shortage_COVID-19_Rapid_Tests _Increase_Demand_Laboratory_Testing_1.html; Sheri Fink, "Maker of Rapid Covid Tests Told Factory to Destroy Inventory," *New York Times*, August 20, 2021, https://www .nytimes.com/2021/08/20/us/abbott-covid-tests.html.

7. "National COVID-19 Testing Implementation Forum," US Department of Health and Human Services, accessed October 2, 2022, https://www.hhs.gov/coronavirus/testing/national-covid-19-testing-implementation-forum/index.html.

8. *Testing Overview, Opening up America Again*, White House, CDC, FDA, 2020, https://s3.documentcloud.org/documents/6878367/Testing-Overview.pdf.

9. *Testing Blueprint, Opening up America Again*, White House, CDC, FDA, 2020, https://www.documentcloud.org/documents/6878645-Testing-Blueprint.html.

10. *Report to Congress: COVID-19 Strategic Testing Plan*, US Department of Health and Human Services, May 24, 2020, https://www.democrats.senate.gov/imo/media/

doc/COVID%20National%20Diagnostics%20Strategy%2005%2024%202020%20v
%20FINAL.pdf.

11. *Testing Blueprint, Opening up America Again, Addendum to the Testing Blueprint*,
White House, CDC, FDA, 2020, http://web.archive.org/web/20200605225747/https:/
www.whitehouse.gov/wp-content/uploads/2020/06/Addendum-to-the-testing-blueprint
-FINAL.pdf.

12. "More Than 90% of COVID Deaths Occurring among Elderly Adults: CDC," ABC
News, https://abcnews.go.com/Health/90-covid-deaths-occurring-elderly-adults-cdc/
story?id=94211121.

13. Apoorva Mandavilli and Catie Edmondson, "Trump Administration Coronavirus Testing Strategy Draws Concerns: 'This Isn't the Hunger Games,'" *New York Times*,
May 25, 2020, https://www.nytimes.com/2020/05/25/health/coronavirus-testing-trump
.html.

14. "HHS Releases COVID-19 Testing Plans from States, Other Jurisdictions," American Hospital Association, August 11, 2020, https://www.aha.org/news/headline/2020
-08-11-hhs-releases-covid-19-testing-plans-states-other-jurisdictions.

15. Peter Baker and Jesse McKinley, "Trump and Cuomo Put Aside Disputes during
White House Meeting," *New York Times*, April 21, 2020, https://www.nytimes.com/
2020/04/21/us/politics/trump-andrew-cuomo-meeting.html.

Chapter 10

1. "Nursing Home Reopening Recommendations for State and Local Officials," Center
for Medicare and Medicaid Services, May 18, 2020, https://www.cms.gov/files/document/
qso-20-30-nh.pdf-0.

2. "Nursing Home Reopening Recommendations" (emphasis added).

3. Maggie Flynn, "HHS Warns against Using Antigen Results for Nursing Home
Cohorting, but Sharply Criticizes State Ban," Skilled Nursing News, October 9, 2020,
https://skillednursingnews.com/2020/10/hhs-warns-against-using-antigen-results-for
-nursing-home-cohorting-but-sharply-criticizes-state-ban/.

4. Her team included Brajendra Singh, Prabasaj Paul, and Hannah Wolford—all
full-time staff at the CDC.

5. "Q: Does the FDA Have Recommendations for Health Care Providers Using
SARS-CoV-2 Diagnostic Tests for Screening Asymptomatic Individuals for COVID-19?,"
General FAQs, US Food and Drug Administration, accessed August 29, 2020, quoted
in https://www.hhs.gov/sites/default/files/prep-act-coverage-for-screening-in-congregate
-settings.pdf (emphasis added).

6. "Updated CLIA SARS-CoV-2 Molecular and Antigen Point of Care Test Enforcement Discretion," CMS, accessed August 29, 2020, https://www.cms.gov/files/document/
clia-poc-ag-test-enforcement-discretion.pdf.

7. "Guidance for PREP Act Coverage for COVID-19 Screening Tests at Nursing
Homes, Assisted Living Facilities, Long-Term-Care Facilities, and Other Congregate
Facilities," US Department of Health and Human Services, August 31, 2020, https://www
.hhs.gov/sites/default/files/prep-act-coverage-for-screening-in-congregate-settings.pdf.

8. Antigen tests rely on detecting a protein component of the virus; they specifically do not amplify a small segment of RNA. With PCR amplification, sensitivity (being able to detect something that is there) is not a problem. For antigen tests, however, sensitivity is the whole game, so incredible effort is needed to go into identifying the exact right antibody for the test, the specific configuration of the gold nanoparticles on the strip, and even the unique type of paper strip (nitrocellulose) to make the system work. There was an enormous amount of sophistication packed into a small, cheap package.

9. Paul Mango, *Warp Speed: Inside the Operation That Beat COVID, the Critics, and the Odds* (New York: Republic Book, 2022).

Chapter 11

1. Peter Navarro, "Anthony Fauci Has Been Wrong about Everything I Have Interacted with Him On: Peter Navarro," *USA Today*, July 14, 2020, https://www.usatoday.com/story/opinion/todaysdebate/2020/07/14/anthony-fauci-wrong-with-me-peter-navarro-editorials-debates/5439374002/.

2. "*Meet the Press*—August 2, 2020," NBC News, https://www.nbcnews.com/meet-the-press/meet-press-august-2-2020-n1235604.

3. "Remarks by President Biden at COVID-19 Response Team's Regular Call with the National Governors Association," White House, December 27, 2021, https://www.whitehouse.gov/briefing-room/speeches-remarks/2021/12/27/remarks-by-president-biden-at-covid-19-response-teams-regular-call-with-the-national-governors-association/.

4. Tomás M. León et al., "COVID-19 Cases and Hospitalizations by COVID-19 Vaccination Status and Previous COVID-19 Diagnosis—California and New York, May–November 2022," *Morbidity and Mortality Weekly Report* 71, no. 4 (2022): 125–31.

5. Scott Atlas, "Specific Notes on Prioritized Testing," unpublished memo, August 2020.

6. *Guidelines, Opening Up America Again*, White House, CDC, April 16, 2020, https://trumpwhitehouse.archives.gov/wp-content/uploads/2020/04/Guidelines-for-Opening-Up-America-Again.pdf.

7. Adrianna Rodriguez, "'This Change in Policy Will Kill': Experts Troubled by CDC Changes to COVID-19 Testing Guidelines," *USA Today*, August 26, 2020, https://www.usatoday.com/story/news/health/2020/08/26/cdc-changes-covid-19-testing-guidelines-will-kill-experts-say/3441828001/.

8. Nick Valencia, Sara Murray, and Kristen Holmes, "CDC Was Pressured 'from the Top Down' to Change Covid-19 Testing Guidance, Official Says," CNNPolitics, August 27, 2020, https://www.cnn.com/2020/08/26/politics/cdc-coronavirus-testing-guidance/index.html.

9. Valencia, Murray, and Holmes.

10. Deborah Birx, email message to Brett Giroir, August 5, 2020.

11. Mango, *Warp Speed*.

12. "Select Subcommittee Releases Initial Findings from Transcribed Interview of Dr. Deborah Birx," Select Subcommittee on the Coronavirus Crisis, October 26, 2021, https://coronavirus.house.gov/news/press-releases/select-subcommittee-releases-initial-findings-transcribed-interview-dr-deborah.

13. "Select Subcommittee Releases Initial Findings from Transcribed Interview of Dr. Deborah Birx," Select Subcommittee, October 26, 2021, https://coronavirus.house.gov/news/press-releases/select-subcommittee-releases-initial-findings-transcribed-interview-dr-deborah.

14. Christian Spencer, "Top Pandemic Official Claims Trump Could Have Saved 130K People from Preventable Deaths," *Hill*, October 27, 2021, https://thehill.com/changing-america/well-being/prevention-cures/578667-trump-could-have-saved-130000-people-from/.

15. "COVID-19 Results Briefing," IHME policy briefing, September 15, 2020, https://www.healthdata.org/sites/default/files/files/Projects/COVID/2021/102_briefing_United_States_of_America_37.pdf.

16. "Trends in Number of COVID-19 Cases and Deaths in the US Reported to CDC, by State/Territory," CDC, accessed October 4, 2022, https://covid.cdc.gov/covid-data-tracker/index.html#trends_dailycases_select_00.

17. Aaron Keller, "The C.D.C. Has New Covid Guidelines. This Is What It Got Wrong," *New York Times*, December 28, 2021, https://www.nytimes.com/2021/12/28/opinion/covid-isolation-guidelines.html.

18. "Daily State-by-State Testing Trends," Johns Hopkins, accessed October 1, 2022, https://coronavirus.jhu.edu/testing/individual-states.

Chapter 12

1. George Santayana, *Reason in Common Sense* (New York: Scribner and Sons, 1905), 284.

2. A fact-based dramatization of the Nipah virus pandemic was the 2011 movie *Contagion*.

3. "Tracking BSL-4 Labs around the World," Global Biolabs Project, accessed October 3, 2022, https://www.globalbiolabs.org/.

4. System components included amplification of all nucleic acids within a sample followed by a more specific amplification with primers for all the major known groups of life (viruses, bacteria, fungi, and others). The products were then sprayed into a mass spectrometer, and the resulting array of mass-spec signatures underwent complex (but automated) signal processing to identify the organism—whatever it was. Because the database encompassed essentially all known microbes that are relevant to humans, specific identification is made through a comparison of the results with the entire library of microbes (essentially all known pathogens and their variants). However, if there is a new microbe in the sample, there would be no match in the database, and *that* would immediately trigger a full-out investigation by infectious disease specialists to determine the identity of the new pathogen.

5. Metzgar et al., "Initial Identification."

6. James Curtis, "Every Marine a Rifleman," *Marine Corps Gazette*, May 2021, 53–53, https://mca-marines.org/wp-content/uploads/0521-Every-Marine-a-Rifleman.pdf.

7. "The Impact of Chronic Underfunding on America's Public Health System: Trends, Risks, and Recommendations, 2020," Trust for America's Health, April 2020, https://www.tfah.org/wp-content/uploads/2020/04/TFAH2020PublicHealthFunding.pdf.

8. "National COVID-19 Testing Implementation Forum."

9. Chris McChesney et al., *The 4 Disciplines of Execution: Achieving Your Wildly Important Goals* (New York: Simon & Schuster, 2021).

10. 42 U.S.C. § 202: Administration and Supervision of Service (2022), https://uscode .house.gov/view.xhtml?req=(title:42%20section:202%20edition:prelim).

11. The public health emergency for the opioid crisis is an exception because that public health emergency will last for years and was more of a call for the prioritization of research, policy, and funding (from the federal level) as opposed to indicating the need for an acute emergency response and short-term deployment of resources. But all other public health emergencies fall squarely in the realm of the ASPR, and the ASPR's leadership related to medical and public health response needs to be formally recognized and affirmed by the secretary.

12. "Emergency Support Function #8—Public Health and Medical Services Annex," FEMA, US Department of Health and Human Services, January 2008, https://www.fema .gov/pdf/emergency/nrf/nrf-esf-08.pdf.

13. "Reviewing COVID-19 Response and Strengthening the WHO's Global Emergency Preparedness and Response, WHO ROADMAP," official communication from Admiral Giroir (US representative to the WHO Executive Board) to the WHO Executive Board, September 2, 2020.

Index

Page numbers in *italics* refer to figures.